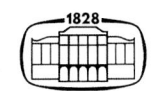

# Pictorial Expression in Psychiatry

## PSYCHIATRIC AND ARTISTIC ANALYSIS

BY *Irene Jakab*, M.D., Ph.D.

AKADÉMIAI KIADÓ, BUDAPEST

*A work based on the collection of patients' art products
at the Psychiatric and Neurological University Hospital
of Pécs, Hungary.*

*Art Advisor:* †*Ferenc Martyn*

*Cover design: Edith Székely*

*Typography: Péter Gábor*

ISBN 963 05 7492 6

© *Irene Jakab, 1998*

*Published by Akadémiai Kiadó
H–1519 Budapest, P.O. Box 245*

*All rights reserved. No part of this book may be reproduced
in a retrieval system, or transmitted in any form or by any means
without the prior permission of the publisher.*

*Printed in Hungary*

# CONTENTS

FOREWORD / 7

PREFACE / 11

INTRODUCTION / 13

A Historical Overview of the Diagnostic
    and Therapeutic Use of Psychiatric Patients'
    Art Products / 13
Recent Developments / 17
Comments on Creativity and Psychiatric
    Art / 23
Future Trends in Research and Application / 24

## Psychiatric and Artistic Evaluation

CLINICAL OBSERVATIONS
AND PRESENTATION OF THE DRAWINGS
AND PAINTINGS / 31

Schizophrenia (Cases 1–12 and 16) / 31
Manic Depression (Cases 13–14) / 118
Alcoholic Hallucinosis (Case 15) / 124
New Case with Long-term Follow-up
    on Outpatient Basis (Case 16) / 129

THE CHARACTERISTICS OF DRAWINGS
AND PAINTINGS OF PSYCHIATRIC PATIENTS
FROM THE ARTISTIC POINT OF VIEW / 158

The Content / 159
    Manifest Content / 159
    Symbolic Content / 160
The Composition / 162
The Style / 162
The Ways of Expression (Technique) / 164
    The Line / 164
    The Creation of Form / 165
    Colors–Effects of the Light / 166
    The Space / 166
    Body Proportions and Movement / 167

SPONTANEITY AND PERIODICITY
OF THE ARTISTIC ACTIVITY,
THEIR RELATIONSHIP TO PSYCHOSIS / 168

DIAGNOSTIC VALUE OF THE PICTORIAL
PRODUCTS / 171

Diagnostic Qualities of the Artworks of Schizophrenics
    / 173
Diagnostic Characteristics of the Works of Manic
    Patients / 175
The Works of a Patient Suffering from Alcoholic
    Hallucinosis: Relationship to the Psychosis / 176

CHARACTERISTICS OF THE REPRESENTATION
OF HALLUCINOSIS / 177

PROGNOSTIC SIGNIFICANCE OF THE STYLE
AND OF THE TECHNICAL QUALITIES / 180

SOME RELATIONSHIPS TO CHILDREN'S
DRAWINGS / 182

CERTAIN RELATIONSHIPS
WITH ARCHAIC DRAWINGS
AND WITH THE DRAWINGS
OF PRIMITIVE PEOPLE / 184

SUMMARY / 187

BIBLIOGRAPHY / 191

# FOREWORD

This book is an updated and enlarged English translation of the first publications of Irene Jakab's French edition, *Dessins et Peintures des Alienes,* 1956, and of German edition, *Zeichnungen und Gemälde der Geisteskranken,* 1956.

This new English edition has added new dimensions to the field of psychiatry and art. Furthermore it includes a new clinical case. This Case 16 describes a patient who was hospitalized for schizophrenia at age 17. After his discharge, he was followed as an outpatient for more than 35 years. He became a professional artist-painter. The review of his paintings from the time of psychosis and recovery to the present adds to the understanding of creativity in mental illness.

Irene Jakab writes about the recent developments of art therapy, creativity, the analysis of psychiatric art, visions of research in the future, and applied research. She also points out that psychotherapy is one of the goals of artistic expression. This will include individual psychotherapy, family therapy, group therapy, as well as art and creative therapies. In the future, Irene Jakab sees that it will be possible for specialists to make consultations by using evolving technology.

One of the many achievements of Irene Jakab, in the field of psychiatry, is the establishment of a clinical psychiatric method using, as the basis, the psychopathology of expression. She also supports the development of art therapy with strong theories and practices.

The pathological intra-psychic process of mental illness brings about the increase of image formations, perceptions, emotions, thoughts and activities. These synthetic functions become heightened or distorted, even if the patient is in a state of consciousness. The possibility of a state, where one's creative abilities are displayed, can be imagined. At that point, the patient's consciousness toward creativity and the continuation of directed activities develop the patient's originality.

With such methods, both the normal consciousness and the pathological consciousness progress centering on creativity. We understand that it is important that the artistic expressions of normal persons, of patients who were thought to be mentally ill, and of artists, can be understood from the viewpoint of psychopathology of expression.

Psychopathology of expression is a field of psychiatry where the expressive activities of human beings and their products are evaluated. Macroscopically, man's expressions of action are included. Normally, however, our field concerns expressions of art such as pictorial art, music, dance, poetry, and literature when mental illness is involved.

This field began in the latter half of the 19th century. Paintings and drawings of the mentally ill drew the attention of physicians in academic circles. French and Italian doctors began writing scholarly papers. H. Prinzhorn laid the foundation for psychopathology of expression. From mental hospitals in various parts of Europe, Prinzhorn collected more than 5,000 paintings and drawings. In 1922 he wrote the book, *Bildnerei der Geisteskranken*. It is widely used for academic analysis of the psychology and the pathology of artistic expression.

In 1956, after World War II, the psychopathology of expression saw resurgence. In France, R. Volmat, published *L'Art Psychopathologique*, a book in which he used materials from a number of collections exhibited at the First World Psychiatric Congress in Paris in 1950.

Irene Jakab's *Zeichnungen und Gemälde der Geisteskranken* was published also in 1956. She presented the results of her research to the world and they may now be read. In 1959 several physicians interested in research, from Europe and America, formed the Société Internationale de Psychopathologie de l'Expression (SIPE). Following the establishment of this Society national societies were founded worldwide, in France, Italy, Germany, Austria, USA, Switzerland, Mexico, Argentina, Brazil, Japan and Korea. Irene Jakab a founding member of the SIPE has an active role as Vice President. Because of the foundations set by the Society of Psychopathology of Expression, new treatments were brought into the academic arena. In 19 6, A. Bader, Switzerland, and L. Navratil, Austria, together published *Zwischen Wahn und Wirklichkeit*.

The paintings, drawings, and sculptures of the mentally ill are used to further the issue of creativity and art therapy. The term art therapy began with A. Hill's publication *Painting Out Illness* 1942 in Britain. Treating chronic tuberculotic patients he used pictorial art production and appreciation of art to stress that life is worth living. Thus a more positive relationship was found between art and medicine. However, at that time, essential psychiatric treatment and significance of art were not yet connected. In 1966, M. Naumburg, USA, wrote *Dynamically Oriented Art Therapy* which received much attention. Following public interest, the practice of art therapy gradually increased. Approaches concerning the theory and practice of art therapy have become multifaceted. There are psychodynamic approaches, humanistic approaches, behavioral, cognitive, developmental approaches, and an eclectic approach. These have developed independently.

At the end of this Foreword, I would like to mention something about myself. Before becoming a psychiatrist, my life as an artist began from my student days. After becoming a medical doctor, I acquired many medical experiences and gained much knowledge. Although I was deeply interested in art and psychiatry, or psychopathology of expression, at that time in Japan, there was no one to teach me, therefore, I had to educate myself. There were those who saw me as a heretic. However, in 1958, an answer to my interests in this field appeared before me; one book by Prinzhorn and another by Irene Jakab. Immediately, I obtained them. Irene Jakab's book was her first edition in German. This has become my life-time favorite book, and it is a joyous celebration to think that presently it is updated and available in English.

Today, there is much interest in psychopathology of expression and art therapy. Specialists such as psychiatrists, clinical psychotherapists, art therapists, occupational therapists, artists, people involved with art, and others have embraced the field.

For all these specialists who have a profound interest in the professional kowledge of this field, I wish that this book will answer your concerns as it did for me. That would make this book a yet more brilliant publication, and a true contribution towards the readers, who all admire Irene Jakab and her works.

As a scholar in this same field, I believe that this pioneering English publication will be welcomed by a large number of readers.

*Yoshihito Tokuda* M.D.

# PREFACE

The case histories and illustrations of my book on the *Drawings and Paintings of the Mentally Ill* published in French and German only (JAKAB 1956) are incorporated in this book. That material, of course, required updating. Many new aspects of the role of the patients' pictorial expression have been discovered since its publication. Although the original book is out of print since many years, it is still quoted in the literature as a pioneering work. Several colleagues have expressed the need for an English edition, in addition to the interest in a Hungarian edition of this book based on a collection of 2,000 artworks of psychiatric patients treated at the Psychiatric and Neurological University Hospital of Pécs (Hungary).

I felt that a new unchanged edition of the same book, although it may be of historical value, would not do justice to the field of psychiatric patients' pictorial expression. Therefore, this new edition is updated incorporating new research and important changes in the role of pictorial expression in psychiatry and art therapy.

In the past, the first use of the patient's art was its value in communicating repressed feelings. The pictorial expression was interpreted by psychiatrists and psychoanalysts similarly to dream interpretations. Only a few such cases were published. Next, following the groundbreaking monography of H. Prinzhorn in 1922, the diagnostic importance of patient art became the new focus of publications. However, until 1956, no works based on large collections were available. Then practically at the same time as the publication of the monograph, *Drawings and Paintings of the Mentally Ill* (Jakab 1956, Budapest: Akadémiai Kiadó), Volmat published a multi-authored book based on the material of patient-art exhibition of the Congress of Psychiatry in Paris in 1956.

After these publications, the interest in the diagnostic and prognostic value of patient-art became widespread and led to extensive research in this area.

Finally, the use of patient-art as a treatment modality led to the development of a new branch of mental health services, the art therapy practiced by specially trained art therapists. The name of Art Therapy was first used by Margaret Naumburg.

I felt the importance to incorporate the new developments in research and clinical practice. A better understanding of psychiatric patients is now achieved by refined diagnostic and prognostic use of their art products. Furthermore, information on the therapeutic use of art, both in individual, and in group practice, based on extensive research and practical experience is incorporated in this new book in order to update the original material.

A new case *Zs. H.* (Case 16) is added to the discussion of the 15 patients in the original book. This patient, who was hospitalized at age 17, was quite talented. At that young age, he felt the need to express his feelings and some of his dreams in drawings and paintings. After his discharge from inpatient status (diagnosis: schizophrenia), he was encouraged to continue to draw and paint. It is now 37 years after his first hospitalization. He has achieved a lifestyle as a painter. He became a member of the local painters' association in Pécs, Hungary, and exhibits yearly with other artists in addition to some one-man exhibits in the last years. Although *Zs. H.* was not enrolled in formal art therapy, he was encouraged to use art expression which, I believe, was a self-healing process for this talented man.

I hope that the publication of this case will encourage therapists and some talented patients to continue to use art in a self-healing process instead of suppressing their talent just to be replaced by the practical demands of daily life.

The use of diagnostic interpretations may serve as a screening method for at-risk populations (from school children to adults in stressful occupations and to those coping with the emotional–social stresses of aging). It could detect early signs of emotional problems, thus help prevent the development of more serious disorders by timely referral for psychological intervention.

Art therapy may be useful beyond the realm of actual mental illness in helping people to cope with the emotional reactions to various stressful situations in their life.

I would like to express my sincere thanks to Professor *Mátyás Trixler,* M.D., Chairman of the Psychiatric and Neurological University Hospital of Pécs, Hungary, for providing access to the remaining pictures of the Reuter collection and to the medical records of the patients presented in this book.

Thanks are due to *Tamás Tényi,* M.D., Assistant Professor, who has facilitated my personal contact with my former patient, Mr. Zs. H. Dr. Tényi accompanied me on several occasions to the home of Mr. Zs. H. (who was his patient during his past brief rehospitalizations), and was helpful in the selection of the paintings reproduced in this book.

Last but not least I am grateful to the Head and Staff of the *Institute of Mental Health and Hygiene,* Pécs, Hungary. They have first called my attention to the artistic activity of Mr. Zs. H. and his recent, successful one-man show of paintings. Mr. Zs. H. is presently under their care as an outpatient.

I hope that the readers will find this book both enjoyable and useful.

*Irene Jakab*

# INTRODUCTION

## A HISTORICAL OVERVIEW OF THE DIAGNOSTIC AND THERAPEUTIC USE OF PSYCHIATRIC PATIENTS' ART PRODUCTS*

The artistic productions of mentally ill patients have aroused the interest of psychiatrists since the beginning of the twentieth century. In the literature we find mostly pathographies which offer a psychiatric analysis of the works of painters who became mentally ill, either to explain the psychological background of their works from the psychoanalytic point of view or to arrive at diagnostic conclusions about the relationship of the symptoms of the disease and the quality of the works (ANDREOLI 1966, BADER 1968, BRÜCKMANN 1932, DELAY, VOLMAT and PICHOT 1959, DRACOULIDES 1953, DROBEC and STROTZKA 1951, DUPRÉ and DEVAUX 1910, EVLACHOW 1937, GOMIRATO and GAMNA 1954, KRETSCHMER 1941, LALO 1943, MANDOLINI 1925, MÖBIUS 1901, NEIMAREVIĆ 1969, ROUX and LAHARIE 1997, SCHNIER 1950, SZILÁGYI 1992). Several authors have studied from this point of view, for example, the works of Van Gogh (JASPERS 1922, MINKOWSKA 1947, RIESE 1926, etc.), mostly from the point of view of the change of style.

In modern times the life and creative works of artists has become again the subject of psychological research. These publications are not called pathographies any more. They may be designated as "meta-biographies" as suggested by GEDO and OREMLAND, as they describe the subjective and objective psychological traits of the artists and their art works. A list of authors and the artists they descibe is given below.

DIGIOVANNI (1990) on Georgia O'Keefe; DIGIOVANNI and MCINTIRE-MANGO (1991) on Bonnard; IN DER BEECK (1975) on Vincent van Gogh and James Ensor; FOY (1991) on Giorgio de Chirico; GEDO (1980) on Picasso; LEWIS and MCLAUGHLIN (1991) on Leonardo da Vinci; RHI (1994) on Lee Choong Sup; STANNARD (1991) on Toulouse-Lautrec; VOLMAT (1991) on van Gogh; and ZERBE (1990) on Berthe Morrisot. The most recent pathography which can be designated as a meta-biography, *Art et Folie au Moyen Age* by ROUX and LAHARIE (1997) provides very interesting data on Opicinus de Canistris, a fourteenth-century monk. The biography and the description and analysis of his unique art work is the result of intensive research with a comprehensive research of these mystical drawings found in the archives of the apostolic library of the Vatican.

MORGENTHALER (1921, 1942), KRIS (1933), and ARNHEIM (1986) are among the pioneers of this science with a background in both psychiatry and art.

* This historical review is based on a detailed presentation at the Budapest Colloquium of the International Society of Psychopathology of Expression (JAKAB 1992).

The work of SIMON (1888) preceded the work by PRINZHORN (1922). RUSH (1812) mentioned in his publications the graphic expressions of psychiatric patients.

After the first extensive description and interpretation of the paintings and drawings of the mentally ill given by PRINZHORN in 1922, a long interval had elapsed until attention was focused again on the graphic expression of the psychiatric patient. Monographs and journal articles, containing extensive bibliographies, are now available on this subject (ANASTASI and FOLEY 1941, AUBIN 1970, BENDER 1952, DRACOULIDES 1953, JAKAB 1956, KRIS 1933, NAUMBURG 1950, PLOKKER 1962, RENNERT 1966, STERN 1923 and VOLMAT 1956).

MACGREGOR (1989), in his extensive review, *"The Discovery of the Art of the Insane"*, gives detailed descriptions of several important collections, as well as an excellent historical review of the first attempts to recognize and to analyze the art of the insane.

The question of the relationship between the drawings and paintings of the mentally ill, the art of primitive people and the trends of modern art has been raised by several anthors.

The expressionists use, according to KRETSCHMER (1941), mechanisms similar to those in the thought processes of primitive people and of schizophrenic patients. The following traits are manifested in their expressions: ambivalence, condensation, and displacement. Several articles in the literature treat surrealism in comparison to the drawings and paintings of the mentally ill (CONRAD 1953, DELAY 1952, DROBEC and STROTZKA 1951, EWALD 1952, EY 1948, FERNANDES 1933, LEHEL 1926, MORGENTHALER 1921, 1942, PFEIFER 1923, ROY 1953, 1958, SCHMIDT-HEINRICH 1953, WEYGANDT 1925, WYSS 1950, ZELDENRUST 1951). According to WERNER (1952), surrealistic painting is a painting of dreams and thus explainable by psychoanalysis. However, the identification of surrealism and primitive art with schizophrenia and the art of dreams is not acceptable to SCHMIDT-HEINRICH (1953). EHRENZWEIG (1948) has established that in classical art the negative forms (the background) have only an unconscious influence while in modern art the free space of the background has a high significance. The choice among the superimposed figures is left to the spectator. According to EHRENZWEIG (1948), "Gestalt"-free interpretation is the artistic way to see the world.

Without any doubt one can establish certain resemblances between the art of the mentally ill and expressionism and surrealism where the painters elaborate visual material arising from the unconscious functions, thus having some relationship to visions and dreams. BAUDOUIN (1929) indicated as the joint trends of dreams and art products, that they both project fantasies. The difference lies in the desire to communicate of those who produce art works. The value of dream-content and of free associations is less significant from the aesthetical point of view than for its role of helping to understand the creator of the artwork.

Before the 20th century, with few exceptions, neither psychiatrists nor art historians were interested in collecting the art works of patients. Nonetheless, one has to ask if some among the painters of earlier works of art, which are admired by us, could have been considered mentally ill. In Gothic times, for example, monsters were often represented in the fine arts, for instance in "les chimères" of the cathedrals and in the pictures of Hieronymus Bosch. BARANYAI (1978) attempted to prove that H. Bosch had used anatomical knowledge of the structure of the eye to represent a multitude of figures in his paintings. This author, an ophthalmologist by profession, gives convincing illustrations from both anatomy books and selected enlarged details of Bosch's paintings. It is a question whether these monsters were inspired by the expression of ecstatic religious concepts of their time, or were the expressions of visions. One cannot solve this problem unless one knows in detail the biography of the artist.

In the recent literature collections of patients' art have been studied from the psychiatric point of view. The most detailed work among these is the classical book by PRINZHORN of 1922 (new edition: 1968). BIEBER and HERKIMER (1947/48), EMERY (1929), FERDIÈRE (1947a,b, 1951), PANETH (1929), REITMAN (1948), UEBERSCHLAG (1936) and YAHN (1950) have published the analysis of drawings and paintings of the mentally ill from an artistic point of view. The monograph of VOLMAT (1956) is based on the analysis of the psychiatric art works presented at the World Congress of Psychiatry in Paris in 1956. It deals essentially with the psychotherapeutic value of patients' art. TÉNYI and TRIXLER (1992) published a collection of poems written by the patients of the Psychiatric and Neurological University Hospital of Pécs, Hungary. Several variations of poetry therapy are used in formal art therapy (HARROWER 1972, PETŐ 1997, TAYAL 1968, TÉNYI and TRIXLER 1992). Highly structured interactive techniques of poetry therapy are Renku as psychotherapy (TAMURA and ASANO 1997) and Haiku therapy of schizophrenics (IMORI 1997). Music therapy is also practiced successfully (HANSER 1997, SAKAUE 1997, YOSHIDA et al. 1994).

Paintings and drawings are the most frequently used art expressions among psychiatric patients. Other art forms such as poems, music and sculptures are less frequently used by them. Sculpture requires access to material: clay, wood, metal, stone, etc. and tools as well as technical knowledge. Therefore it is less frequently used by patients, unless they participate in art therapy where a well-equipped studio is at their disposal, and technical assistance is also available if needed. Exceptions in creative achievement are some monumental buildings of unique and great ornamental value which were produced single-handed by their creators who worked for decades to accomplish such psycho-architectural monuments (JAKAB 1978). The documentary film *'Imaginary Dwellings'* by Sandoz (1976) shows these exceptionally beautiful and interesting buildings. The film was produced as a collaborative work of FERDIÈRE (1976), BEHRENDS (1976) and JAKAB (1976), each describing one of the buildings. An introduction and final conclusion were written by JAKAB (1978). JAKAB assisted in the editing in addition to writing part of the script.

According to BILLIG and BURTON-BRADLEY (1975), art plays a significant and intimate role in the life of the preliterate society. It concerns the entire community but only selected individuals participate in the making of art works. "The artist has a message to convey ... therefore [he must] be 'readable' and understandable to his public."

Archaeologists use artifacts, drawings (e.g., cave drawings and other ritual, graphic expressions by primitive people) and remnants of different architectural constructions in interpreting and understanding past cultures and lifestyles. Similarly, we may use the development and changes in the style of art works by psychotic patients, as psycho-archaeological artifacts (especially series of works produced over time by the same person) through which the past can be reconstructed, the present may be understood and the future treatment may be planned with more accuracy. For instance, we may understand the psychiatric processes of adult persons by reviewing their childhood drawings, if any were preserved by the family (JAKAB 1996).

Artists had been preoccupied with the expression of strong feelings, and of distorted or morbid emotions, long before psychiatrists discovered the usefulness of art products in the understanding of such feelings in their patients. Since 1937, a series of 'Crying Women' were painted by Picasso (ELGAR and MAIULLARD 1956). The strong emotion is represented in an ideographic manner. Broken lines of the contours and features, giant tears and bewildered eyes out of place and out of proportion, instead of a bland photographical reproduction of their features serve to represent the effect of emotion on the 'Crying Woman'. The distortions, masterfully exaggerated, convey the intensity and disintegrating force of the emotion.

The copper etching of Albrecht Dürer entitled 'Melancholia', of 1514 (HAMMAN 1935), depicts the hopeless stare of a depressed woman. Vincent Van Gogh's 'Old Man Worrying' (SHAPIRO 1958) is sitting on a chair, bent over with his bald head resting on both fists with his face buried. The background is a bare brick wall. The lonely suffering is expressed by the body position and the lack of any details in the milieu to soften this effect. Salvador Dalí's surrealistic combination of human figures and objects gives a strong ideographic representation of emotions and ideas in his painting called 'Premonition of the Civil War' (ROY 1953).

In a lithography poster in 1945, Kokoschka (BULTMANN 1960) represents Christ reaching down from the cross towards the children. The following inscription is on the cross: "In Memory of the Children of Europe Who Have to Die of Cold and Hunger This Christmas". The strong feelings of the painter are expressed in his work not only through the traditional pictorial media but also through the added words. This method is often used also by patients when they feel that neither the words nor the graphic expression alone can convey their feelings.

Verbal aberrations of psychiatric patients are well known, such as schizophasia, echolalia, and other diagnostic characteristics. Diagnostic traits in the graphic expression of patients often parallel these pathological verbal expressions (ASSAEL 1990, BADER 1971, 1972, IN DER BEECK 1966, JAKAB 1969a, MÜLLER-THALHEIM 1975, NAVRATIL 1965, 1978, RENNERT 1966, ROUX 1991, TOKUDA 1986, WIART 1967). BILLIG and BURTON-BRADLEY (1975) have described special criteria for the diagnostic signs in the art of schizophrenic patients in Papua New Guinea. By analyzing the spatial structure of schizophrenic patients' art works, they found analogies with the disintegrating reality relationships caused by their illness. MOUSSONG-KOVÁCS (1992) calls attention to the temporo-spatial orientation in pictorial expression as a diagnostic criterion.

An analysis of patients' art from the point of view of the fine arts criteria brings a different dimension to the evaluation of patients' art by acknowledging that the criteria used in the fine arts can be applied to a formal analysis of the style of even those art products which do not have great aesthetical appeal or great value in terms of the fine arts. Among the pictorial elements, the style, line, composition, contrasts, are used as guidelines in evaluating the art products of patients (JAKAB 1956).

The attitudes of professional painters and psychiatric patients differ greatly in one aspect, namely in the "animation of the created figures". Patients often treat their art products as if they had a life of their own. This attitude is quite different from the intentions of some modern painters to let their emotions guide their hands and see later what the production will become, for example, in the case of Jackson Pollock, when the artist allows a free flow of unconscious drives to guide his pictorial expression. The schizophrenic patient often invests the power of guidance into the painted object, or person, and waits for the message, like a slave of the very person whom he has created.

A pictorial balance of objects, decorative elements or figurative elements, and colors characterizes the paintings with aesthetical value in the fine arts. The lack of this balance in pathological art is one of the major differences between "normal" and "pathological" art.

The content of patients' art may be interpreted best in collaboration with the patient, who may reveal the latent content and who may produce relevant associations leading to meaningful insight into the dynamics of the illness.

Artists consciously experiment with colors. They use "cool" or "warm" colors and shading through soft or harsh light to emphasize their subject. The emotionally disturbed patient frequently reaches instinctively for the "most appropriate" color combination to produce an increased impact on the viewer, heightening by means of colors the unusual emotions expressed in their works. The colors used by depressed children in their spontaneous drawings were purple, gray and dark brown, while black was used in the drawings of depressed adults (JAKAB 1967). RIESE (1959) studied the aging process from a color-psychological point of view. VOLMAT, WIART and USAL (1967) describe the use of colors as communication and information. EMERY (1929) discusses the intepretation of color in occupational therapy.

STEWART and BAXTER (1969), in a detailed statistical study of the reaction to drawings by elementary school children, established no ethnic preference for a specific color among Black, Latin, and Anglo children. There was a strong preference for color in all groups. Similarly, in a study on children's aesthetical choices, school children, from ages 6 to 18 years, selected color over monochrome renderings of the same pictures (JAKAB 1969b).

## RECENT DEVELOPMENTS

The study of *special patient groups* produced research on the characteristic style and content of various disorders other than schizophrenia.

Among the few authors who have studied the drawings and paintings of alcoholic patients, NAVRATIL (1965) has published findings of a figure drawing test in chronic alcoholism.

In several publications based on extensive case material, HÁRDI provided a phenomenological analysis of alcoholism in the light of dynamic drawing sequences collected throughout extended periods of follow-up, from acute to chronic and deteriorated states with diagnostically relevant fluctuations in content and style of the same gestalt produced by individual patients. At first, Hárdi's (1968) method was based on the analysis of human figure drawings. Later, Hárdi (1990) also extended his research to the study of drawing sequences of animals. A comprehensive review of his long-term follow-up of alcoholic patients has been published recently (Hárdi 1992).

Tayal (1969) called attention to the fact that the occurrence of "visual thought images" and their significance in suicidal communication are the least studied areas. The lack of such diagnostic studies of depressed patients' art work is in contrast to the extensive number of publications about the symptoms and signs of clinical significance in the communication of suicidal ideation and intent (DeLong and Robbins 1961, Menninger 1938, Motto and Green 1958, Pokorny 1960, Robbins et al. 1959, Schneer et al. 1961, Stone 1975, Yessler et al. 1961).

It may help to understand these works as expressions of the cultural societal role of art in their own time, similar to the criteria set forth by Billig and Burton-Bradley (1978) about the role and characteristics of tribal art in New Guinea. These authors make clear the differences between tribal art and art produced by native patients (mostly schizophrenics) in a psychotic state.

Billig and Burton-Bradley (1975), in their masterful work *Cross-Cultural Studies of Psychotic Graphics from New Guinea*, help us to understand both western and non-western psychopathology. The study of psychopathological art in New Guinea has a most specific advantage from the point of view of "lack of outside influences" since there is an almost complete cultural isolation due to that country's geography where villages and towns are cut off from the outside world by the non-existence of roads. "Neighboring villages cannot communicate with each other since people in each village among the two million people of New Guinea may speak one of 700 different languages (languages *not* dialects)." Billig and Burton-Bradley explain that the inherent difficulties in understanding the schizophrenic patients' language is greatly increased if it becomes necessary to translate the local "place talk" distorted by psychotic disintegration.

At the beginning of a psychosis, culture-bound delusions may be difficult to differentiate from prevailing cultural beliefs. Control by spirit-beings, or magic concept, may be a part of a paranoid delusion or part of a cultural belief, making it essential to base the diagnosis of schizophrenia rather on the structure of the disorder than on the content of delusions (Billig 1968, Billig and Burton-Bradley 1978).

Both verbal psychotherapy and art therapy are products of our century. Both are tools in the treatment of psychiatric patients. Both methods are rather ill defined.

The therapeutic value of art was recognized by Pinel (quoted from MacGregor 1989). He advised the staff of the two psychiatric hospitals in Paris (the Bicêtre for women and the Salpetrière for men) to encourage patients to draw, and to give them materials to be used for artistic expression as this would calm them and help their recovery.

The therapeutic use of art was first cultivated by psychiatrists and psychologists in Europe; in France, mostly by Freudian psychoanalysts while in Switzerland, mostly by Jungian analysts. JACOBI (1964, 1969, 1971) published a large collection of paintings discussed according to the Jungian interpretation of the patients' dreams and free associations.

In the United States, a new movement, Art Therapy, has surged in this century (KRAMER 1974, NAUMBURG 1950, 1953, ULMAN 1971). Art therapy is provided by specially trained therapists, who have a background both in art and in psychology. Several colleges offer degree programs in the field of art therapy.

The *American Journal of Art Therapy*, devoted exclusively to articles on art therapy, is a fine resource in this field.

The *Japanese Bulletin of Art Therapy* is a scholarly publication in Japanese in this field.

In September 1997 the first issue of the *International Journal of Art Therapy* has been published under the patronage of the World Psychiatric Association.

The proceedings of the national and international congresses organized by the American Society of Psychopathology of Expression are reflecting the up-to-date development of research in art diagnosis and art therapy.

*Over the past decades, new methods have been devised and special patient populations have been addressed as recipients of art psychotherapy.*

Just as verbal psychotherapy has progressed from essentially individual therapy to group therapy in our century, the use of art has also progressed from individual diagnostic evaluation to the therapeutic use of art, both in *individual* cases, *and* as a method of *group art therapy*.

Clinicians developed deferent techniques, for example: The use of Ikebana method of sculpturing with flowers (NUCHO 1986); the composite drawing method (IJUIN 1992); puppetry (IRWIN and SHAPIRO 1975); the landscape montage technique (KAITO 1994); TOKUDA (1997) gives a broader overview of therapeutic topos and their background dynamics.

Next, a new art therapy form has evolved, *family art therapy*, as practiced by KWIATKOWSKA (1971), RUBIN and IRWIN (1975). Other authors have reported their work with special groups of patients: STEWART (1968) studied the tactile aesthetic perceptions of blind children. TÉNYI and TRIXLER (1996) found unique characteristics in the drawings of Hungarian Gypsies, as they showed both culturally determined magical beliefs and pathological magical thinking. LAING (1975) revealed typical traits in the paintings of sado-masochists.

JAKAB (1990b) used the method of video-art-therapy for family art diagnosis with further technical refinement. In this case, the family art evaluation has been conducted with the help of videotaping the sessions; during a session of replaying the videotape to the family members, their interaction and the meaning of the art products were interpreted. In this case the art diagnostic and therapeutic intervention has been based on three 90-minute-long videotape sessions with the patient and the family. The patient, a 12-year-old girl, suffered from anorexia nervosa. Her family consists of both parents and her 21-year-old mentally retarded and autistic brother.

During the first 90-minute-session several sheets of different color, colored crayons, as well as plasticine for modelling were available. The representations of the following themes were requested:

1. Free subject (draw anything you want).
2. Draw a person.
3. Draw a person of the opposite sex.
4. Draw a picture of yourself.
5. Draw a picture of your family.

During the second videotape session the following assignments were given:
1. Draw a picture of happiness.
2. Draw a picture of sadness.
3. Draw a picture of love.
4. Draw a picture of hate.
5. Draw a picture of anger.

At the end of this session the family jointly drew a large mural on a sheet of brown paper attached to the wall. They chose the subject, a landscape by the river where they had a picnic in the past. They also assigned the drawing of the various details to each other.

During the third session which was also videotaped we replayed for the family a 60-minute videotape which was the edited version of the two previous sessions. During this session we discussed not only the meaning of the art products but also the relationship of the family members to each other. This proved to be of therapeutic value.

The subjects of the drawings and the order in which they were requested was determined by Jakab. In order to facilitate the verbal interaction and to arrive at some interpretations, Jakab and her assistant (Rubin) made comments during the sessions and asked questions related to the drawings which were affixed to the blackboard. Each family member was asked to comment on his/her own drawings and on those of the other family members. This led to several meaningful insights.

STONE (1969) formed a group of *"mute" patients*. Methods of painting with or near the patients, talking with them, requesting and obtaining written or pictorial answers have proven useful in establishing trust and in ventilating pent-up emotions. Stone's patients have "graduated" to verbal art psychotherapy following the positive experience in the interaction between them and the therapist, and in that of the group members among themselves.

HALBREICH (1978) uses a *nonverbal dialogue* in the treatment of schizophrenic patients. He bases his method on NAUMBURG's (1966) assumption that almost every individual has a latent capacity to project his inner conflicts into visual form.

*Dialogue drawing* between spouses is described by WADESON in marriage counseling. Lilla HÁRDI (1992) describes the progress of psychoanalysis as seen in her patients' paintings.

RUBIN, MAGNUSSEN and BAR (1975) describe a two-year period of treatment of a young man with dysfluency (stuttering). They emphasize the diagnostic and therapeutic value of art, especially the value of "family symbols". They used several modalities in sequence: art diagnosis, group art therapy, joint mother–child sessions, family art evaluation, and family art therapy.

ASSAEL (1990) used spontaneous painting as a means of communication in group art therapy.

ASSAEL, GABBAY and ROSEMAN (1975) described the method of spontaneous drawing in groups for artistically talented patients with failure to communicate. It facilitated the process of establishing contact with reality and brought about resocialization.

MÜLLER-THALHEIM (1975) describes the regulative mechanisms activated in schizophrenia which serve the reconstruction of the ego. He wonders "whether these regulations to maintain or reconstruct psychic balance may not be ubiquitous and may not constitute one of the sources of creativity". As he discusses the self-healing tendencies of creativity, he describes the self-healing process as being "orderly, relieving, connecting ... and of pleasurable nature within the entire breadth of creativity". MÜLLER-THALHEIM (1975) quotes BADER (1972): "All this appears to the creative being as an everlasting ritual of exorcism, whereby he tries to bear and survive the unbearable tensions of its condition."

LUCAS (1991) found that among the many types of psychotherapy, *Art Group Psychotherapy* (AGP) has gradually become one of the most appealing and valuable methods of therapy.

MATERAZZI (1990) uses *psycho-cine*, a modality of helping patients to produce films with a content relevant to their emotional problems. The patients in the group select the topic, write the script, and produce the film, acting in it and directing it. They may get technical assistance in the production phase. The process helps them acquire both ego-integration and social integration.

BADER (1972), in the film production by patients, mixes acting and animated characters. This method fosters symptom relief, and group cohesion among patients.

RUBIN and IRWIN (1975), in their paper *"Art and Drama: Parts of a Puzzle"*, describe their use of both art and drama in diagnostic interviews with children and adolescent outpatients. These combined methods enhance the opportunity for more fully understanding the child.

STONE (1975) uses sequential graphic gestalt production in art psychotherapy, where the client is requested to produce several drawings in rapid succession, while sharing the activity with the art therapist. From among the spontaneously created pictures one is selected as "stimulus painting" symbolizing a possible latent conflict or anxiety, and the client is requested to draw several more pictures rapidly in two or three minutes, in a sequence, which depict the theme or possible action suggested by the first painting. It is emphasized that an ending, climax or solution must be drawn to extend the meaning of the originally portrayed problem. This helps to complete the incomplete gestalt and to bring closure to long-standing conflicts. The client is requested to place the entire graphic sequence in order of completion, study it, and create a written dialogue for the principal symbols and figures. The patient is further requested to write the dialogue in the first person singular, present tense for all subjects. This is important to aid in making contact with personal feelings and meanings.

Drawing the accelerated graphic sequences helped the clients gain some measure of confidence and emotional mastery over threatening dreams or anxieties.

In a variation of Stone's Sequential Graphic Gestalt method, HARDING and JONES (1975), quoted by STONE (1975), have utilized an opaque projector to greatly enlarge the client's 7" × 9" stimulus dream pictures for stage sets during carefully structured gestalt "art–psychotherapy–psychodramas".

In verbal psychotherapy, the interaction is essentially between patient and therapist. In art therapy and art psychotherapy, the interaction is extended to the connection between the art product, the patient and the psychiatrist.

In some instances, without an interpretation,

the patient may experience a *catharsis* during the spontaneous production of the art work. Several patients have reported being relieved of the anxiety and fear of their "persecutor" and frightening nightmares and hallucinations after they have expressed these graphically.

It is well known that in mildly stressful situations, such as while sitting in meetings, many people resort to doodlings as a spontaneous mechanism to relieve tension (HALLIDAY 1981). This may be regarded as a minor catharsis and self-therapy (JAKAB 1990a).

In art therapy catharsis may also be achieved. Nonetheless, in some cases dwelling on the memory of events which caused major stress may actually increase the anxiety. VAN DER KOLK et al. (1985) found that psychotherapy of patients with posttraumatic stress disorder is often not successful because it may increase the level of anxiety.

A paper to be well remembered is UHLIN's article (1971) on the possible negative effect of art therapy on children with perceptual neurological handicap. He wrote: "the child with neurological handicap is one of the notable and exceptional few for whom art has not performed its vital service". "... Such a child often suffers an extreme distortion in the perceptual process which may impair his ability to even close a line to produce a form. We may say that he does not experience or 'see' as others".

If any attempt is made to use art materials in the rehabilitation of neurologically impaired children, we must first ascertain that they do not suffer from such symptoms as space agnosia or constructive apraxia, because for those subjects the expectation of using art materials appropriately for communication may be very frustrating. In LEHTINEN's definition (quoted by UHLIN 1969a), they are 'perceptually handicapped'. They require other methods of rehabilitation than art therapy.

Art works are viewed by many therapists as media of communication. The communication through art media takes place between two poles: the *'communicator'* (the patient) who intends (or does not intend!) to communicate and the *recipient* (the therapist) who understands or assumes to understand the intellectual and emotional message of the communicator. JAKAB (1986) requested drawings from a cardiac transplant patient and his family as a form of special communication of their feelings before, during, and after the transplant. These drawings brought into consciousness feelings they had not clearly perceived during the actual major stress of facing the life or death situation.

The effects of major environmental events are reflected in the drawings and paintings of the survivors. BRAUNER and BRAUNER (1994) describe drawings and paintings of children who have survived the holocaust and atrocities of wars in different countries. YAMANAKA (1986) published dramatic case studies of children who survived the great Hanshin earthquake and who expressed their impressions and feelings in drawing. Group art therapy with survivors of the Hiroshima atomic bomb is presented by YAMAGUCHI (1995, 1997).

Drawings and paintings of patients who suffered severe personal abuse (aggression or sexual abuse) were described by IRWIN (1981) and by JAKAB (1994b).

The importance of general socio-cultural factors in psychopathology are described by JILEK (1995). NUCHO (1986) reports on the influence on art of the social changes in Latvia after the collapse of the Soviet Union.

Often, the verbal therapy is conducted by a person different from the one doing the art therapy. These therapies must be coordinated (JAKAB 1968). If the goal of the treatment is expression of unconscious emotions and feelings, that should be allowed both in free associations of the verbal therapy and in the graphic expression. On the other hand, if the goal of therapy is supportive and reality oriented, then the expression of bizarre and unsettling emotions should be discouraged in the graphic expression as well as in the verbal therapy sessions.

## COMMENTS ON CREATIVITY AND PSYCHIATRIC ART

Various theories on the nature of creativity have been advanced in relation to master works of fine arts and also in relation to psychiatric art (FOY 1968, 1971, 1990, JAKAB 1979).

The relationship of the creative talent to the neurotic and psychotic state is often questioned. The classical statement that in art "a regression in the service of the ego" takes place (KRIS 1952) is one of the most accepted theories. Regarding art products by patients, several examples point to the fact that the artistic talent is not produced by the psychosis but its expression might become more efficient through the reduction of inhibitions. Lonnie, a 15-year-old talented boy with severe borderline psychosis, represented himself as an anthropomorph tree, while he experienced a state of depersonalization proving that his creative ability remained unaffected during this episode (JAKAB and HOWARD 1971).

A comparison of the technical methods and styles used by artists and those used by psychiatric patients (JAKAB 1969a) reveals that both groups use the following techniques to express very strong or distorted emotions: condensation, unconnected body parts, floating figures, hierarchic perspective, transparency, direct psychomotor expressions, exaggeration, antithesis of elements, non-figurative abstractions and stereotyped representations.

In several cases, the creative talent of schizophrenic patients seems to lose its originality and their art work becomes stereotyped or disintegrated as the illness progresses to chronic states (DAX 1953, FERDIÈRE 1947a,b, 1951).

DRACOULIDES (1952) correctly states that the artistic talent has to exist as a previous condition in order to allow the production of really artistic creations as a sublimation.

RAPAPORT (1968), who studied the art of mentally retarded persons, attempts to explain the contrast of the low mental development and the high artistic ability of some retarded children. He applied the term of "gifted retarded" to those whose creative intelligence far surpasses their IQ measured by psychological tests. TYSZKIEWICZ (1975) demonstrated unexpected values in the art of mentally retarded children. KLÄGER (1992, 1993) presents impressive art works by mentally retarded persons.

FISCHER, in 1969, established a biological model of creativity. He contends that 'normality', 'creativity' and 'schizophrenia' represent states of increasing arousal and, therefore, can be conceived as lying on a continuum:

"Creativity is an excited-exalted state of arousal with a characteristic increase in both *data content* and *rate of data processing*. The acute schizophrenic state is marked by an even higher level of arousal, but the increase in data content is not matched by a corresponding increase in the rate of data processing. The creative state is conducive to the evolution of novel relations and new meaning, whereas the schizophrenic 'jammed computer' state itself interferes—through 'protective inhibition' and a narrowing of the field of attention—with the individual's symbolic interpretation of his own central nervous system activity."

It is uncanny how accurately Fischer has compared the workings of a pathological mind to a 'jammed computer' and the occurrence of 'protective inhibition' in such a computer. Recently, a computer program simulation experience has been carried out which proves that 'overload of information' leads to 'confused processing and to inhibition' (HOFFMAN 1987, 1992).

## FUTURE TRENDS IN RESEARCH AND APPLICATION

It is evident that the development of psychological and psychiatric theories about psychopathology have had an impact on the use of the art of psychotic or neurotic patients in the diagnosis and treatment of their illness.

The development of technology in the second half of this century has had a great impact on the medical sciences, as well as on the fine arts. To mention just a few highlights, the use of refined laboratory techniques in genetics and other diagnostic medical fields is now taken for granted. The use of X rays, for instance, in the art field is also taken for granted in revealing the different layers of the "overpainted" art works. The spectrometric analysis of color, pigment, and background material is well accepted in the circles of art critics and art evaluators, and it is used also to detect forgeries.

I would like to provide here a comparison between art forgery and "forgery" in the art expression of psychiatric patients.

When we talk about forgery in art, it usually means that an artist of reasonable talent copies art works of other artists, well enough to pass it off as the original, thus trying to reproduce the style, the content and the colors of the painting that has been copied. Modern technological methods can identify such forgeries.

In the patients' art products, 'forgery' has a very different meaning. I would call the dissimulation of symptoms a forgery, when a patient deliberately uses art expression to conceal feelings, or to express feelings he/she does not have, wanting to appear "more sick" or "less sick" than he/she is. This applies to patients with some sophistication in art expression and in psychology, who "know" what the therapist would "see" in their art work, and therefore produce something they want the therapist to see. For example, one patient, who desired to remain hospitalized after recovery, produced 'schizophrenic-like drawings', although he did not show clinical symptoms of psychosis any more. Because the stresses of his life were too great, he felt entitled to be "kept in the hospital". He has produced a number of drawings very similar to the schizophrenic patients' drawings which he has seen on the ward; nonetheless, these were compositions in which pathological vignettes were randomly introduced and appeared alien to the total composition. The patient was not a good forger. The artificial madness was revealed not only in the drawings themselves, but also in the patient's behavior in which he tried to imitate the behavior of psychotic patients without actually being able to give the impression of genuine behavior.

Depressive patients sometimes intend to disguise their depression. This is especially evident at times when they want to be discharged from the hospital or discontinue their treatment and medication while they are still depressed. In such cases, the patients may have the energy to put on a cheerful demeanor. They change the drawing style from gloomy, depressed subjects to more "happy-looking" pictures. Nonetheless, in such 'forgery', it is often quite easy to discover the underlying depression by the relative size of the different elements in the composition, the visual asymmetries, or obsessive symmetries (defenses), and the use of colors usually on the more somber side. Sometimes, however, the patients, trying to fake health, use inappropriately bright colors and sharp contrasts. Naturally, the interpretation of art work has to be paralleled by the clinical observation and interpretation of the verbal behavior as part of the patient's total behavior. Depressive patients are inclined to dissimulate at the point in their treatment when their energy level and psychomotor activity has increased, while suicidal ideation still persists. They are in great danger of accomplishing such acts. Thus, their suddenly changed and potentially misleading art works must be assessed very critically.

The technological development in medicine, and to a lesser degree in psychiatry, has progressed towards the use of computerized expert systems in diagnosis and treatment decisions. These systems are used as "consultants" in diagnostic evaluation.

Although the first artificial intelligence expert system in psychiatry was designed for a computerized interpretation of the *Minnesota Multi-Phasic Personality Inventory (MMPI)* test, there was a long gap before other computerized evaluations have been designed for psychiatric diagnosis. Furthermore, the few psychiatric expert systems designed up to now are rarely used.

It is conceivable that a well-designed expert system for the interpretation of art works from the point of view of composition, style, content and color could be of use in the future for putting art diagnosis on a more scientific basis as well as making it available to professionals in the field of general medicine or psychology who are not specifically trained in art interpretation or art therapy. It could be used as a diagnostic tool by the general practitioner and as an evaluative tool in multi-disciplinary teams. Naturally, these expert systems can supply only guidelines for diagnosis and treatment while the final decision remains in the hands of the mental health professional who uses them. They are not meant to replace the professional but to serve as 'consultants'. They could become a useful diagnostic and treatment advisory tool in the future.

In 1987 and 1992, HOFFMAN described a very interesting use of neural nets in computer simulation of complex neural systems, which is a model of associative memory and gestalt-seeking during cognition. What is fascinating about this report is that the perturbations imposed on such computer simulations caused catastrophic breakdowns of the neural-net functions. The resulting "cognitive disturbances" assumed two forms: one "schizophrenic-like" and the other "manic-like". The schizophrenic-like form was induced by memory overload and resulted in misperceptions, loose associations, and also parasitic processing states that pathologically controlled the flow of associations. The manic-like form was caused by increased randomness of neural activity, which induced "jumps" from one gestalt to another. The relationship between this differential model of psychotic disturbances and other studies of schizophrenia and mania was explored by the author. This model could certainly help us understand the mechanisms acting in the human brain when such psychiatric disorders become clinically manifested.

Maybe psychiatry could be credited with a "treatment for crazy computers" used in early days of computer dysfunction, namely the "electric shock treatment" *(ECT)*. Now, five decades after CERLETTI and BINI's (1938) introduction of the electric shock, we still do not know why schizophrenics improve and depression subsides after ECT. Neither is it clear how it "cured computers".

*The inevitable progress of technology should be no substitute for the compassionate, sensitive and creative approach of mental health workers toward their patients. In the healing profession, we are the ones responsible for the humane and caring relationship to our patients. Our duty is to use the technology in the best interest of the patient. The pursuit of basic and applied clinical research in our field is essential for the long-range goals of refining our diagnostic skills and increasing the range of our therapeutic interventions.*

❧

*The past* is an era of pioneers in art-diagnosis, art therapy as well as in the study of creativity underlying the artistic expression.

*The present* is a refinement of the diagnostic methods through systematic research and of the therapeutic activities through the introduction of family therapy and group therapy and their variations in art drama, and psycho-cinè. The impact of art therapy is enhanced in homogeneous groups of patients regarding the nature of their illness; e.g., alcoholic patients, non-verbal patients, artistically talented patients with verbal communication disorder, etc.

*The future* holds ongoing research potential in all aspects of our field. It also has the potentials for developing new approaches by utilizing the up-to-date technology of expert systems to make the expertise of specialists more widely available than the person-to-person consultation.

*The material in this book is based on the paintings and drawings of the collection of artworks produced by patients treated between 1920 and 1959 at the Psychiatric and Neurological University Hospital of Pécs, Hungary.* This collection includes about two thousand paintings and drawings of which we have selected a small number to be reproduced in this book.

The special value of this collection is in the

long-term observation of the clinical course of the illness of our patients and of their artistic work during and after hospitalization. Most of these patients were hospitalized for years or even decades before the advent of psychotropic medications.

Some patients received electric shock treatment which caused transitory memory deficits and as a consequence regression in the style of their artworks to a childlike product. Others who were treated by lobotomy showed no regression in their artwork after surgery.

The majority of drawings and paintings date from the time when the former Chairman, Professor Camillo Reuter (1874–1954), was the head of the department. These are the years between 1918 and 1946. Dr. Reuter, a psychiatrist and connoisseur of the graphic arts, was interested in the artistic works of patients. It is due to him that this large collection has been preserved. He followed the preparation of this book with great interest and assisted in the selection of drawings and paintings to be reproduced in it. We are most grateful for his advice.

This author joined the Psychiatric and Neurological University Hospital of Pécs in 1947.

Some of the patients whose works are described in this book were still hospitalized at that time. The case histories of these patients were updated by this author, with ongoing progress notes and references to their artistic activity regarding the works produced after 1947. Furthermore, the present English edition contains an additional case history (Case 16) of a patient who was hospitalized as a teenager from 7 January 1959 to 23 March 1959. After successful treatment with electric shock he was discharged and his follow-up continues on an outpatient basis to the present. His talent was evident already before his psychosis and he became a professional painter after his discharge from the hospital.

In accordance with the psychiatric literature, we found that the majority of patients who painted and drew were schizophrenics. Those who suffered from manic depressive psychosis produced drawings and paintings only in the manic phase. Finally, one of our patients, who suffered from alcoholic hallucinosis, drew the images of his visions. We have included only art works produced spontaneously (and not as the result of art-therapeutic intervention).

In the following pages we present the case histories of our subjects. Based on the data recorded in the case histories, we propose to analyze from a dual point of view, both psychiatric and artistic, the drawings and paintings in this collection. The artists who produced these drawings and paintings all suffered from psychotic states during their hospitalization.

It has to be mentioned here that among the patients who have been treated at our hospital there were no famous painters or sculptors. This observation is true even for those patients who had taken courses at the Academy of Fine Arts.

I want to express my special thanks to the late Ferenc Martyn*—a good friend and expert theoretician of art interpretation—for his help in the artistic analysis of the works of our patients. I am deeply impressed by his generous contribution. Without his advice the artistic interpretation of the collection would have been much less elaborate.

---

* Ferenc Martyn (1899–1986) was a painter of international fame. Several of his works—paintings, drawings and sculptures—are now permanently housed and exhibited at the Martyn Museum in Pécs, Hungary.

# Psychiatric and Artistic
# Evaluation

# CLINICAL OBSERVATIONS AND PRESENTATION OF THE DRAWINGS AND PAINTINGS

## SCHIZOPHRENIA

### Case 1 — L. I.

*Date of birth*: 21 February 1902
*Occupation*: Student at the Technological University
*Diagnosis*: Schizophrenia
He was treated at the Psychiatric and Neurological University Hospital of Pécs, Hungary, with some interruptions from 4 December 1923 to 29 March 1925.
*Family history*: No relevant illness.
*Personal history*: The patient became withdrawn and introverted at the age of sixteen when he was preoccupied with meditations. At the same time, he became agitated, mostly at night, and disturbed his family. In the upper grades of high school, it was observed that the scholastic work of this previously quite conscientious and gifted, diligent youngster had declined. At that time he occasionally had hallucinations. At the age of seventeen, he ran away and disappeared for four months, influenced by ideas of persecution. At the age of twenty-one he was hospitalized because of an attempted suicide and ideas of persecution, aggressivity, and severe psychomotor agitation.
*At admission* to the hospital his behavior was confused. He gave irrelevant answers to questions and declared that he had come here to draw. At the same time he held his belt like a pencil and made gestures with his hand on the table, as if drawing.
*Medical and neurological examination* revealed no pathological sign. Bordet–Wassermann reaction (for syphilis) was negative. The patient was pale and had a circumscribed red spot on each cheek. We mention this because he frequently adorned the region of the cheeks on his drawings with a circle or star in the area where his red spots were.
The patient was agitated, restless and excitable. His speech was incoherent. His attention span was diminished while at the same time it was difficult to engage his attention by outside stimuli. He expressed megalomanic and persecutionary ideas at the same time as hypochondriac delusions.
*Course of illness*: His family tried to return him to his home several times, but he had to be brought back to the hospital each time because of agitation and hostile behavior. Once he attacked the members of his family with a pair of scissors.
During this hospitalization, the patient declared one day that he was in Tibet and liked to be there very much since he had the possibility of abandoning himself to his meditations.

His behavior was variable, sometimes bizarre, at other times stereotyped. His speech was incoherent and his voice had bizarre inflections. In the same sentence, some syllables were spoken with a strong voice, while others were barely audible whispers. He did not disclose the subject of his vivid hallucinations. Sometimes he was in a state of catatonic stupor. At times he was very agitated. He chased the other patients out of their beds, and threw the bed linen, pillows and blankets onto the floor. He ripped off his shirt and ran around naked in the corridor. Then he suddenly stopped to balance himself on one leg with closed eyes until he fell down.

The patient both drew and wrote a great deal. He wrote "scripts" for plays for the theater, "pamphlets", "novels", and a large number of letters. In his written works, in addition to well-composed phrases, there are also strings of words without meaning and even whole "letters" which are only pure strings of meaningless words. Similar characteristics may be observed in his drawings some of which are expressive, executed very precisely, while others are only scribblings.

Here are some passages from his "novel" entitled "Álmos" (may be translated as The Sleepy One—or it may be the name of a Hungarian chieftain):

"The music of the military chapel spreads sadly over the markets and the boulevards.

Cecelia, the young Ingenueengineer, drags herself sadly over slippery stones. She trots abandoned on the fluid and blackish asphalt, sometimes counting her money to reassure herself that it has not fallen on the sidewalk.

He was employed at the Board of an aviation society and served mostly between Wien and 'Buynosayresz'? He was still a precocious child at twenty-nine years of age." ...

"Álmos has dedicated all his time to the very famous Union named after the happiness evoked from Cecile. It stimulated Cecile's spring soul for the buds to open up!! And the diligent work also produced its special result. Cecile has been promoted in an instant to woman arch-engineer at the polytechnical school in Wien, and they have already cut through the cloudy skies together over the express wings towards the rich capital of 'B:ulynos # Aijdesz', with white gloves on their hands. En route, they kissed over and over and they arrived at the capital tired by the 'parfumeros rouge kisses'. The mayor of the city has been waiting in an airplaneboat for the rare-distinguished engineer-aviator-sub-engineer guests!

After the lunch, both were permeated by the sweet, sweet, sweet, sweet, sweet, sweet, sweet, sweet warmth of new aromatic kisses."

The short story "Peter" written by the patient is the following:

"The milk stood there on the table. The little mother traipsed sadly and quietly through the old worm-eaten door which squeaked pitifully on its tight ungreased hinges.

She straightened her faded greenish-black head scarf that she wore over her forehead over the graying thick locks so these would lie back from her eyes and nose and not disturb her. She was an old wrinkled little thing. The new modern rubber shoes on her feet did not fit at all, also the rings on the well cared for colorful thin fingers did not fit. Her son, the hopeless Peter, lazed around the table and in the garden chairs. His hair was a blonde unparted funny thing which has always hung in thick locks into his face, sometimes into his eye, near his ear ...

Mary was a beautiful girl with chalk-white face and coal-black hair, twenty years old. The love of Peter. She hurried with dreaming steps along the Papst Street directly to Peter. She entered. The little mother received her, aunt Ancsura who held together with jealously yellowish shimmering hairpins of bone ... her unkempt hair in an unskilled way ...

Peter was shy, strange, and held the girl's hand, grabbing it avidly and kissed her also... He was not embarrassed, and Mary came to him also without embarrassment; nonetheless, she was a light blooded little woman. A fresh short-skirted soul-sending-feelings of a woman who was there to the pleasure of the whole city through her excellent manners, skillful dance rhythms and sparkling speeches—her conversation ...

Peter frequented the university, the faculty of law. But now he skipped it and lies around the house.

They kissed with the girl instinctful and heated, wild and laughing loudly with laughing laughter, with sensual pleasure, warm, soft, moving around, moving, touching, in feverish rings bejeweled, let down, stupid, lost half-drunken, not desiring just giving, did he kiss ...

But this was a kiss on the lips. Soundless. A scheme like a happy Calvary of love. Of this kiss originated a prayer, a mute dying veiled love-prayer, kiss; simpler, cooler, dying, tired kiss ... It was beautiful so.

The head of death of the moon slumbered sleepily through the curtains. The girl and the boy scared looked at the window sill as if they had understood and sighed loudly ... Soon storm-clouds have covered their triple faces...

He writes ... It was written by Baron L.P.I. from Borsod Architect Candidate."

As the inventor of an operetta, the patient has invented names. For the composer of the musical score, he gave another unknown name and in addition he also wrote the name of Béla Bartók.

"THE CORVETTE

Operetta in three acts.

First scene.

Fine dark heavy furniture of noble wood in the room. The mirror smooth oakwood parquet which was cleaned with white Tekla is covered with dark green Persian carpets. From the Roman type arched windows hang light sea-green thin silk house curtains. The light comes through four windows ... The desk is of ebony, three standing nut-wood cabinets with feet, also three in number—all good things are three heavy, upholstered green chairs. An inkwell decorated with diamonds just as the pencil and pen holder; flord amoür x molin rouge x,,, vaera violett '"very sweet, pleasant, one can drink it with heavenly smell the pale falling blue: (cobalt): blue as forget-me-nots light wallpaper ... Electrical imitation of candles—chandelier, quartz lights which shine like diamonds, strengthen the day- and evening light.—The operetta's actors are dressed very simply, nonetheless hyper modern, in the fashion of the latest French style.

| Andreas | The Corvette |
| Michael | The father of Corvette |
| Hermine | The fiancée of Corvette |
| Irene | The young girl |

I. (Act I)

*Andreas*: Does he hold in his hand the "Új Nemzedék" (the title of a newspaper)? He reads news about the Navy. All his sensory organs vibrate nervously, he scrutinizes every single little truly Hungarian sentence from the overall fine modern, very elegant military marine journal!

... I. e.: ... A "submarine boat", 3, —destroyer found happily a harbor on the land of the French colony New Caledonia ... The staff of the torpedo-boat destroyer were to the last one unharmed and also the commandant of the ship Corvet Andrea Tor. Tor has surprised the Caledonian marine office with a new torpedo-boat-discovery ...

*Michael*: And you are certainly well instructed about all this, isn't it true? My dear little son Andreas? Follow this so that you can make your way soon with the next ship ...

*Hermine*: (Storms into the blue salon charmed but with disturbed face and falls into the arms of her fiancée the Corvette): As I see, my dear Andreas, you have become a strong Corvette since I have seen you the last time, you look good. You have become nice. Show me your face, your mouth, the sweet arch of your lips, your matte pale white beautifully powdered chin. For how long have I not kissed them! Oh for how long have I not given you compliments my only beautiful Andreas, my sweet Corvette! Your face is pale like a foam-white violet, your chest is thin like the lagoons which spread on the edges of the Danish fjords. Ah, you are sicker than before!?! Heal thyself, care for yourself—allow me to treat you—Andreas ... my faithful sweetheart, lover what's happening to you? Hey? Ah, are you a waste? My angel my soul my stupidity, my everything Andry, my dear angel. Answer! I am waiting for your musical words, why have you abandoned your beautiful kissing being. Oh you unhappy youngster, are you Lieutenant or Corvette? Maybe you could be major, general, field marshall, if you only would not abandon me you bohemian youngster. You are crying. You are moaning. You are desiring me. I know it well. I don't understand. I have asked the heaven in prayer that no harm should befall you!

*Irene*: We are also sad about you, Corvette Andreas Torr. Stutter and handle what weighs on you, what hurts your gourmand lips. Come with me, I will make you happy, Irene, the siren the young blessed and modest ... Come let's go, let us leave all sadness, everything only everything which can be sad ... Irene, still poor will save you, the proud, shred your worries, break the cabinets the ones that separate me from you ... Do not kiss my hands, my mouth, my shoulders, my chin, do not lick my wrinkled face forever without cause. Do not abandon my carefree beautiful life moaning, laughing, singing, disgusting! ...

*Andreas*: As French Corvette I tell you you have lost my flower, my mandoline; I ask you hopelessly also on Pengő money. I search for you desperately my Hermine, my foam-white mink. Wait for me my little figure-girl, my feminine dawn, with dew on your beautiful girlish face; there at the end wait, rest my expensive creme, deep below far from here from the periphery of smoke here on the back of the sweet orchids, azaleas, goldenrods, here ... yes ... sweet ... kiss on the balcony ...

*Michael*: Go now my little Pajodom. Little brave young woman Hermine—the service boils over ... Go far away from here, Irene and Hermine, my beautiful dove, far, far, far, far ... over the moat of the castle on the cordon and undulating fields ..."

Some of the patient's letters contain only a meaningless chain of words.

"I have no time, I beg you, I go away. Zábó and Mussolini are aggressive men. They look at me with an ordinary left hand. Karl Veidal. Crayon from Pozsony, Wilhelm Pozsony. One shilling. Painter Megyeri. I don't need Uncle William. The county Bihar was big. I bemoan the Ferdinand. 29, the Ferdinand. Terrible, terrible. And what do they take me for? Terrible hero of the county of Pozsony. Because this land, every land, on which I am the dirt, old man, the Hungarian state. The Hungarian merchandise 'VAJDESZ'. We don't know what is wrong with him. Things, I arrive to Pécs, in Schilling-Pécs, Swiss Frank to Pécs. Big house. Things also to Pécs the most infuriating."

The patient often requested paper and pencil to draw. Sometimes he only scribbled, at other times he wrote bizarre letters of the alphabet which he called "roman letters".

He draws his autoportrait and the portraits of other patients.

His products are stereotyped. Sometimes he covers the whole surface in a few minutes. At other times he works minutiously and slowly. He usually writes the names of persons whom he wants to represent in the drawings. The patient has also produced some oil paintings. During his hospitalization he drew hundreds of pictures on cigarette paper.

He repeats the same subject for weeks and then changes to a new subject, which is again repeated in the same stereotyped manner, sometimes for months. For example, he draws innumerable samples of maps of Hungary.

He shows his drawings proudly and brags about them, but does not give away any of them as gifts. He answers only briefly to questions while he is drawing, without interrupting his work.

He prefers to represent important political people and well-known actresses. He writes the names of one of these persons at the margin of his stereotyped drawings, which are totally lacking any resemblance to the persons he pretends to have represented. His bizarre associations are reflected sometimes in the motivation of the names he has chosen. A man with a tall hat (cylinder) on his head suggests to the patient, by alliteration, the name of the film actor Psylander. (This explanation was given by the patient himself.)

To the question why he always repeats the same faces, he answers: "That is interesting, I have never realized that." He does not realize either that his figures are nudes because "there is a cross or a necklace on the lady". Rarely, he also draws animals and objects such as shoes or slippers. On some of his drawings, which represent figures or portraits, he writes his own name completed by such title as "prince of ...", "count of ...", "film actor".

He asked the staff for journals "to study the futuristic style" which he wants to assimilate.

He recognizes his preference for figures "barely clothed". Sometimes he kisses his pencils. He only rarely gives any explanation about his drawings. The geographic maps are sprinkled with drawings of irrelevant objects such as a toothbrush, a glass, a shoe, a cup, etc., or

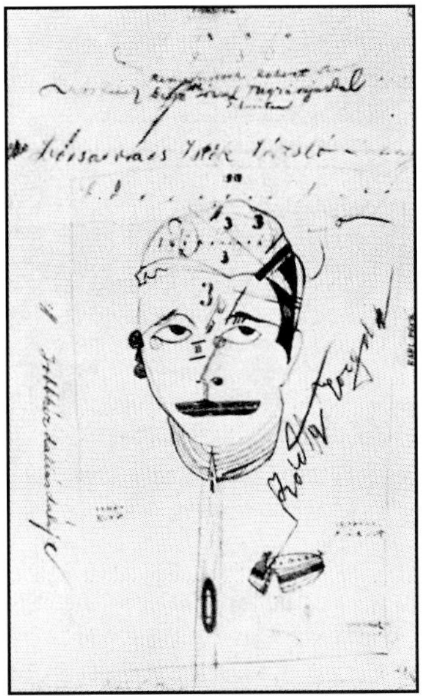

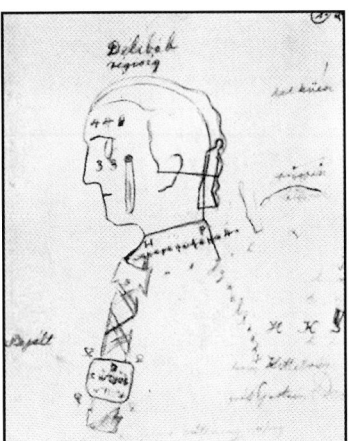

\* All measurements are given in centimeters.

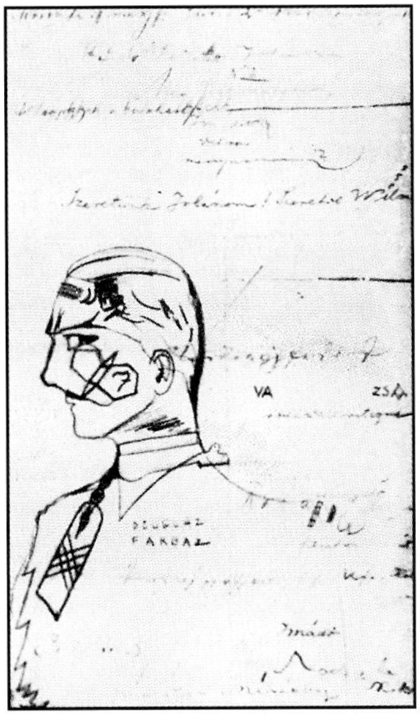

Case 1 - Fig. 1
Pencil drawing. 20x12.5\*

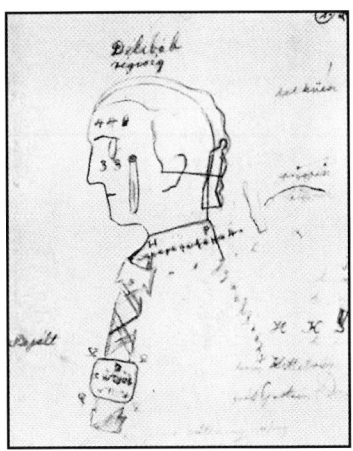

Case 1 - Fig. 3
Pencil drawing. 19x15

Case 1 - Fig. 2
Pencil drawing. 20x12.5

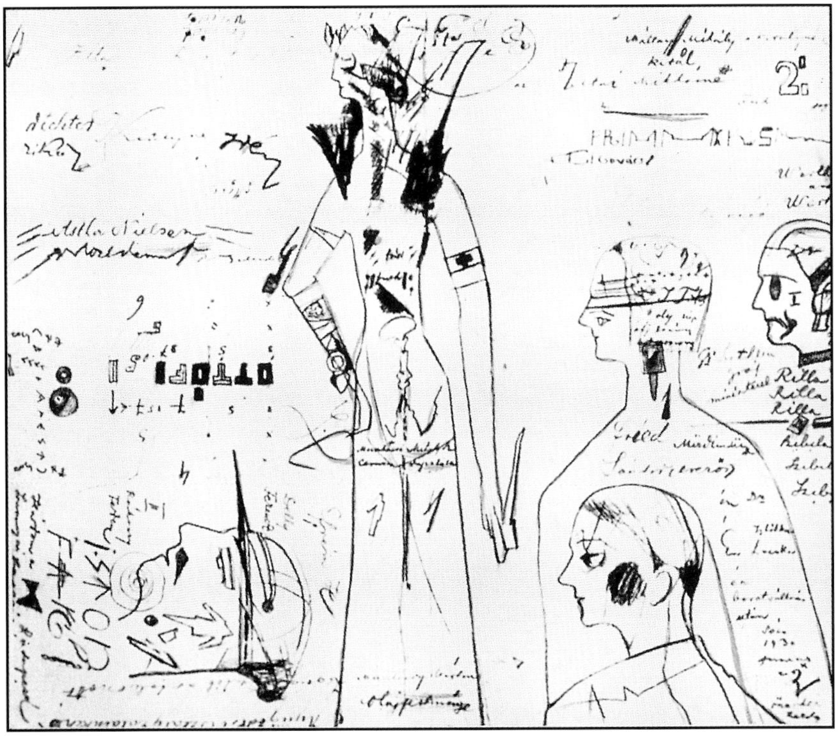

Case 1 - Fig. 4
Pencil drawing. 20x25

36

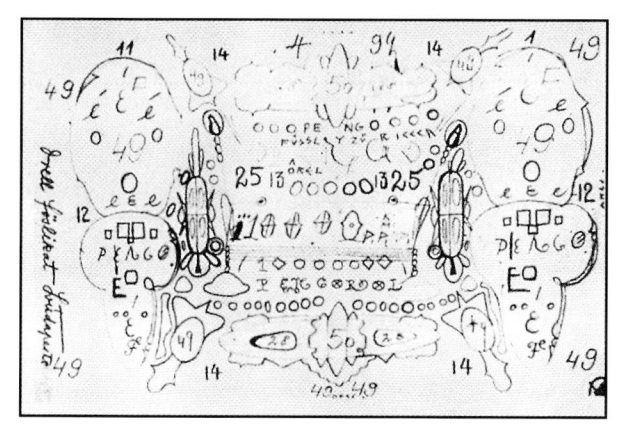

Case 1 - Fig. 5
Pencil drawing. 10.5x17

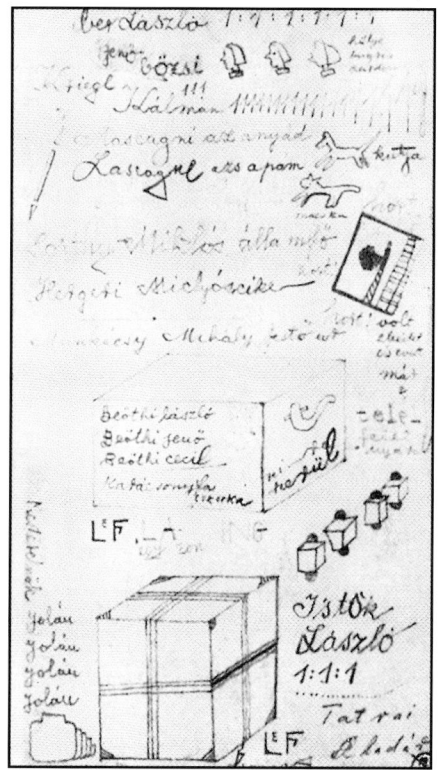

Case 1 - Fig. 6
Pencil drawing. 15x8.5

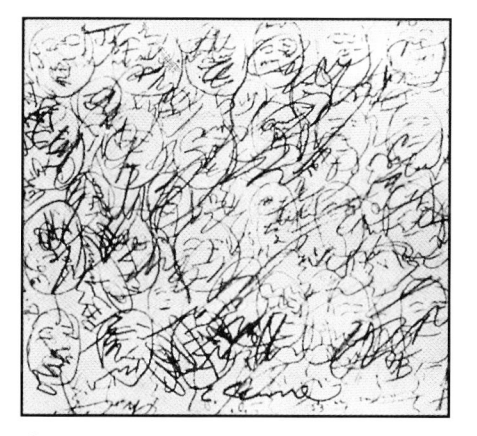

Case 1 - Fig. 7
Pencil drawing. 14.5x17

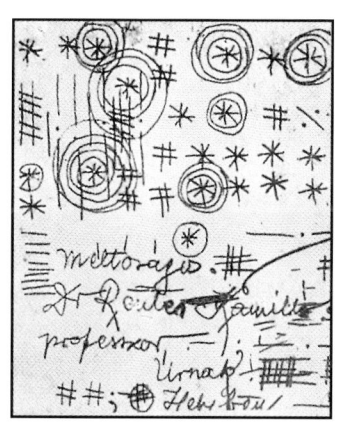

Case 1 - Fig. 8
Pencil drawing. 17x14.5

37

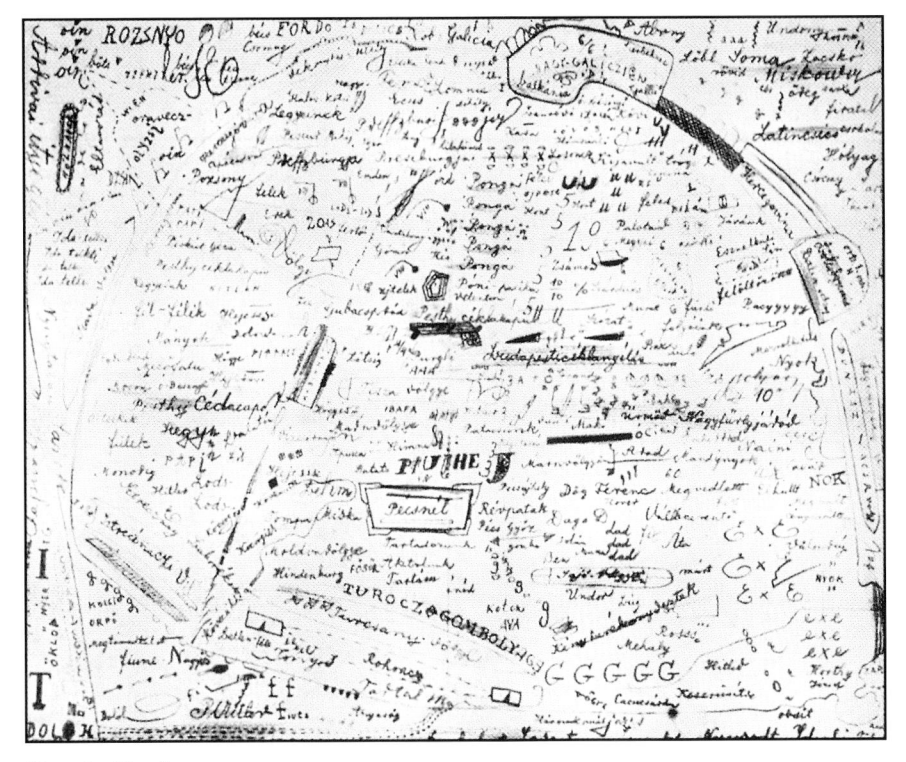

Case 1 - Fig. 9
Pencil drawing. 17x21

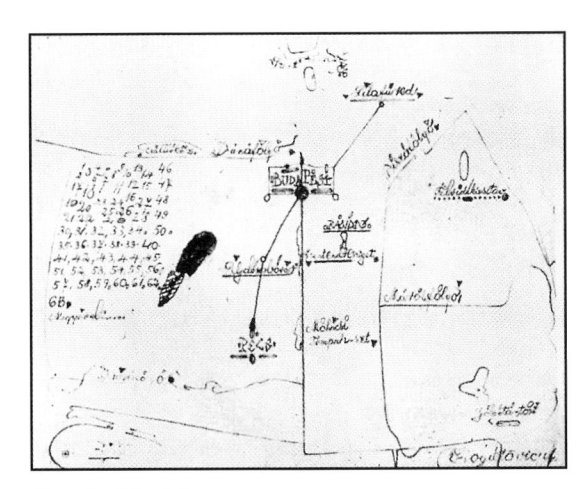

Case 1 - Fig. 10
Pencil drawing. 17x21

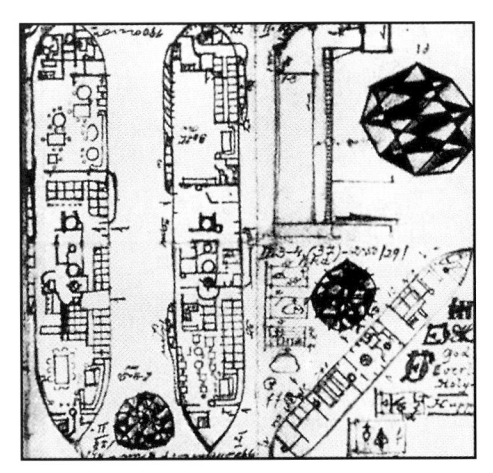

Case 1 - Fig. 11
Pencil drawing. 10x10

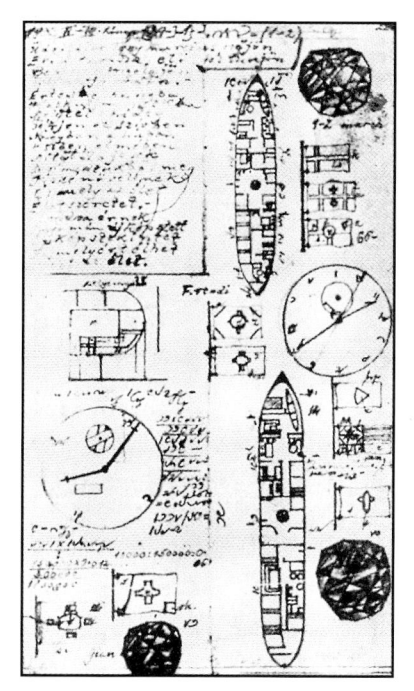

Case 1 - Fig. 12
Pencil drawing. 21x13

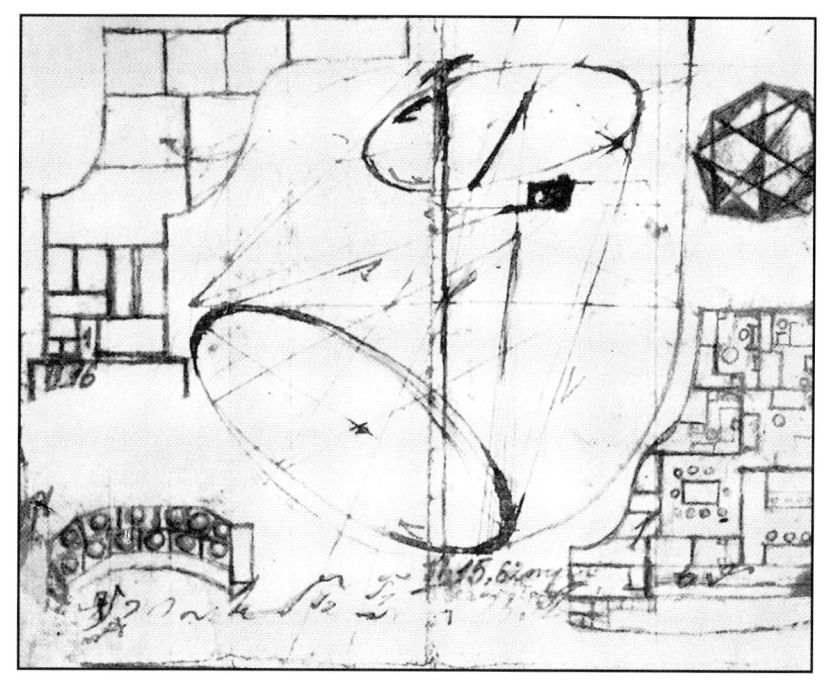

Case 1 - Fig. 13
Pencil drawing. 10x12.5

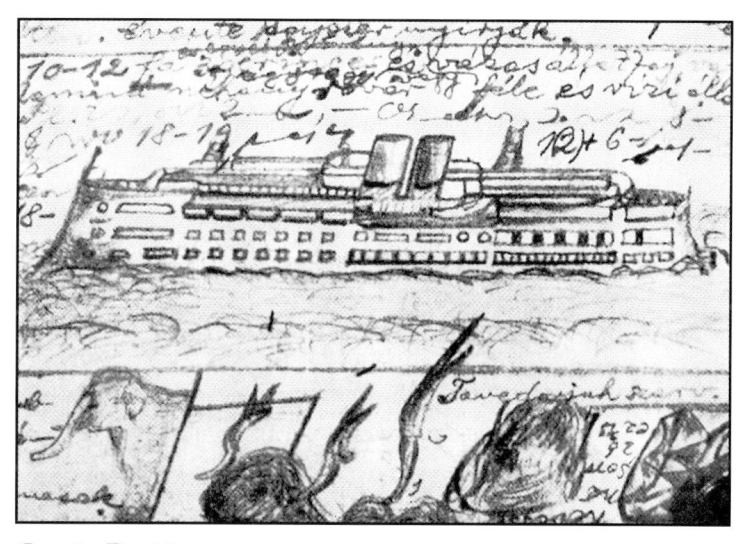

Case 1 - Fig. 14
Pencil drawing. 8.5x14.5

39

written over with words without any meaning. He scribbles a lot over the walls and even on the clothing of other patients. He also drew portraits of the other patients and produced some oil paintings.

*The drawings of L. I. can be classified into four groups.*

*In the first group* the surfaces of the sheets are filled with words, letters, numbers, heads and figures without any relationship to each other. One could compare these works to the incoherent language (word salad) of schizophrenic patients. The heads are generally drawn in profile. Sometimes the lines are almost invisible while others are traced and retraced with energy, producing vast bizarre angles from which the different parts of the face and head emerge. On the hair and on other parts of the face, he draws letters, words, numbers, and lines including geometrical figures (*Figs 1* to *3*). On one of these works, in addition to the letters, words, numbers, and four heads, we find the figure of a woman. Below the hips, the following is written by the patient: "Pencil Drawing by Mihály Munkácsy". This is a pornographic drawing showing the genital organs in an almost anatomical fashion (*Fig. 4*). *Figure 5* could be classified as one of his bizarre drawings composed of lines and numbers arranged in an ornamental way, evoking the sketch of a paper currency (1920's bank note). *Figure 6* may be considered a graphic equivalent of incoherent verbalizations. It consists of numbers and stereotyped repetition of letters, geometrical forms, and faces without any systematic composition. Finally, *Fig. 7*, where a great number of heads are surrounded by circles and crosses, could be used as an example of pure stereotypy in the same way as *Fig. 8* which consists of a great number of stars, traced monotonously and scribbled over with lines on the whole surface.

*The second group* of his drawings is made up by "the geographical map of Hungary" repeated indefinitely. Naturally, these drawings are by no means precise maps. The localities are situated at the wrong places from the geographical point of view. Their whole surface, both inside and outside of the unrealistic borders marked by him, is sprinkled with words and numbers. The letters and words adjacent to each other are often nothing but stereotyped repetitions. In *Fig. 9*, the associations of words are determined by homophony, that is by similar sounds of pronunciation, such as: "pati, papi, fél, félek, fülek". (Translation: pati—a word without meaning in Hungarian (schizophasia); papi—daddy; fél—he is scared; félek—I am scared; fülek—the ears; Fülek—a place in former Hungary.)

On one of his maps he wrote the names of only a small number of localities and completed the square-shaped space by numbers from 1 to 63. If he skips one number, he completes the chain by adding the skipped number between the lines. This great number of digits has no relationship whatever to the map *(Fig. 10)*. This method of juxtaposition of unrelated details reminds us of the method of drawing of a patient of ZSAKÓ (1908) who drew pictures of incomprehensible sketches adjacent to images of churches in the classical style.

*The third group* of his drawings could be designated as "engineering drawings" of machines. On these drawings the stereotyped repetition of details is also evident. Others in this group

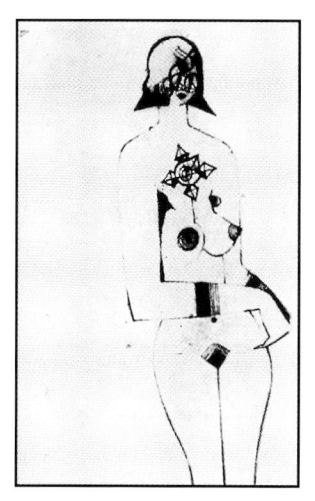

Case 1 - Fig. 15a
Pencil drawing. 14.5x8.5

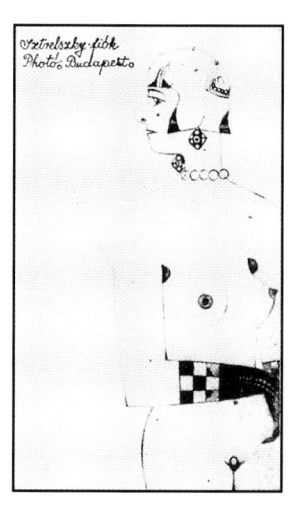

Case 1 - Fig. 15b
Pencil drawing. 10.5x7

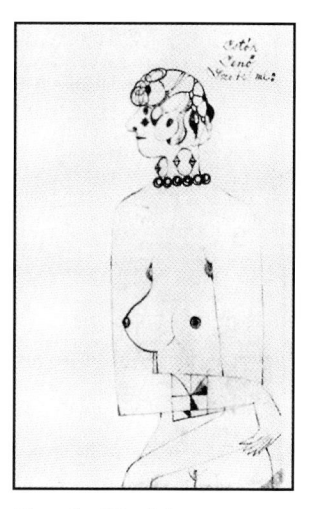

Case 1 - Fig. 15c
Pencil drawing. 14.5x8.5

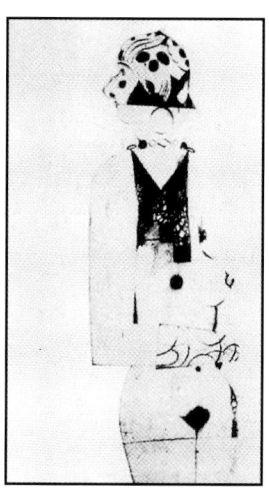

Case 1 - Fig. 15d
Pencil drawing. 14.5x8.5

are only a fantastic superposition of projections of different geometrical forms. Around some of these one can find words in shorthand *(Figs 11 to 14)*. While he produces these drawings with precision and minute details, tracing the lines with a ruler, he sometimes sketches bizarre monsters on the border of the paper *(Fig. 14)*. We may assume that when his attention was not sufficiently concentrated on the drawing it allowed the surfacing of hallucinations.

*The fourth group* of our patient's works is made up of figurative drawings of pornographic nature. These are mostly nude women, very stereotypically drawn, represented from the head to the middle of the thigh; the breasts and genital organs are highly accentuated. These figures are almost identical, as if produced in series. Only the ornaments and jewelry allow one to distinguish between them. The representation of different hairstyles shows a bizarre variety, from being traced in a few lines, to the minute execution of hair styles or ornaments produced by geometrical figures or wavy lines. At other times the hair appears as a dark cap *(Figs 15a to 15d)*. He also composed a large number of pornographic scenes, naked women and men, with the same extravagant hair arrangements. He gives the title to all these drawings (too obscene to be reproduced) "Hercules and his wife". On some of these drawings he also writes his own name and the names of actresses of his time.

Most of these nude pictures are labelled with the first name of a well-known contemporary actress.

On rare occasions, when he draws male figures, he represents them either in military attire or dressed in the fashion of the turn of the century. At other times, he draws only the head of males covered by a military cap. The way of drawing the hairstyle of males is identical to

41

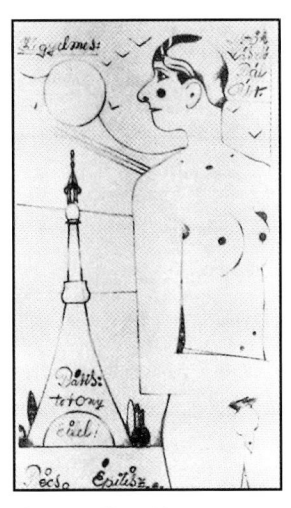

that of the females *(Figs 16a, 16b)*. One of the male figures has female breasts. Here we should mention that, according to his medical record, the patient occasionally had a nightmare about being a hermaphrodite. Beside this male figure with the breast, he wrote his own name and he drew a picture of a tower on which he wrote the words: "Paris, Tour Eifel (!)" *(Fig. 16a)*.

We find in this fourth group of his drawings certain pictures which are essentially abstract, symbolic, and very characteristic of his style. Namely, in a kind of frame similar to a torpedo, representing a female figure, he draws a female head, more or less ornamented. A variety of linked geometrical forms (squares and circles) indicate the limbs. The genital organs of these

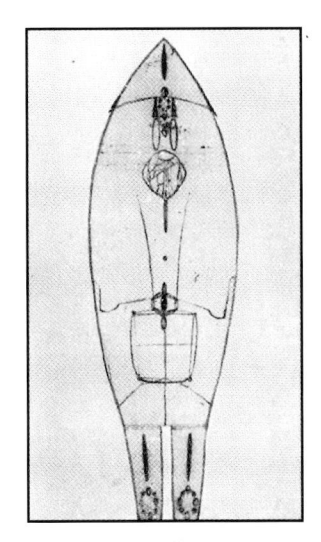

Case 1 - Fig. 16a
Pencil drawing. 14.5x8.5

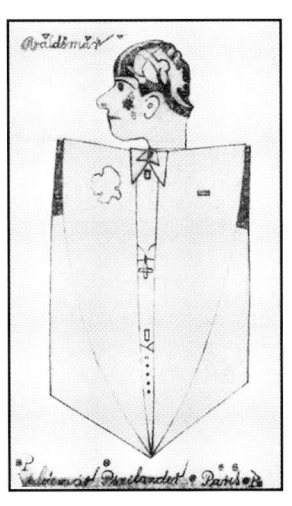

Case 1 - Fig. 16b
Pencil drawing. 14.5x8.5

Case 1 - Fig. 17a
Pencil drawing. 14.5x8.5

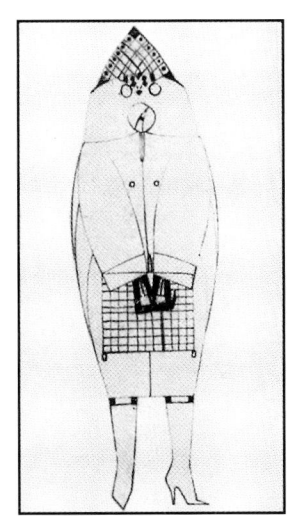

Case 1 - Fig. 17b
Pencil drawing. 14.5x8.5

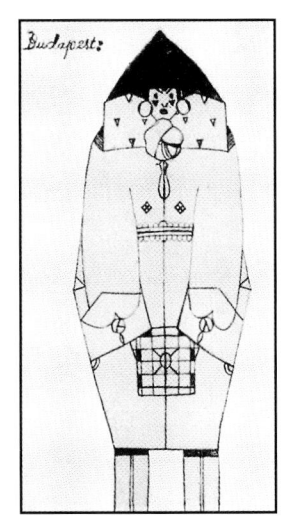

Case 1 - Fig. 17c
Pencil drawing. 14.5x8.5

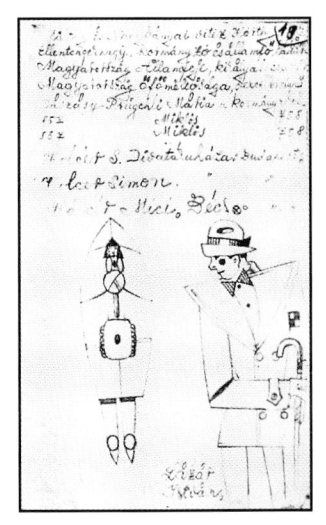

Case 1 - Fig. 17d
Pencil drawing. 14.5x8.5

figures are also symbolically accentuated. On these figures we see a large variety of ornamental elements *(Figs 17a* to *17d)*. On the right of one of these "torpedo females" he drew a man, fully dressed, who looks at her provokingly *(Fig. 17d)*.

We can establish that *L. I.* repeats in the third and fourth group of his drawings a single form. In the fourth group this is similar to a torpedo, to an almond, or to a leaf of a plant. He indicates the longitudinal axis on these forms by dividing them fully or partially. Inside of these frames he draws the details with strong lines. He arranges the details in strikingly strong marks on the female figures.

In the models of machines he uses the same technique. Actually, the "machines" are nothing but the graphic repetition of detached pieces of an imaginary machine, repeated graphically in a stereotyped fashion.

His human figures are usually presented in frontal view while the head may be in profile, as in Egyptian reliefs. The hairstyle is like a helmet. The hands are only rarely representsed and are always the weakest part of the drawing, as compared to other details.

*L. I.*'s compositions are restricted in form. He expresses himself by homogeneous unaccented lines drawn in a manneristic fashion. Sometimes his marks barely touch the paper. At other times he practically pierces the paper. Within the boundaries of the figure, certain surfaces are filled in vigorously in black pencil. The lack of middle values in his drawings gives a "graphic" character, without fine nuances.

He painted on a canvas a Madonna with Child. He also made a sketch of it in pencil *(Fig. 18)*.

In this drawing, around the eyes of the Madonna is a bizarre ornamental motif similar to the petals of a flower. The body of the Madonna as well as that of the Child are primitive, badly executed without appropriate proportions and depth.

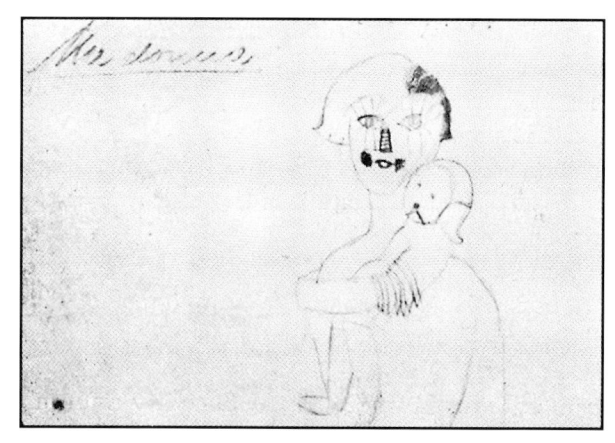

Case 1 - Fig. 18
Pencil drawing. 11x15

# Case 2 — L. L.

*Date of birth*: 26 July 1879
*Occupation*: Notary public in the office of the mayor
*Diagnosis*: Schizophrenia

He was hospitalized at the Psychiatric and Neurological University Hospital of Pécs from 1915 to 1947 when he was transferred to an asylum.

*Personal history*: According to his medical record, already while he was working in the community, as secretary of the mayor, he was interested in literature and wrote poems. He enlisted as a volunteer during World War I and was discharged from the military after being hospitalized.

*The medical and neurological examination* revealed no pathology. Bordet–Wassermann reaction was negative.

*Course of illness*: In the first few years of his hospitalization his mood was pleasant; later he became depressed. He suffered constantly from ideas of reference and megalomanic delusions and hallucinations. "Everybody observes him." "He is the son of God and could be an emperor." "His fiancées are members of the aristocracy." The content of his paranoid ideas during the depressive phase are mostly about being poisoned. He complains that people are burning his head and keep stabbing him with needles. "One has stolen him from the world" and they have exchanged him for somebody else. He must undo the sins of that individual by being brought to the hospital.

He desires to occupy himself with metaphysical problems. He writes several letters in which he implores the bishop and other notables to free him. He also writes similar letters to the editors of journals. His behavior is sometimes stereotyped and negativistic. He uses bizarre and affected gestures. He mixes into his speech neologisms and neophrases. He is not interested in his environment and does not get into contact with the other patients, the nursing staff or physicians. He draws and writes a great deal. Toward the end of his hospitalization he became more and more inactive.

His letters, poems and short stories are actually at many places only strings of incomprehensible words. An example follows from a letter written by him 13 January 1927:

"Mr. Chevalier (noble man)! I shall remain one or two days in the day room of the patients and I shall not eat in order to be recognized (found). I will not eat because here I am always in contact, above me there is a Jewess. This one, because of her magnetism, attracts every man to herself and lives off heads. Like the horse which takes his food from a feed bag hanging on his head. We must all be brave heroes, this is why the emperors, the people, and the inventors have sacrificed their treasures, their strength, and their fortune. The ones who live on the brain and the heart of the man without defense are either unbearable factors on this earth of orphans or they do not have the right to live.

They must kill themselves by suicide or present themselves to the hangman. This house is a place of American torture. In Budapest they have seen that I was saved. Nonetheless because that was the war, from the train station József-város (one of the boroughs of Budapest) to Olsanica, I have to end through a mysterious calvary, the procedures of the police. (Interrogation by a detective.)

Believe me, you have illusions. You are cheating each other gradually. As soon as you liberate me I shall have the key and a beautiful suit like I had once. One can approach the little ones at her 'children's parties' pretty and honest and then we shall live up to the most beautiful stations among the free men. The friend of R. G. bestows upon us her childhood toys. The disgusting and horrible are not motivated. Capitulate! Adieu!"

In the following we quote a few more passages from another letter written by the patient in 1938.

"Excellency! Mr. Professor!

It is unbelievable to me that this clinic of nervous and mental illnesses is the work of masters who want to take by force the heads of intellectuals and that the high commanding office of the war has trusted these patient assassins with the bodies carried and hospitalized here.

An invisible machine destroys and extinguishes my healthy body and there is not a soul to whom I could reveal my horrible situation.

Excellency! Mr. Professor!

The God Mars and his regiment of stars have no pity on the human body; on the contrary, he plays with the life and death of mankind. We are all here under the sun as toys, the puppets of these Gods who have discovered the method of stopping the human heart and who cause the obstacles to the resurrection of the body.

But if all creatures on earth are nothing for this divinity, that doesn't mean that an officer—like yourself, Excellency—who is placed at the head of a similar institute could not observe the disasters which occur in front of his eyes, the inhumanities and the injustices that jump at one's eyes because, in that case, in all creatures a hope founded on the goodness and justice of God stops and justifies the supposition that we are here on this Hungarian earth in a house-of-murder, in a room that destroys the Hungarian race where the physician plays at treating the sick, wringing their neck while smiling.

Excellency! Since the year of 1930 I have sent to the office of the director poems, drawings and other little things. I have given them to the office not to never see them again, but to get out of here with them into the life and finally to use them myself. Please return them to me, I beg you, so that I can copy them in ink.

I am very tired, nonetheless capable of making an existence for myself just the way I have done it several times here (I have not eaten anything for two to three days, thinking that this way, as a civilized man and a gentleman, I could become free). But if your Excellency, Mr. Professor, will not listen to my request, and will not treat me accordingly, then either I shall break the windows in the corridor or I will strangle myself. *I don't wait any longer!*

Produced in Pécs, the 2nd of October 1938 (in the evening)
with high respect
L. L."

The patient frequently draws portraits of children. On any little piece of paper he can put his hands on, he draws human heads. He never explains any of the subjects of his drawings. He keeps them jealously and shows them only from a distance. Once he said: "These are my illuminations that I have made myself." He draws the same figures in a stereotyped fashion. Regarding two of these portraits, he states that they are political personalities. Sometimes he asks for illustrated postal cards to copy them. He refuses vehemently to show us his uncompleted drawings or his poems. Once he submitted to us (the hospital staff) a drawing with the request to send it to the editors. He denies having learned to draw, but recognizes that he enjoyed drawing during high school and during the time he was a public servant. He also copies portraits from journals. He is satisfied with his drawings and brags about them and expects them to be praised.

He folds the paper along the longitudinal axis and fills the whole space at his disposition with heads and human figures stacked on top of each other, similar to totem poles. Some figures lean directly on the head of the figure underneath. This distribution and the folding of the paper in a longitudinal fashion is reminiscent of the legal documents which he was used to while working. In the drawings in which he completes the head with a body and extremities those are usually very small and quite ridiculous. The heads are monstrous, ugly and repulsive. The nose is in the shape of an elephant trunk, a shovel or a beak. His drawings have a disquieting and menacing effect, except those copied from elsewhere. The first figure at the top of *Fig. 19* is interesting because of the bizarre distortion of the body and of the extremities. According to the marginal note, this is a "footbath". The patient attempts by the representation of the horizontal lines below the head the optical illusion of water. On the same *Fig. 19*, in the upper right-hand corner we see the motif of the mustache repeated on the body. The remarkable aspects of the human figure to the right and underneath are the nose and the right arm, which are drawn as parallel appendages.

In *Fig. 20* there are six heads of different sizes on very small bodies. The horizontal bending of the legs of the creature in the right upper corner accentuates the fantastic aspect of this drawing.

His portraits show formidable eyes with a disquieting look. In *Fig. 21* we do not find the monstrous grimace of the other works. Nonetheless the flattened forehead gives a disquieting expression to the eyes of the attached profiles of this Janus-face which are identical on both sides of this bizarre creature. The body and the neck are formed by two lozenges. The extremities are sketched in an unskilled way. In *Fig. 22*, besides the people, two little birds appear top left, and a little train similar to a child's toy is drawn on the side of the figure at bottom right. These motifs are drawn in childish fashion. The figure in the middle of the right column is standing, with feet resembling those of a duck, on the head of the figure underneath. That is how the convexity of the head is molded over by the feet which are arched. The beard reaching to the floor on the person in the top right corner is of the same length as the whole length of this human figure. One has to remark, nonetheless, that in relationship to the size of the head, the beard is of normal length. It is only the disproportionately small body and extremities that give this beard an aspect of reaching down almost to the feet. The patient entitled this page: "The little men of miracle".

We may assume that part of these works are—only arbitrarily transformed—reproductions of illustrations from journals. Another group of drawings appears to express hallucinations. Without doubt, the male and female figures of *Fig. 23* may be classified in this category.

Case 2 - Fig. 19
Pencil drawing. 34x21

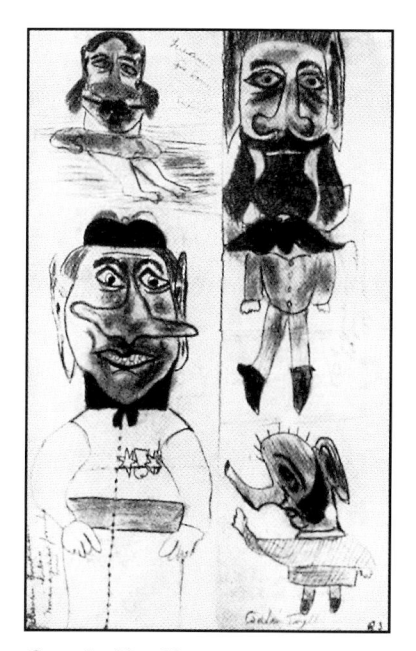

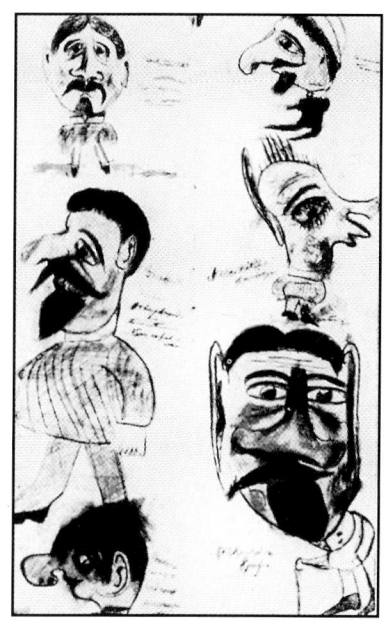

Case 2 - Fig. 20
Pencil drawing. 34x21

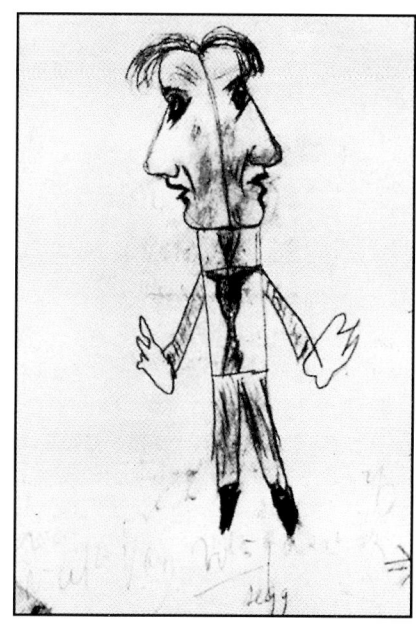

Case 2 - Fig. 21
Pencil drawing. 14.5x10

The legs of the upper right figure are bent at the knees in a right angle (possibly because of lack of space). The fingers and toes are like fans and the nose is like a snout. The characteristic aspects of the woman presented on the right are: a large, almond shaped eye, a long nose, and a disproportionately small body. Her hair is plaited into two thin braids. These two figures appear almost as if they were painted rather than drawn. Their tone is uniform without any three-dimensional aspect. In *Fig. 25* on the bottom left is a creature (similar to the one in *Fig. 23*) who holds, in his single hand, an extraordinarily long cigarette. On the top of the same half of the paper, a man with a conventional face is smoking a cigarette. Possibly this has inspired the bizarre representation of the smoker below, as part of an illusion. The thin neck of this magical smoker supports a head on which the nose has the form of a beak. This figure appears like a silhouette. One of his legs is bent, in a right angle, along the edge on the bottom of the page like a kind of pedestal. This representation is unconventional and is original in the utilization of space. The figure in the middle with a conventional face has a small chest, with a necktie which ends unexpectedly in a vague dark shape, similar to a shoe. The left arm of this figure hangs down and ends in a barely sketched hand with four fingers, while the right arm raised abruptly to the side, up to the level of the ears, ends in a hand almost five times larger than the left hand. The right arm is actually not attached to the body and gives the impression of emerging from the shoe.

The drawings of this patient *(L. L.)* are ste-

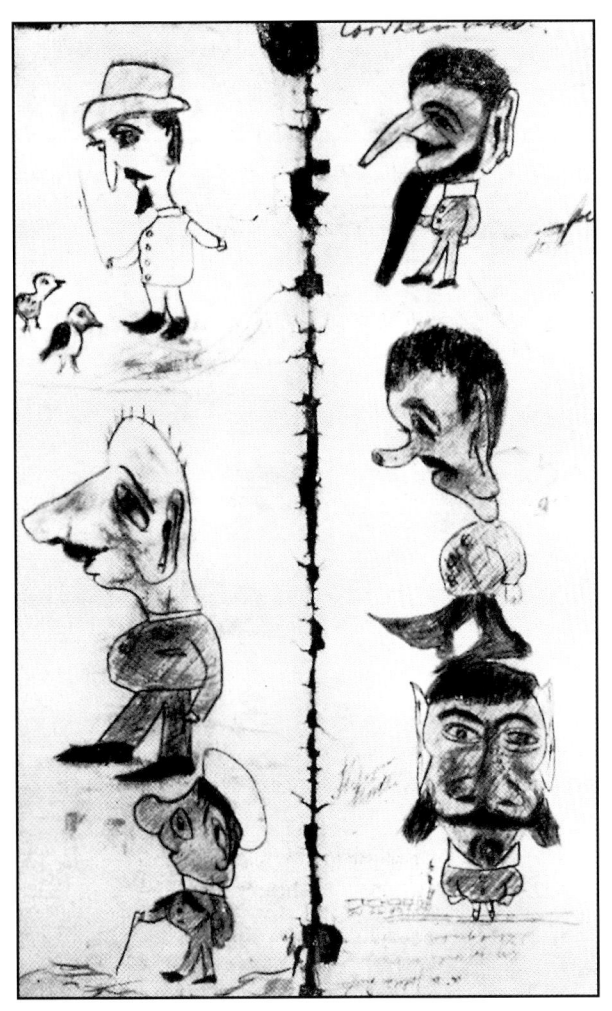

Case 2 - Fig. 22
Pencil drawing. 34x21

of the human figures are not yet present. Among the drawings made in 1933 *(Fig. 24)*, the proportions correspond to reality. These portraits were copied from illustrations in a journal.

Among some of his hundreds of drawings there is only one which represents buildings *(Fig. 26)* which is undoubtedly a copy of an illustration from a magazine.

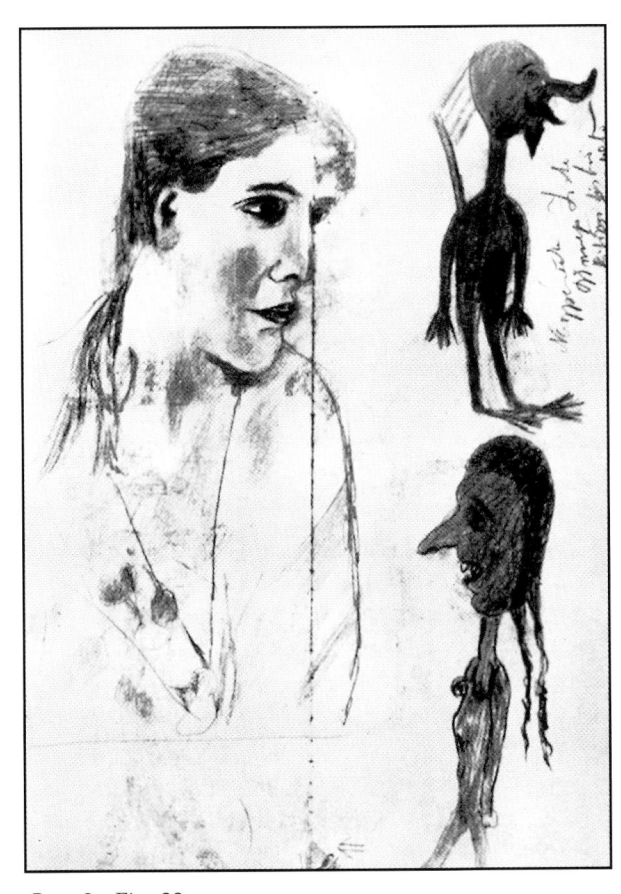

Case 2 - Fig. 23
Pencil drawing. 29.5x21

reotyped. The lines are homogeneous. The details which he wants to accentuate are expressed by dark shading and mostly by outsize proportions.

At the beginning of his illness, the repulsiveness and the lack of proportion among the parts

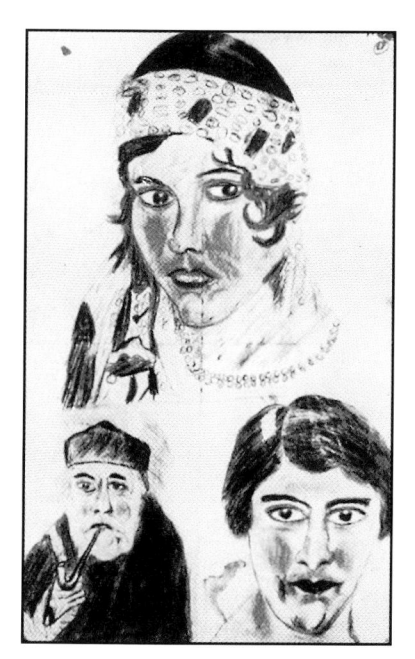

Case 2 - Fig. 24
Pencil drawing. 29.5x21

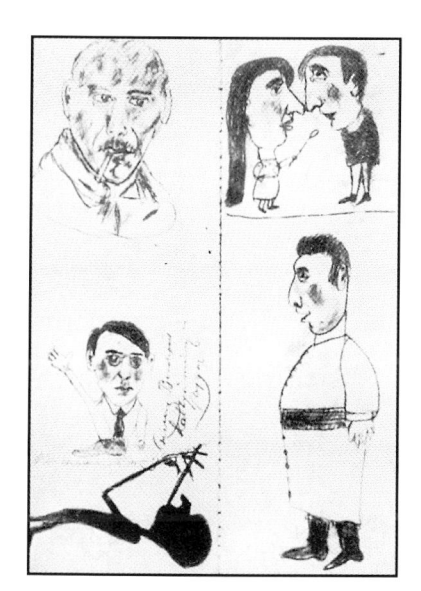

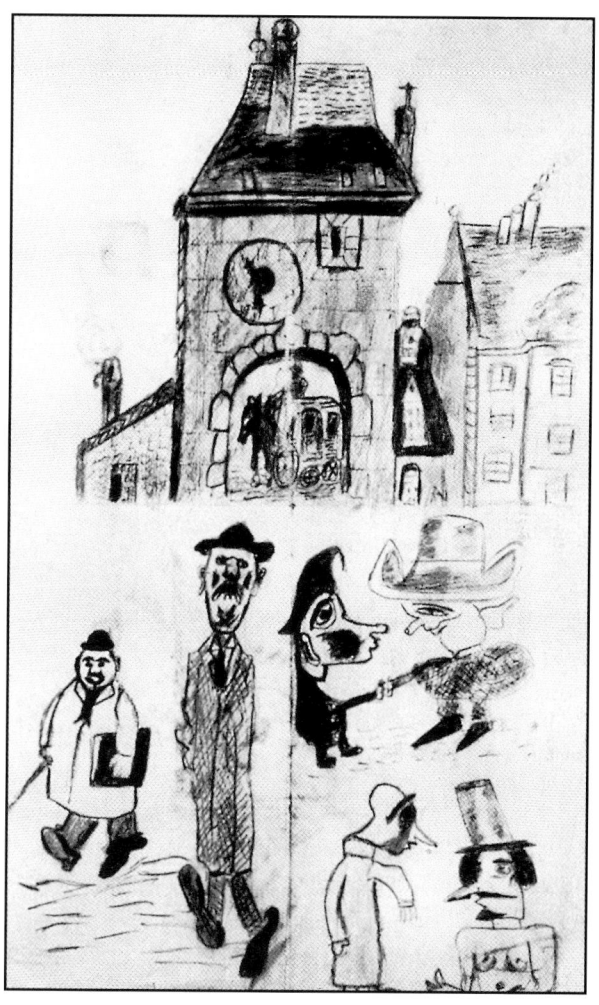

Case 2 - Fig. 26
Pencil drawing. 34x21

Case 2 - Fig. 25
Pencil drawing. 34x21

49

## Case 3 — Mrs. A. P.

*Date of birth*: 15 September 1912
*Occupation*: Sculptor
*Diagnosis*: Schizophrenia

She was treated at the Psychiatric and Neurological University Hospital of Pécs from 27 August 1947 to 9 September 1949 with an interruption of two months.

*Family history*: The father, a professional violinist, died at the age of 72. The mother died at the age of 70 of pulmonary embolism. She had a "romantic personality" with the ambition to give an artistic education to all her children. A sister of the great-grandmother on the paternal side died in a mental hospital. The maternal grandfather possessed a talent for painting and drawing. Among the ten siblings, five are still alive. Three died in infancy. One sister who was an artist/painter died of dysentery in Africa. The five surviving siblings are the following: 1. H., an artisan, 2. A., a movie producer, 3. M., a cellist, 4. M., a house painter; however, he makes his living by selling his oil paintings. 5. A., a commercial artist.

*Personal history*: Transitory stuttering caused by a frightening experience at the age of three or four years. After four years of middle school she continued her education in a high school for talented children, and then at the Academy of the Fine Arts in Budapest. She also attended for one year the École des Beaux Arts in Paris. A sculpture of hers, a bust entitled "Meditation", was successfully exhibited. She was always a loner. At the age of 20 she married a man who had an engineering degree. They had two children.

Beginning in 1940, she became extremely jealous of her husband, without cause. "Her deceased mother appeared to her in the form of a phantom on top of her husband's head. She is followed in the streets. The hair dresser burns her hair at the command of her husband." She threatened the members of her family. She was admitted to a psychiatric hospital from which she was discharged after three months in an improved state, following electric shock treatment.

After returning to her home, she gave "long moral sermons" to her husband during the night. Her speech was totally confused. In 1946 a new set of electric shocks remained ineffective. She threatened to kill her family and used very obscene language in the presence of her children.

Because of her aggressive behavior and agitation, she was hospitalized at this university hospital.

*At admission*, the medical and neurological examination revealed no pathology. The Bordet–Wassermann reaction was negative both in the blood and in the spinal fluid.

*Psychiatric evaluation*: Her affect was very labile. She had ideas of persecution; she thought that everything was changed in her environment. She was convinced that her husband had married her because he knew she would become mentally ill and that on this ground he could easily divorce her.

She wanted to convince us at all costs that she was "not insane" and "did not come from a family with inherited illness". She said that all her problems were caused by her husband and his family. She was preoccupied with spiritism, keeping a contact with the spirit of her mother who tells her "all the good things that she has hidden in her soul". The mother sent her messages according to which there was no need to celebrate a mass for her after death; she followed this "advice". In her "dreams" she often saw her mother dying. Once her mother appeared to her in the shape of a devil with horns. The devil could take on the appearance of her mother and, disguised as such, talk to her.

During her hospitalization she was frequently very agitated and ran screaming from room to room. At other times she remained motionless for awhile, then suddenly stood up, making gestures as if pushing something away from herself. During these episodes she was screaming and lamenting loudly. If we asked her what she had seen, she shuddered and said, "That is none of your business". She was afraid that she would be murdered by the staff, or by her husband. One evening she asked how it is possible that she saw one of the nurses at two ends of the corridor at the same time. She frequently thought of her children and expressed a desire to see them. She drew very often and also made little statues out of breadcrumbs. She hid her works in her bed, and showed them only rarely. Frequently she was in a state of agitation at which times she attacked those who approached her and spat on them. Her husband took her home for a trial visit for a few days, but it was impossible to keep her because of her agitated state. She burned her husband's professional books, saying that "he has no use for them".

*At the time of readmission*, the physical and neurological evaluation was also negative. However, the patient was much more agitated and aggressive than before and suffering from delusions of persecution.

*On 26 August, 1949, a bilateral prefrontal lobotomy was performed.* Following this her behavior became calm and she did not express any more ideas of persecution. She was agitated only one night.

*Six months after she was discharged* from the hospital, we received a letter from her husband who reassured us that her behavior was good at home and that she had started to produce sculptures again, as she had done "before her illness".

During her illness she drew mainly children's figures in the secessionist style. She worked with great care and detail on the legs and shoes, while the drawing of the hand is less skilled. The other details and the faces are quite stereotyped. Among her drawings, the one shown in *Fig. 27* is the most delicately executed. However, in this picture the little girl has four legs, each completed with great care and precision. We can say the same regarding *Fig. 28* in which, at the edge of the rock, there is a young couple apparently looking at a pretty little village in the valley. These figures are shown from the back. The woman has five legs, each drawn with the same precise technique. In no way does it give the impression that the patient, while looking for the best solution, has left the unfinished sketches of legs beside the other.

*Figures 29* and *30* are original compositions. On the neck of both torsos, a heart shape is attached while a little cupid, standing or kneeling in front of the statue, works on it with hammer and chisel. Undoubtedly these drawings have a symbolical meaning.

The heads are possibly self-portraits. Underneath this drawing, which is full of repressed emotion, the motif of the floor parquet is drawn with contrasting sterile impassivity. On the same pages other unrelated figures are drawn as well. On one page we can see a leg, while on

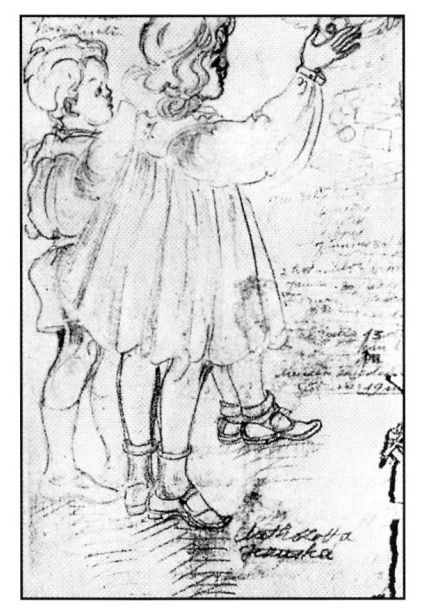

Case 3 - Fig. 27
Pencil drawing. 21x14

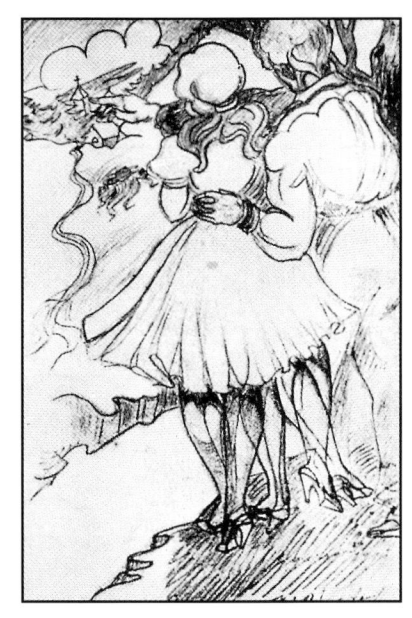

Case 3 - Fig. 28
Pencil drawing. 21x14

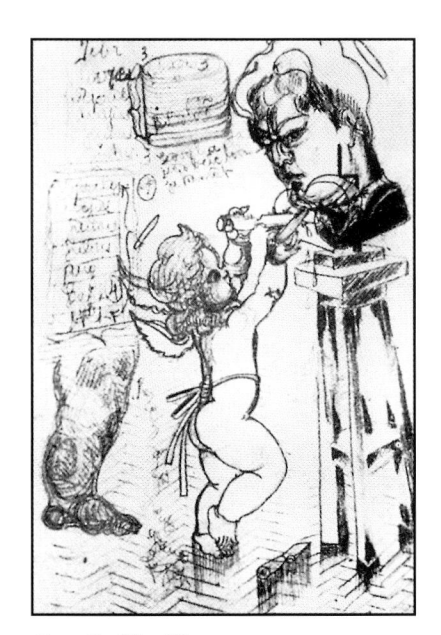

Case 3 - Fig. 29
Pencil drawing. 21x14

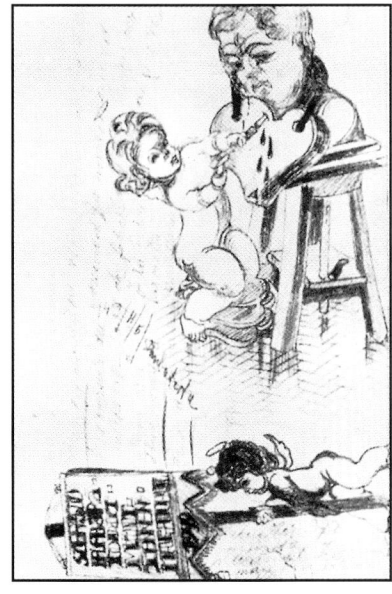

Case 3 - Fig. 30
Pencil drawing. 21x14

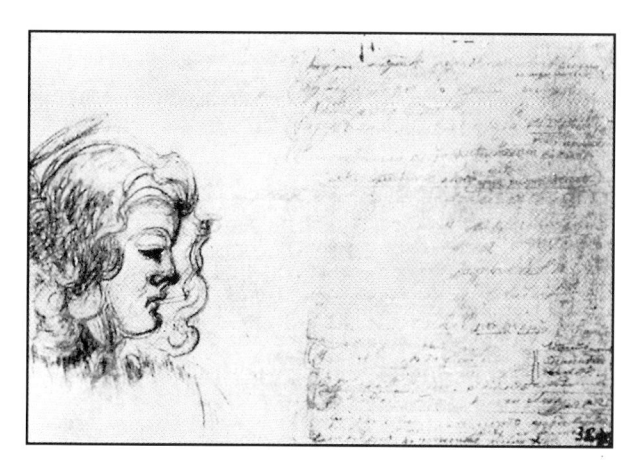

Case 3 - Fig. 31
Pencil drawing. 21x14

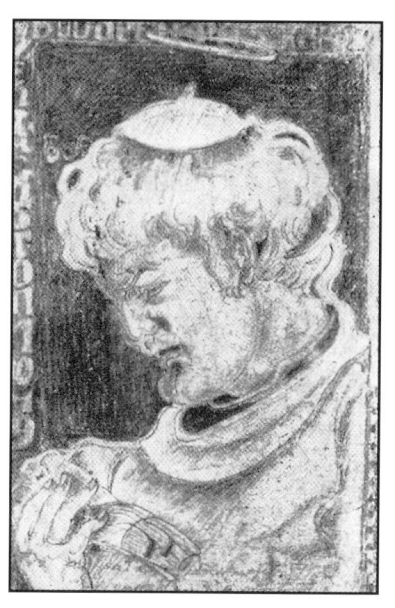

Case 3 - Fig. 32
Pencil drawing. 21x14

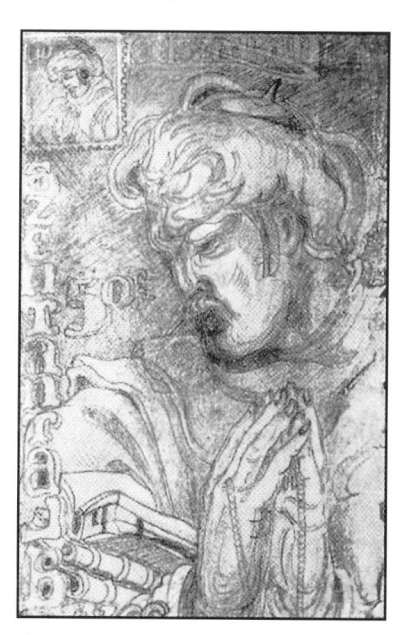

Case 3 - Fig. 33
Pencil drawing. 21x14

the other another little cupid holding up a frame with confused inscriptions. Both the faces on the bust and those of the little cupids resemble each other. *Figure 31* is a self-portrait with a cigarette between her lips (it, indeed, resembles the patient). The smoke of the cigarette rises in spirals and merges with the locks of her hair. The head is crowned with a halo.

Some of her drawings are presented in the form of postage stamps, with an indented borderline. The subjects of these "stamps" for example are curious and bizarre saints. In *Figs 32* and *33*, she represents Saint Anthony, the delineation being rather weak. The hair style is drawn the same way as those of the female heads.

*Figure 34* represents a state of rage. The patient has blackened, with an impulsive gesture, the place of the eye on this profile because she was unable to render the desired expression. This is documented by the following words: "Has the mirror of the soul been done successfully? No." Nonetheless, this strong emotion has

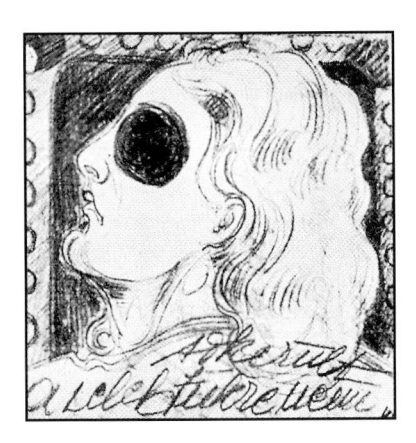

Case 3 - Fig. 34
Pencil drawing.
10x11

from her other drawings, except for the collar of the shirt which shows her typical style of drawing.

*Figure 36* is a typical sample of the way in which the patient fills the space with different unrelated sketches. Two female figures are rendered in the form of statues; nonetheless, they give no three-dimensional impression. On the hips and lower extremities of the upright figure the detailed use of light and shadows is in contrast with the impoverished plasticity of the small arms and the disproportionate breasts. By turning around the same page by 180 degrees, we see two feet with different shoes on them, and the drawing of a child. The child wears shorts and folded-down socks. His legs are much better drawn than the other body parts. Also the details of the other, unattached feet are drawn with care.

not hindered her from surrounding this picture with a minutiously elaborated, indented border, like the border of postage stamps. The portrait of a young man in *Fig. 35* differs in style

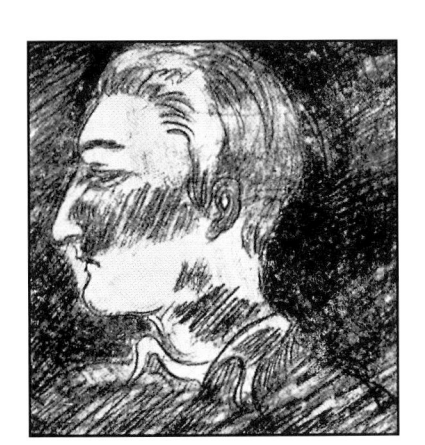

Case 3 - Fig. 35
Pencil drawing. 10x11

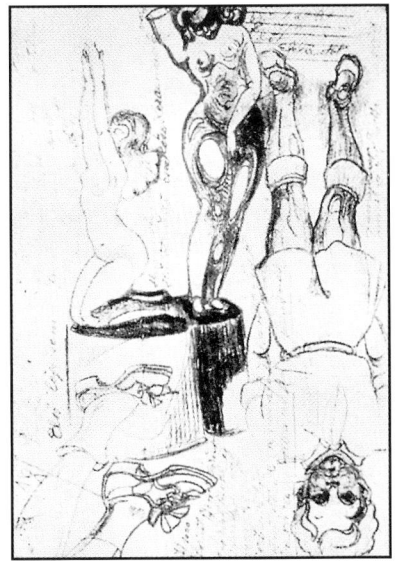

Case 3 - Fig. 36
Pencil drawing. 21x14

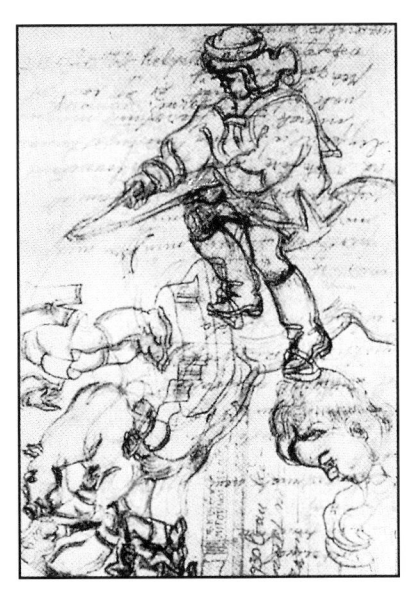

Case 3 - Fig. 37
Pencil drawing. 21x14

In *Fig. 37*, we find, as in the drawings of some of our other patients, bizarre figures on the margin of the sheet, with no relationship to the principal figures of the composition. In the left lower corner a child is sitting, or crouching, in front of a horse—or the head of a horse without a body—with open mouth, which appears to touch the face and the cap of the child as if whispering something or trying to bite. The question remains open whether we should interpret this scene as a symbolical expression, or should consider it as the representation of a hallucination. The principal figure of this composition is a child on a horse, the animal being only vaguely sketched and added later.

This author had the opportunity in May 1956 to visit Mrs. A. P. in her home. This was seven years after her lobotomy. She lives in a household with her husband, her children, and her mother-in-law. She helps with the household chores and cleans her room.

Whenever possible, nonetheless, she withdraws into her room, quite distanced from her family. Here she lives as if in a fairy-tale world among drawings and paintings. The walls of her room are full of drawings of different sizes. Generally she uses papers of 35 × 40 centimeters. She has sewn together, with thread, her drawings in such a way that they produce a frieze. She also works in colored crayon and aquarelles. She has produced several fairy-tale illustrations, as she says, these were drawn for her children. However, many of them are "just brain waves". In these pictures we see unusual, disquieting landscapes. Forests, plant-motifs which are dissolved into wavy lines, trees, rivers, and brooks. Many times they are just part of a blue-green background. Sometimes she also uses lighter and more lively colors. In other very colorful drawings she illustrates small scenes with several adults and children. Some of these are nativity scenes. Others are playing children, or children engaged in some light work, or groups of children dancing and singing. Her pictures representing dancing ballerinas have a pleasant dynamic effect. She says she has drawn these as studies because she likes to draw legs. She thinks that her pictures are "very bad". Nonetheless, she cannot use all her talent for making statues, since she does not get any material for sculpture from her family. In a picture of "Hansel and Gretel" we can recognize the portraits of her children and the witch is a recognizable portrait of her mother-in-law. She admits this and tells us that in general the childrens' portraits represent her own children.

Her delusions remain unchanged. She complains that her children were killed; immediately after this statement she brags that her daughter is a good student and has talent for drawing. She is distrustful of her family and tells us that they are enemies with bad intentions; she has become "crazy" because of them. When we asked her to donate one or two pictures to us, she declined saying that "they are very bad and must be burned". She added that she has hung the pictures only to cover the walls because the paint was already quite damaged.

She shows some drawings made by her fifteen-year-old daughter whom she has taught herself. On these we see similar "baroque style figures" as we have seen in the patient's own artwork; however, the daughter's work is more balanced with calmer lines. The pictures of the child are also of a more pleasant mood. Her ten-year-old son also draws, but in a very different style. His figures are much more rigid and have angular contours.

Later we found out from her relatives that after our visit the patient had taken all of her pictures from the walls and had hidden them very carefully. She was anxious about our visit, thinking that she had convinced us that she was mentally ill and that we recognized her "brain ghosts" that she represented with green paint. And she assumed that, based on her drawings, we would want to hospitalize her again in a psychiatric department. After she hid her pictures she became again more reassured. The family provided us with a few pictures that she had produced in the last year. Of these we are reproducing two. *Figure 38* is part of the Hansel and Gretel series of her fairy tale illustrations. Gretel comes from the house and meets the witch. The gingerbread house is drawn with good perspective. The witch arrives leaning on her cane and has a frightening facial expression as she approaches the girl. In the right foreground we see a fir tree the trunk and the branches of which are unusually shaped as if broken into pieces. These lines are nonetheless put together in such a way that they convey the shape of the trunk and the bark of the tree. It is an ink drawing and partially done with a feather. Through its dark color it differs from the other pictures of the series, possibly because of the threatening character of the scene that the patient wanted to convey.

*Figure 39* is done part in aquarelle, part with colored crayons.

The picture is complete in itself and belongs to a small series. It can be seen that originally, at least as far as the landscape is concerned, the whole was a unified composition. Nevertheless, later it was divided into two halves by an indented double line. In this way, the roof of the oven-like building hangs over from the left to the right side and a branch of the fir tree from the right continues on the left side. The middle of the whole picture is filled with green grass on which three children's figures are represented. Nonetheless, they belong to two different fairy tales. On the left half we see a scene from Hansel and Gretel, while on the right half there are Little Red Riding Hood and the wolf. Little Red Riding Hood comes with a basket in her hand and encounters the wolf whose tongue is lolling out. The wolf is white and its stylized representation reminds us of a hound. In the background we can see sketches of a forest. The dark and black tree trunks stand in contrast with the light colorings of the children. The branches produce quite bizarre arabesques in space. On the right side the forest is more colorful and the tree trunks are yellowish red with brown stripes.

Her relatives also showed us her drawings made soon after the lobotomy. These are naturalistic representations, mostly of her former home, occasionally with children playing in the rooms. According to her mother-in-law, the representations of the furnishings are done with photographic accuracy.

We observed that after the lobotomy her delusions persisted; however, the accompanying affect has disappeared. Thus, Mrs. *A. P.* is able to live with her relatives although she is still autistic and withdrawn. Her artistic drive is unchanged, possibly even increased as compared to the time before her lobotomy. In the first times following the surgery, her pictures were naturalistic. Later they became increasingly more symbolic. In these pictures we find characteristic signs of schizophrenia, that is bizarreness, fantastic convoluted lines, and possibly representations of hallucinations. As far as we can tell, there is an improvement in her

Case 3 - Fig. 38
Ink drawing. 18x21

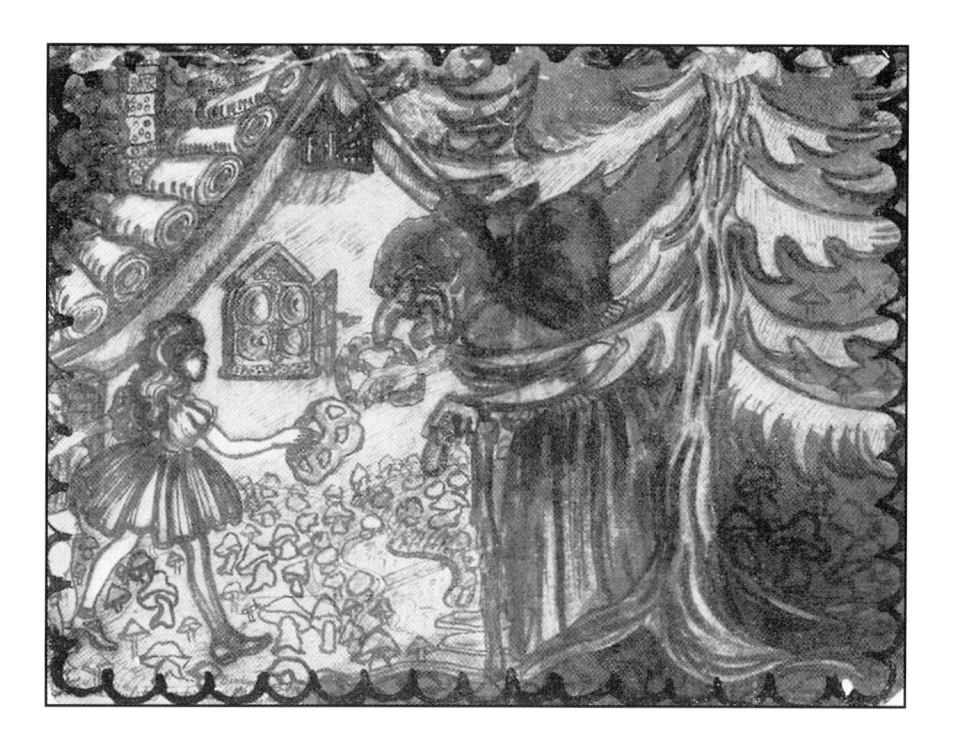

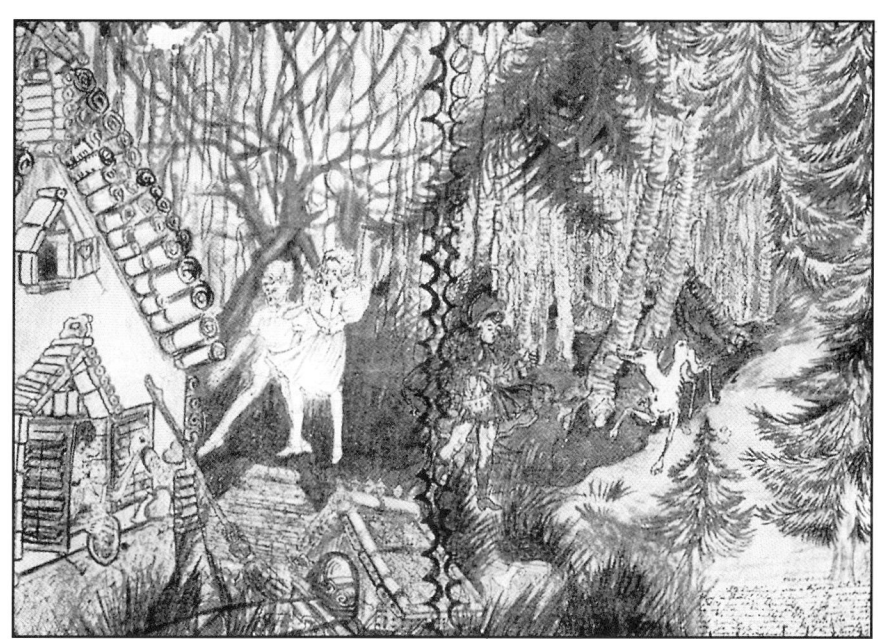

Case 3 - Fig. 39
Aquarelle and colored crayon. 58x86

pictorial ability following the lobotomy as now she is able to produce compositions while earlier she only sketched individual details. The elements of the composition are related and show small groups of figures although she still produces individual drawings, but in a series they are part of scenes. Instead of expressing herself in bizarre and abstract symbols, she uses the subjects of her fairy-tale world. In these works her individual method of representation is clearly visible.

## Case 4 — *L. T.*

*Date of birth*: 20 December 1899
*Occupation*: Schoolteacher
*Diagnosis*: Schizophrenia

He was hospitalized at the Psychiatric and Neurological University Hospital of Pécs from 1 December 1939 to 14 November 1948, when he was transferred to an asylum.

*Family history*: One sister is an alcoholic. Otherwise, unremarkable.

*Personal history*: No previous illness. He interrupted his studies at the age of seventeen, being drafted as a soldier in World War I. He was discharged from the military after six months of service because of "a fever of the nerves". During this illness he was unconscious for ten days. [This was during the great epidemic of 'Influenza' (Encephalitis A) in Europe.] After his convalescence he became fearful and withdrew not only from strangers, but also from his own parents. He hid his food and ate it in secret by himself. In spite of this unusual behavior, he completed his studies and was employed as a teacher. He was subjected to disciplinary actions at work and changed jobs frequently. In 1924 he registered at the Academy of Fine Arts and at the National Conservatory of Music in Budapest. He liked painting and playing the violin.

In 1932 he was admitted for the first time to a psychiatric hospital in Budapest because of loitering. He did not eat regularly and stayed in bed for days at a time. After he left his last position as a teacher, he worked as a physical laborer, a gardener. At that time he also drew and wrote profusely. From time to time he hid himself at home in the basement and in other places.

He was treated repeatedly at the Psychiatric and Neurological University Hospital of Szeged, several times between 1936 and 1938. His diagnosis at that hospital was schizophrenia. From his medical record of that time, it becomes evident that he distrusted everybody, ate very little, and was silent and depressed most of the time. It appeared to him that the whole world was making fun of him. One day for an interval of six hours he took up a strange position on a chair with his legs folded underneath the chair and the head bent forward so as to practically reach the floor. He had ideas of persecution and stated that his wife was influenced by strangers. Between his two hospitalizations he lived the life of a vagabond. Sometimes he even wandered for hundreds of kilometers, for example, from Szeged to Budapest. After he returned to Szeged he did not dare to enter the hospital "because his clothing was not clean". His behavior was modest, somewhat embarrassed, and manneristic. His answers were garbled and unrelated to the subject at hand. He began drawing only during his third hospitalization in Szeged.

One day he was sent to the surgical department accompanied by a nurse and he escaped by throwing sand into the eyes of the nurse. He was brought back to the hospital and gave the following explanation: "I planned this excursion for a long time because one has a need for movement and I judged that the time had come to effectuate this."

Sometimes he could not speak "because of something that strangles my throat and, at these moments, I hear myself talking inside".

His visual acuity on the right eye was 5/50 and on the left 5/15, with correction right: 5/8 and left: 5/15. At the hospital in Szeged he received a series of Cardiazol shock treatments (Cardiazol, a drug given intravenously, produces epileptic seizures—like those produced by electric shock) and also a series of insulin shock treatments.

*At admission* to the university hospital in Pécs there were no medical, or neurological, pathological signs. Bordet–Wassermann reaction was negative.

*Psychiatric evaluation*: He suffers from ideas of persecution; it is mostly his wife who "mobilized the whole village against him". His face is void of expression (bland) and his gestures are impoverished. He remains motionless for hours with his face pressed against the window, gazing into the distance, with arms crossed behind his back. If one talks to him, he shudders, turns around and answers the questions willingly, but soon changes the conversation to the history of his life which he repeats indefatigably. There are gaps in the continuity of his story. References to his delusions become evident. His associations are restricted. His memory is satisfactory. His mood is bland.

He is quite withdrawn and has no contact with the other patients or the staff. He often walks up and down the corridor, with his sketchbook in hand, searching for a place where he can work. He draws a lot. He declares that he loves to draw the patients and that "it is a pity that they escape because one could make interesting pictures". He boasts of having many clients, and of having to do their pictures on order. Sometimes he excuses himself because, he says, "it would not be the same if he should show the pictures to us at this moment because his clients have kept them for themselves". Nevertheless, he often shows his works with pleasure, although he never gives any of them away as a gift. He asks the patients and the physicians to pose for him as models. He also copies some of the pictures hanging on the wall.

He works at length on his drawings, sometimes for weeks on end. His drawings become more and more smudged towards the end of his illness and they are transformed into superimposed spots, with unrecognizable forms, and completely incomprehensible dense grids. Once he ran out of the black color and therefore he tried to explain that he has two kinds of black, the warm black such as that of the charcoal settled inside of an oil lamp, and a cold black such as black ivory. He likes to draw the view from the window. As his illness progresses he becomes taciturn, and is interested only in his drawings. His answers, his spontaneous speech, and his scribblings are not understandable.

One day before the national holiday of the 15th of March, he wrote two or three patriotic poems with colored crayons in alternating lines of red and green "because tomorrow is a national holiday". (The colors of the Hungarian flag are red, white and green.)

At Eastertime he draws compositions characteristic of that holiday.

L. T. works for a long time on his drawings. His favorite subjects are wooded landscapes or forests, human figures or faces, and some battle scenes. In addition to his pencil drawings and ink drawings he also works with pastels and in aquarelle. His behavior is manneristic. He draws the contours by making small disconnected traces.

His pictures are, in general, smeared and some of them are as if woven of black lines. If he produces aquarelles he superimposes patches on patches until the forms are obliterated. Mostly during the last phase of his illness, his pictures have become increasingly more meaningless. He does not always fill the whole surface at his disposal. He often works on several different subjects on the same page without any relationship among them, and without the intention of creating a unified composition.

One can interpret as a sign of stereotypy the three portraits of a man, which are identically drawn: they have a pipe between their lips and their head is covered by a hat *(Fig. 40)*. The colors of these are also identical. On another sheet we see the repetition of a sitting male figure in two copies, one sketched in crayon, the other painted in aquarelle *(Fig. 41)*. Above them are miniature landscapes.

The "two men on horseback" *(Fig. 42)*, a composition of vague silhouettes in a dusk-like atmosphere, has no distinguished contours. The foreshortening of the road at the end of the painting gives the illusion of depth.

*Figure 43*, characterized by his expressive style, is a gentle representation of an idyllic scene in which the persons are dressed in the fashion of the turn of the century.

On the margins of his drawings he often represents small bizarre scenes, and in addition he sometimes writes a text as well. For example, in *Fig. 44* a man leans on his desk with his eyes fixed on a small train and on the telephone poles quite primitively represented. The following sentence refers to this: "Why does the railroad guard salute the train which zooms by in front of him?"

On his small drawings, he completely neglects the laws of perspective and traces unskilled continuous lines.

In *Fig. 45* two principal figures sitting in two corners of the paper are executed in a stereotyped fashion. Small portraits, a window and written text fill the space between them.

During his illness he returns frequently to two subjects: 1. The view of the city of Pécs, 2. Battle scenes. In these two groups, one can follow the psychological deterioration both in the composition and in the execution of the drawings. Below some drawings framed in a round or square format, he writes the name of some boroughs of the city of Pécs without the least resemblance not only to that part of the city which he has named, but to a city landscape at all. One no longer finds any form. In *Fig. 46a*, one of his last drawings, by a spot in the form of a peak, he gives the impression of a bell tower. This impression may be justified by another landscape previously drawn by him in a similar composition in which the silhouette of a church and bell tower are recognizable *(Fig. 46b)*.

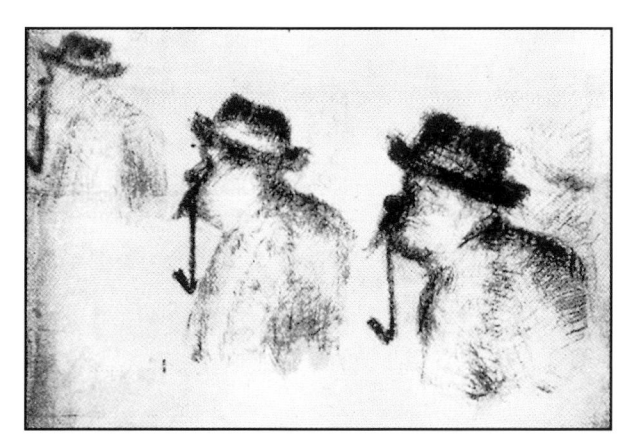

Case 4 - Fig. 40
Colored crayon. 31x45

In *Fig. 46c* only unequal patches of red and violet are in a square-shaped frame formed by lines of unequal size and by touches of the brush, producing dots of different sizes. Dur-

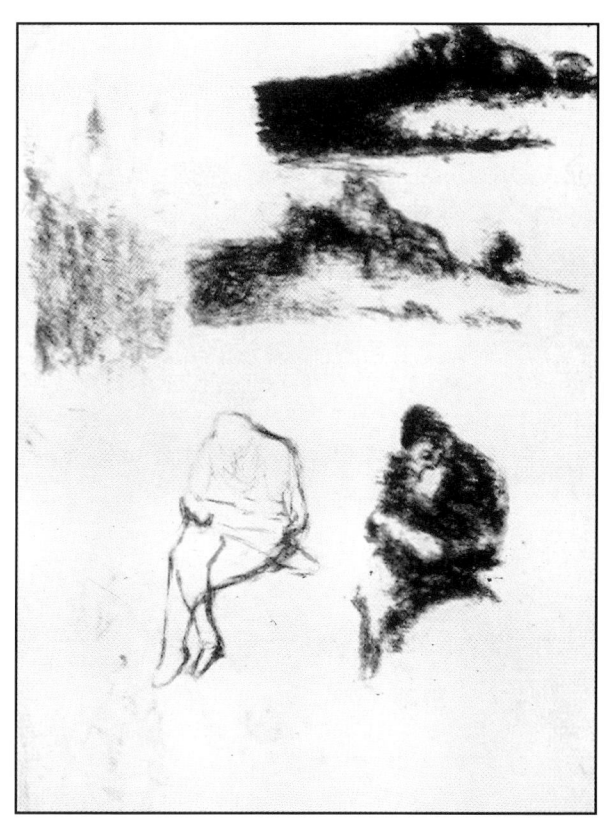

Case 4 - Fig. 41
Aquarelle and colored crayon. 30x21

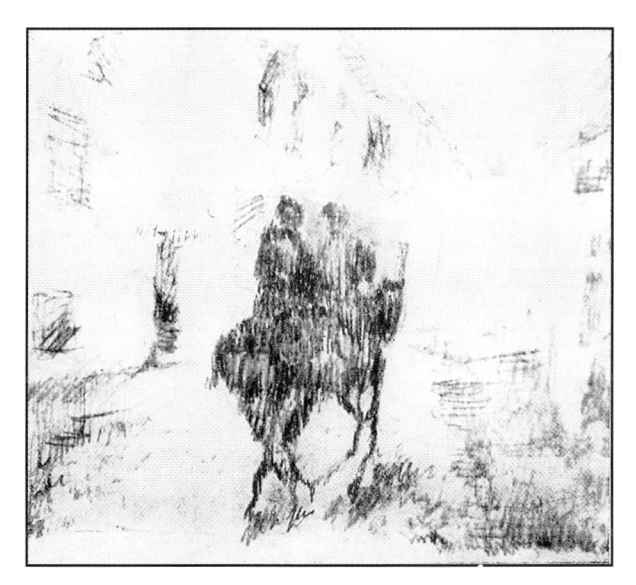

Case 4 - Fig. 42
Pencil drawing. 19x21

ing the course of the schizophrenic process, the patient had lost not only the memory of an elementary composition, but also his formerly acquired technique. This picture reflects the rigidity of his mind in the last burned-out phase of his illness.

In contrast, *Fig. 47*, a composition in pastel, which he produced soon after his admission to the hospital, represents an easily recognizable part of the city. The colored parts in the foreground give the impression of two-dimensional trees and, in the lower part of the page, the wavy

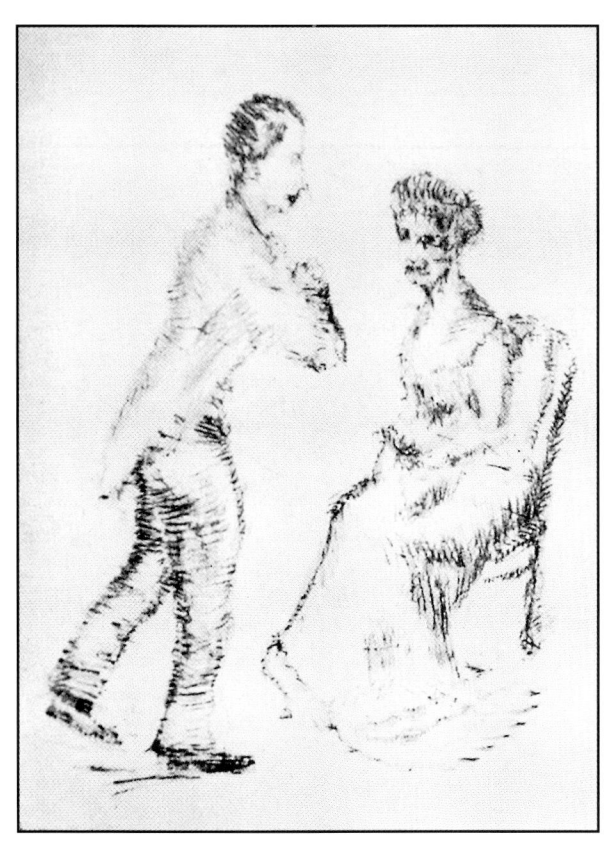

Case 4 - Fig. 43
Pencil drawing. 27x21

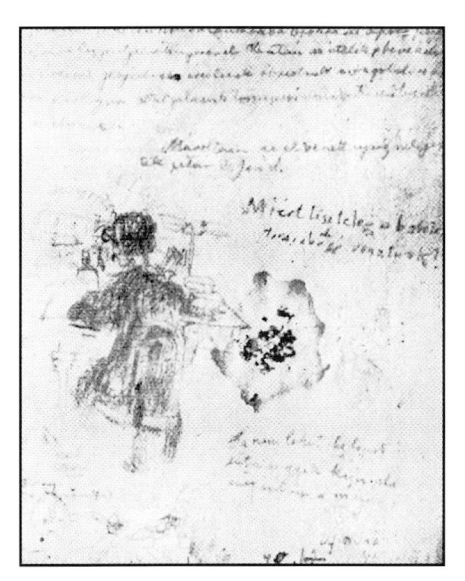

Case 4 - Fig. 44
Pencil drawing. 15x11

Case 4 - Fig. 45
Pencil drawing. 15.5x14

lines are unrelated to the other details of the picture. Finally, the right corner on the bottom was left completely white. This produces the effect of incompleteness and a lack of balance in the composition.

In *Figs 48* to *50*, he represents in colored pencil battle scenes, the charges of the cavalry, with evidently quite a lot of dynamism without representing the figures in detail and even without precise contours. The colors are combined in a lively and original harmony. *Figure 51*, produced a few years later, is done in black crayon

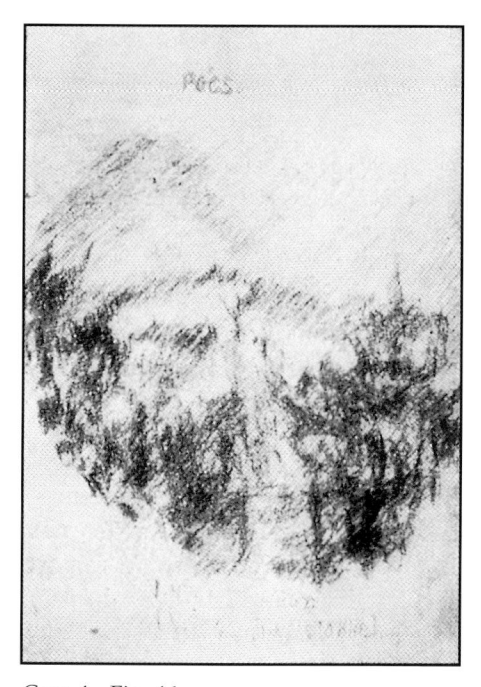

Case 4 - Fig. 46a
Pencil drawing. 29.5x21

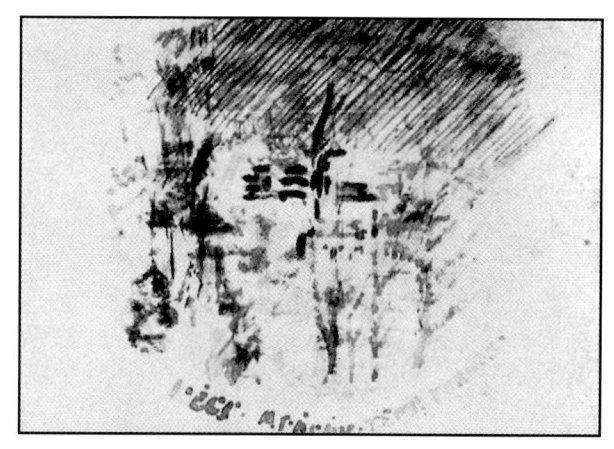

Case 4 - Fig. 46b
Aquarelle. 15x21

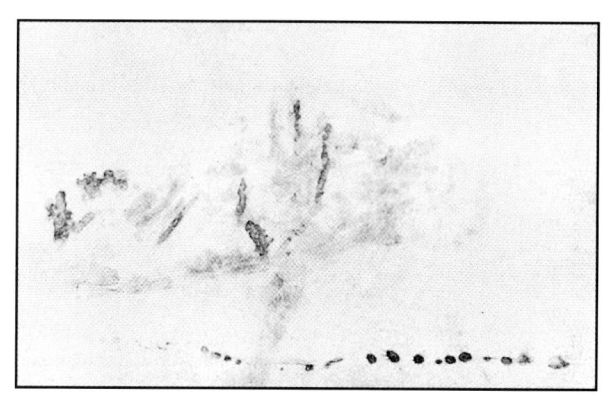

Case 4 - Fig. 46c
Aquarelle. 15x20

and evokes an impression of a battle scene. An interesting feature of this picture is a small armored figure in the left upper corner with a saber in his hand, who floats in the air among the clouds (the God of War?). In the right upper corner, a little man "in nightshirt" stands among the clouds; maybe it is a caricature of the patient himself. Since the patient gave no explanation we cannot decide whether this is a representation of a vision or only a symbolical figure.

In *Figs 52a* and *52b* we see exercises in the letters of the alphabet, as done in school books. He adds, as illustrations, some small landscapes done in Chinese ink. *Figure 53* is an aquarelle painting of a market scene.

L. T. has real artistic talent. His work is personal and coherent. His talent is mediocre. He developed his style only by systematic exercises. He works on his subjects with minutious scrupulosity, according to his ability. He approaches his subject with tenderness and develops it slowly into an impressionistic effect. The patient is consistent in his concept and

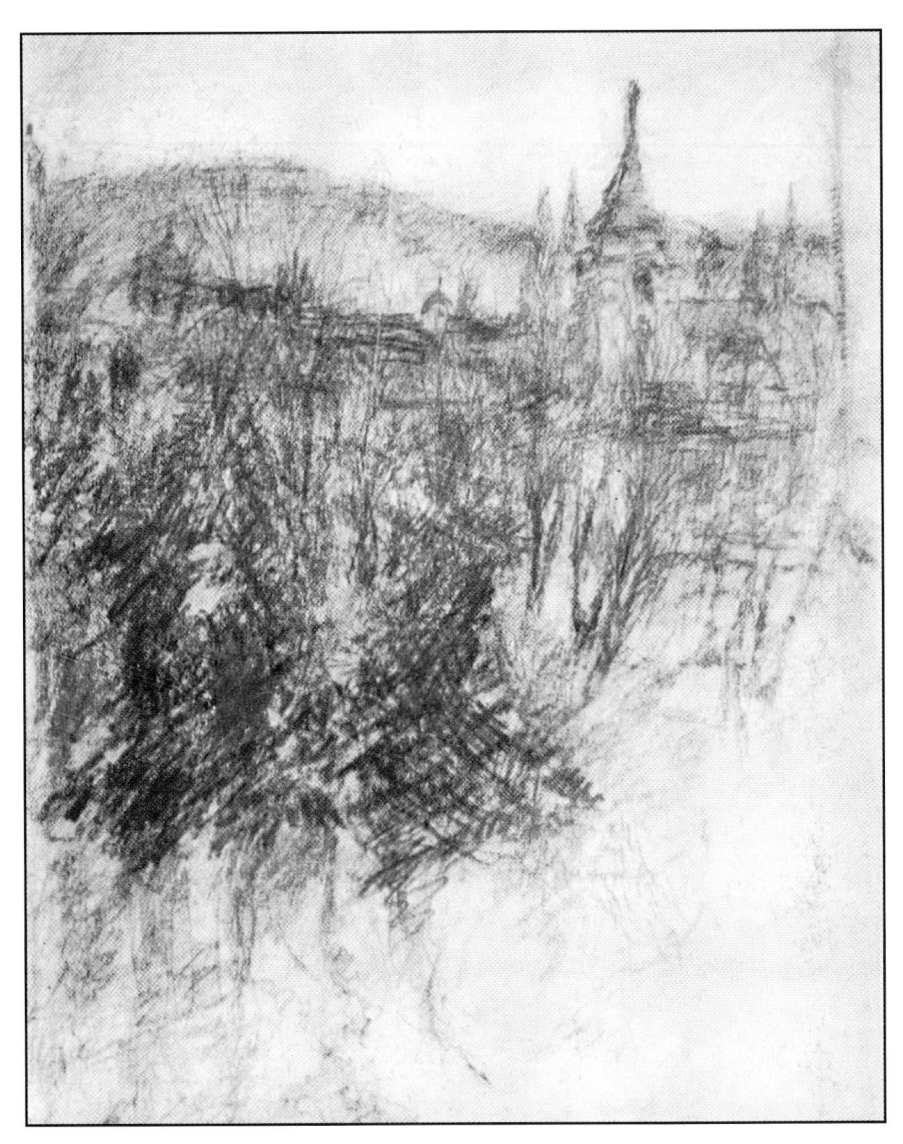

Case 4 - Fig. 47
Colored crayon. 30x21

Case 4 - Fig. 48
Colored crayon. 21x30

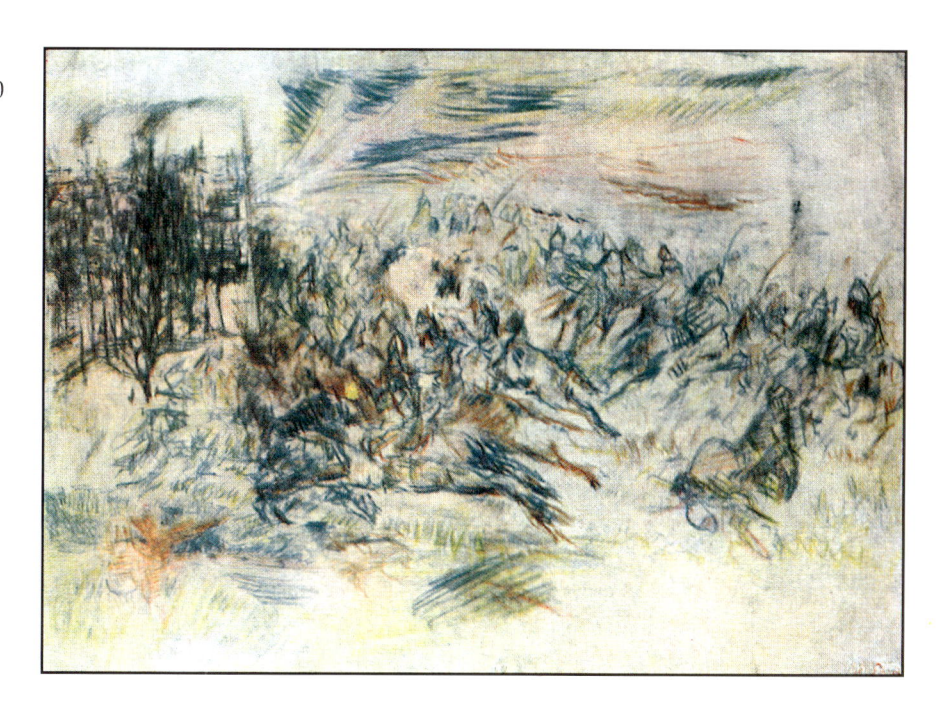

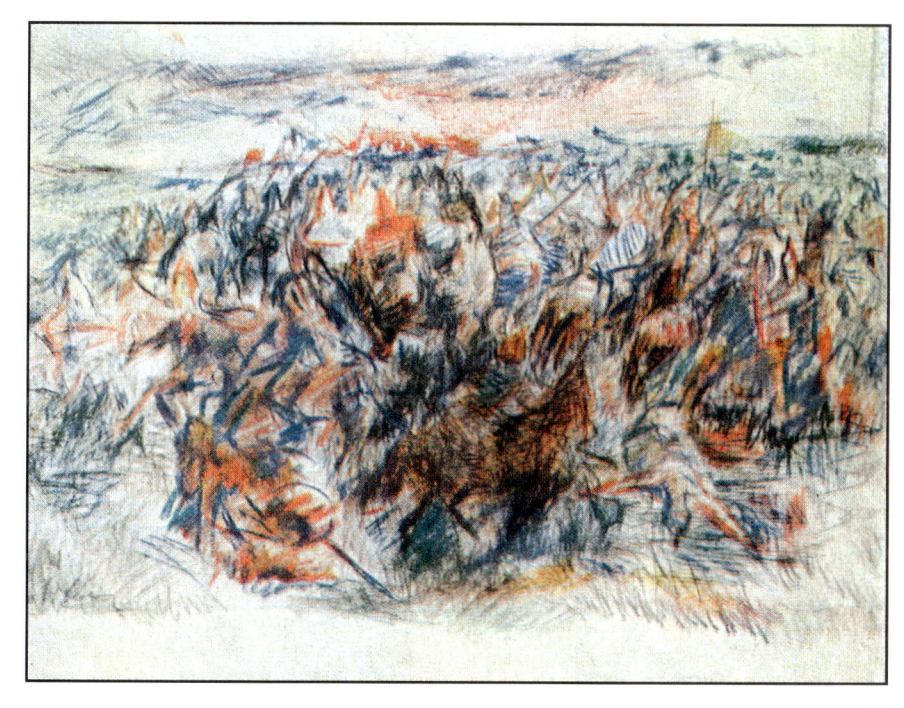

Case 4 - Fig. 49
Colored crayon. 17x21

65

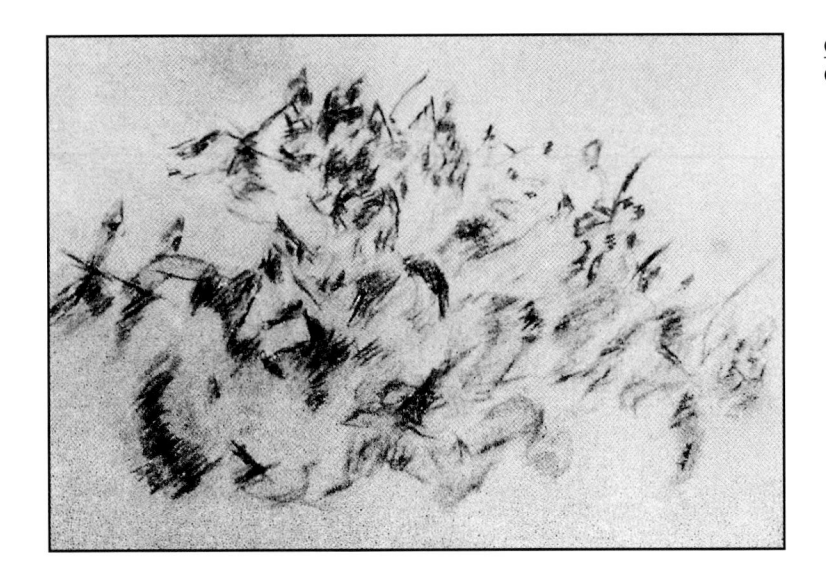

Case 4 - Fig. 50
Colored crayon. 21x30

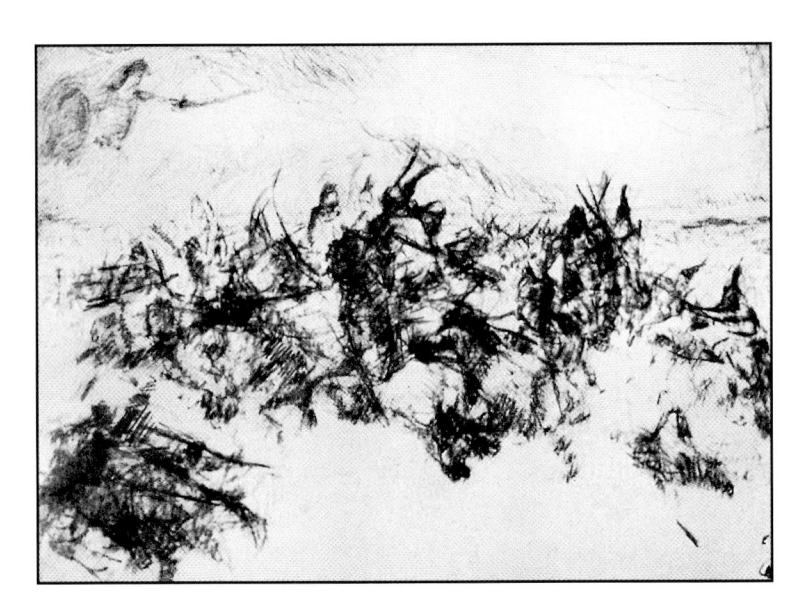

Case 4 - Fig. 51
Pencil drawing. 21x30

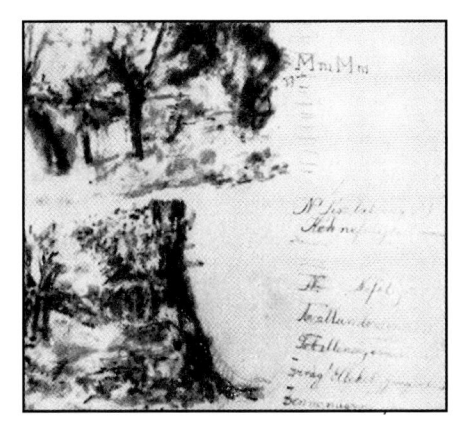

Case 4 - Fig. 52a
Ink drawing. 21x30

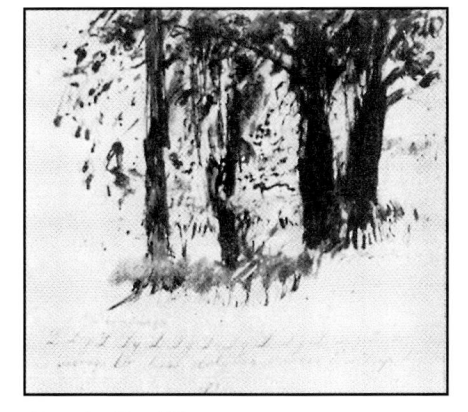

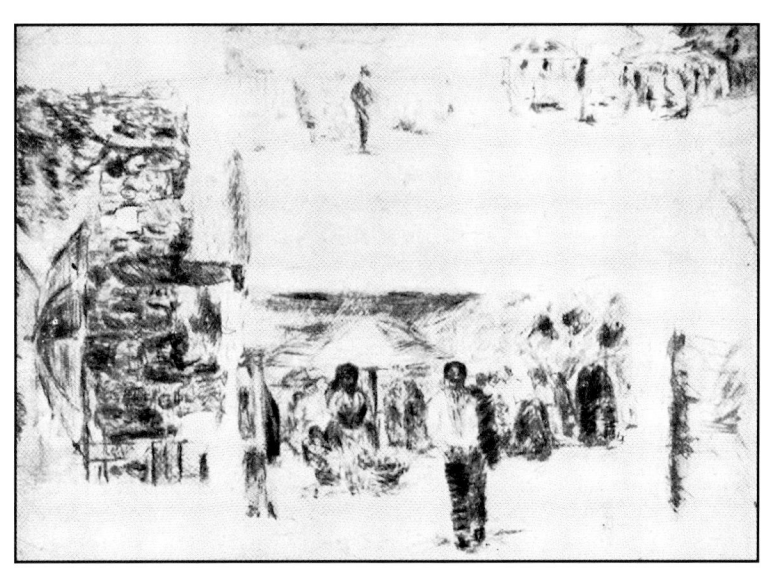

Case 4 - Fig. 53
Aquarelle. 21x30

Case 4 - Fig. 52b
Ink drawing. 21x30

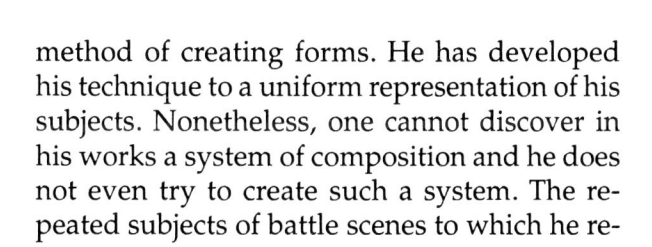

method of creating forms. He has developed his technique to a uniform representation of his subjects. Nonetheless, one cannot discover in his works a system of composition and he does not even try to create such a system. The repeated subjects of battle scenes to which he returns frequently can be explained, possibly, by his personal memories of participating in World War I. On the other hand, he is also inspired by his environment and produces studies of other patients and of the landscape seen from his window.

His representation is neither graphic nor pictorial. The short broken lines do not define contours; however, he tries to give shape seeking forms through these broken lines. The fragments of lines or colored patches, the results of careful studies, give the impression of a timid dreamlike atmosphere. His talent and the modest results reflect a fearful state. The repetition and continuity of the small details have a specific value that could gain the attention even of connoisseurs.

67

# Case 5 — A. J.

*Date of birth*: 1 January 1880
*Occupation*: Businessman
*Diagnosis*: Schizophrenia
He was hospitalized from 1910 to 6 May 1946 at the Psychiatric and Neurological University Hospital of Pécs.

*Family history*: Unremarkable.

*Personal history*: The patient had always been sensitive and withdrawn. He became increasingly distracted, was unable to pay attention to his work and became depressed. Sometimes he had the impression that his head did not belong to him. He had a hypochondriac delusion: he was a hermaphrodite and could never be cured; at work he must cover his head with a towel: then he would be able to solve the most difficult problems, and be capable of any intellectual achievement.

*Medical and neurological examination* is unremarkable. Bordet–Wassermann reaction is negative.

*Psychiatric evaluation*: Attention span is diminished and volatile. His affect is labile. Although formally his thought processes are adequate, his statements are erroneous under the influence of his delusions.

*Progress of the illness*: His behavior becomes bizarre and his associations are increasingly more incoherent. He also has ideas of persecution and coenesthopathic hallucinations. He feels that in his guts there are mice and requests to have an incision made in his anus to kill the mice with a pointed knife, or, to introduce a net of steel and trap them. At other times he fasts two to three days in an attempt to attract the mice through the rectum with sugared milk. He is sometimes agitated and in a bad mood.

In 1922, twelve years following his hospitalization, for the first time the patient asked the nurses for paints to "draw what I experience". He said that his drawings were "fantasies born of my brain". Among the first of his works he drew a bridge and underneath that a portrait of one of the nurses he liked. He declared that he already had talent in his childhood, but lost it because he had to occupy himself with other things and, mostly because "others have sucked up" his talent. He draws "machines" with pleasure and explains their function.

One day he drew squares on the steps of the staircase of the hospital. In the middle of the squares he wrote numbers from 65 to 80. A figure similar to a cannon bearing the inscription, "cultural section" is aimed at the squares. He gives the following explanation: "One has to kill every man between the ages of 65 and 80."

He is preoccupied with inventions that he presents graphically in his drawings. He gives the name of "Window Key" to the majority of his "inventions". (The pass key which opens windows and doors at the hospital.)

From time to time he paints nude human figures. Other times he refuses to draw, under the pretext that he must make statistics or that he is writing his autobiography. Another time he "draws his biography and that of his family". About one of these pictures he declares that all these "represent the keys to the gray Navy ships". On another drawing he represents his adoptive mother on a catafalque and states: "They have pierced her with a dagger and have mutilated her, but all this is nothing else but the keys to the gray Naval ships."

For drawing paper he uses old journals and other already printed sheets. He draws over the text and around it, as if it were a blank sheet of paper, without being disturbed by the printed text.

*His drawings can be divided into two groups.*
*In the first group* we find unusual constructions of machines of a geometrical character. One cannot guess what their function may be. The patient's fantastic ideas that inspired these works are expressed in the words of the text that he adds. "The flying train" represented in *Fig. 54* is nothing but an old couch underneath which there are "motors". His "agricultural machines" *(Fig. 55)* are geometrical figures, stereotyped and monotonous in form, and filled with meticulously repeated motifs.

*The second group* of his works is made up of interesting drawings representing human figures which, according to his added writings, are members of his family.

The human figures are characterized by a large head with distorted faces on a small trunk. Their sizes show no relationship to perspective. Nonetheless, the children are always represented as smaller than the adults.

In *Fig. 56*, in a "picture frame" he drew in the middle of the composition the large figure of a priest. Around this he arranged eight female figures with small arms and drawn only from the head to the hips. Their faces, with close-set eyes, are similar to each other. The hairstyle and clothing correspond to the style of the turn of the century. The individual figures are separated from each other and decorated by an ornamental motif. Beside each of the figures the patient wrote their name and their relationship to the family.

*Figure 57* is very curious. It represents a woman who is dressed except that her breasts are naked. An unproportionally small child and a chamber pot are on the right side. The text added by the patient is the following: "A girl, a boy, I ask for help".

The patient represents his family on a large-sized colored picture *(Fig. 58)*. In the foreground, in front of a landscape several figures are standing or sitting. They are disproportionate and badly drawn; two of these figures appear to float in the air. In the upper right corner a priest is preaching from the pulpit. Underneath him a woman receives, in an opened bag, pieces of gold that fall from the pulpit. On the left side there is a group of soldiers and above them are two cannons. A house without foreshortening constitutes a second level behind these figures. Nonetheless, the shingles are executed minutiously. On the left side between the branches of the tree is a head of a woman with blue hair. Further in the back, at the bottom of the hills surrounded by a row of trees, we can see a cultivated field, also represented without perspective. We can also distinguish here two human figures and a small house. Finally, a blue strip, decorated by small orange colored lines (the moon?, the sun?) closes up the upper margin of the picture. On the slopes a vineyard is represented mostly by blue and green triangles with rounded angles—the colors are poor and so are the forms. The colors are completely unreal and selected arbitrarily. The patient paints the roofs of the houses sometimes in red, sometimes in blue. The basic color of the picture is blue and the hills are also of the same color. This picture has no visual balance. It is evident that this patient works either inspired by a sudden idea or he gets into a monotonous stereotypy.

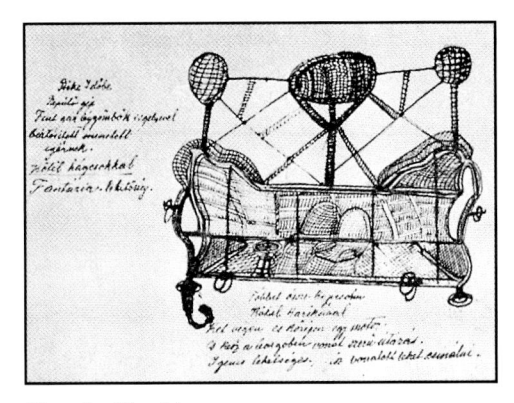

Case 5 - Fig. 54
Pen and colored crayon. 20.5x34

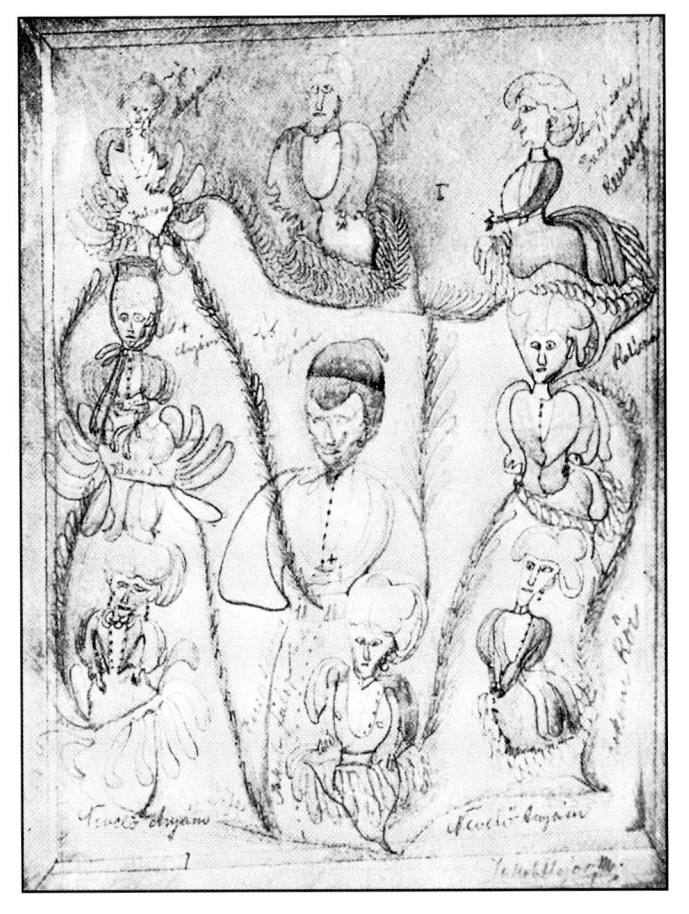

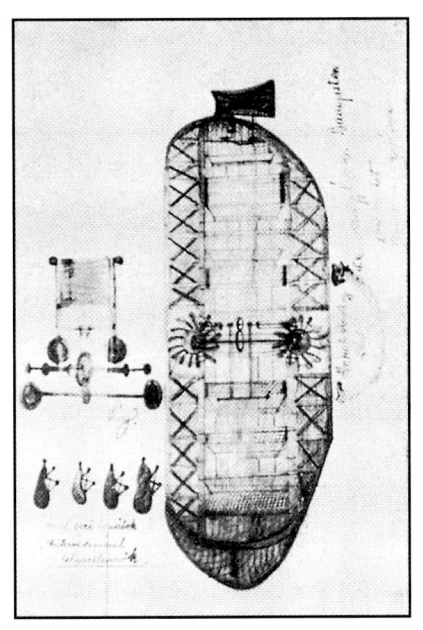

Case 5 - Fig. 55
Pencil drawing. 35x22

Case 5 - Fig. 56
Pencil drawing. 38x25

On *Fig. 59* we see behind the trees on the left a wall and on the trees a huge primitively drawn bird. On the right side we can see, in a row, a compact line of six human figures who are—a curious fact—well dressed, but with bare feet. One can find such curious representations also on some of his other drawings.

We can find an explanation of these representations in the following words written by the patient on *Fig. 60*, which represents a man dressed, but barefoot, and a pair of shoes beside him. "Is it permitted to do this? This one has taken them away." On the same page there is an incomplete description of a person and an inventory of pieces of clothing, probably taken away from the patient on the day of his hospitalization.

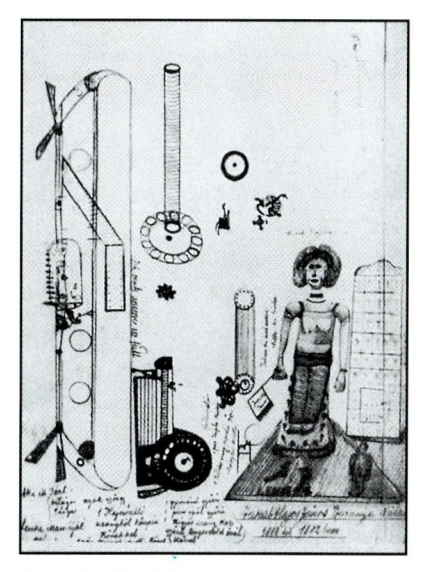

<u>Case 5</u> - Fig. 57
Pencil drawing. 35x28

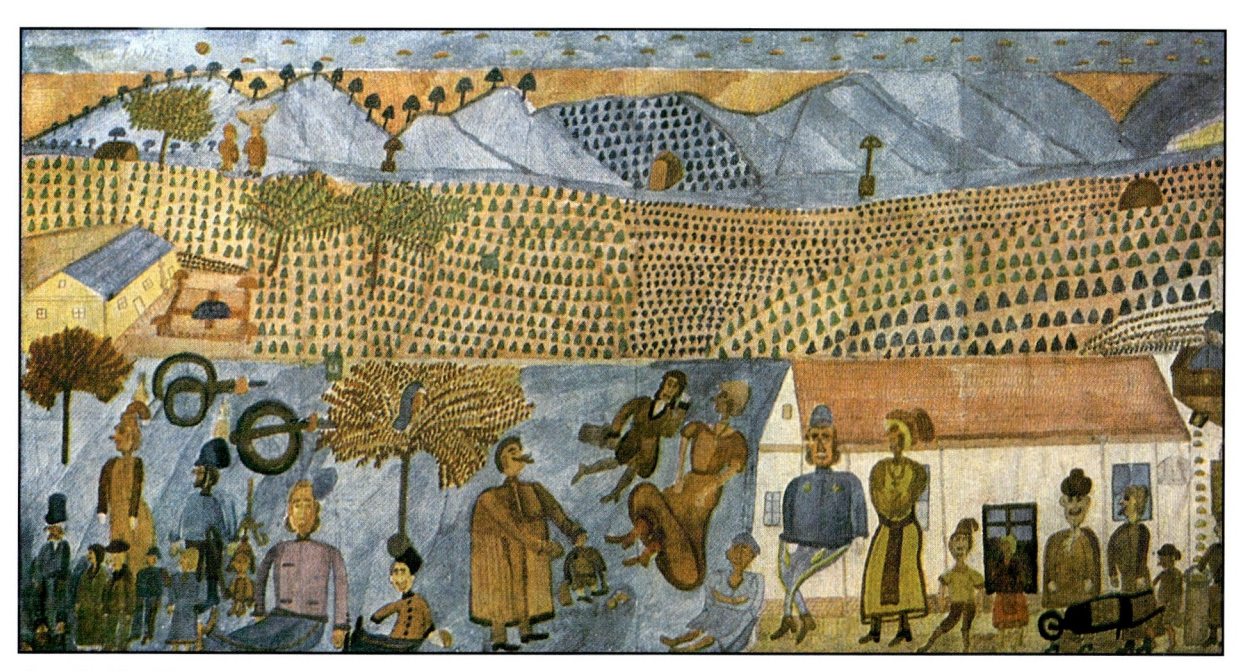

<u>Case 5</u> - Fig. 58
Aquarelle. 46x89

71

Case 5 - Fig. 59
Pencil drawing. 11.5x30

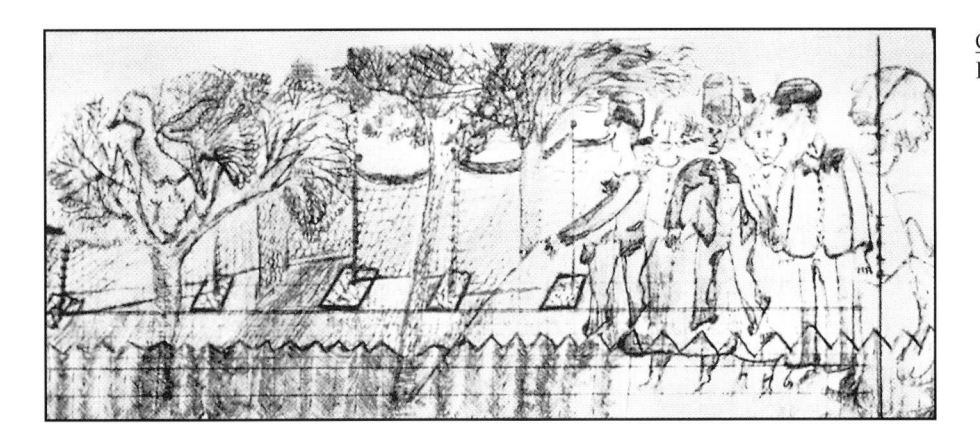

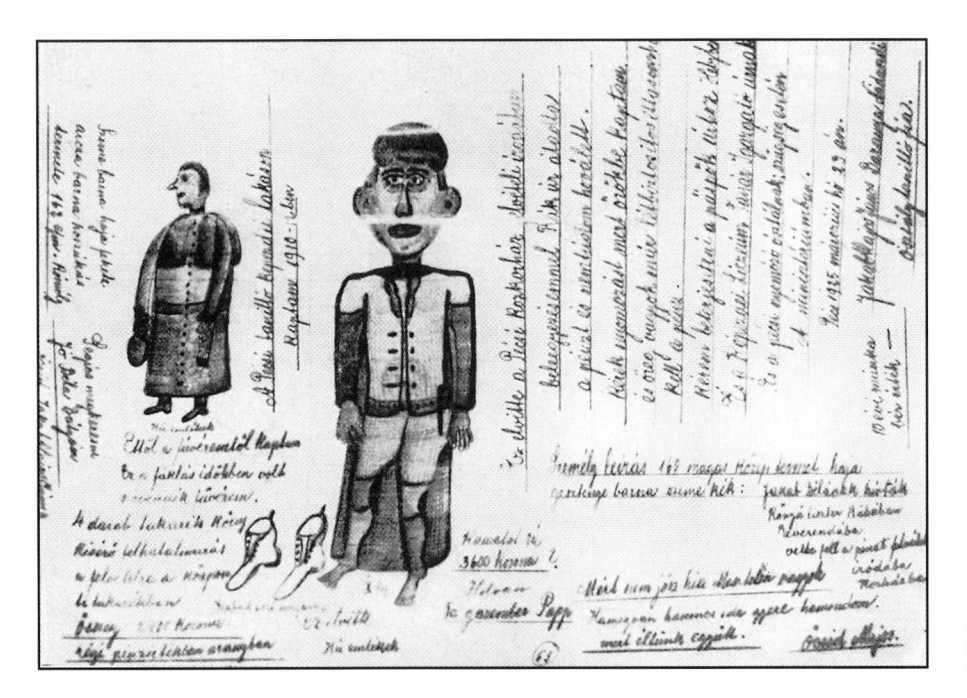

Case 5 - Fig. 60
Pencil drawing. 25x35

*Figure 61* is colored and bizarre. The principal figures, two small figures, stand on a paved terrace and between them is a huge piece of fruit. The background is made up of the hilly banks of a river. On this side of the river, on top of the hill a huge unreal-looking bird, from the world of fairy tales, is poised. The colors of this picture are as individually selected as in his other paintings. The sky is represented by a straight blue band with orange-colored half

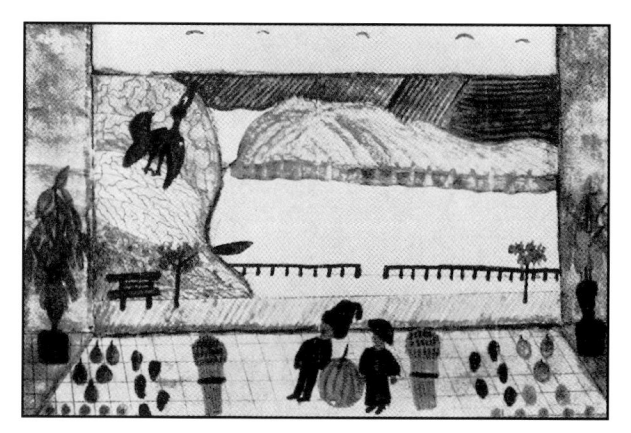

Case 5 - Fig. 61
Aquarelle. 28.5x40

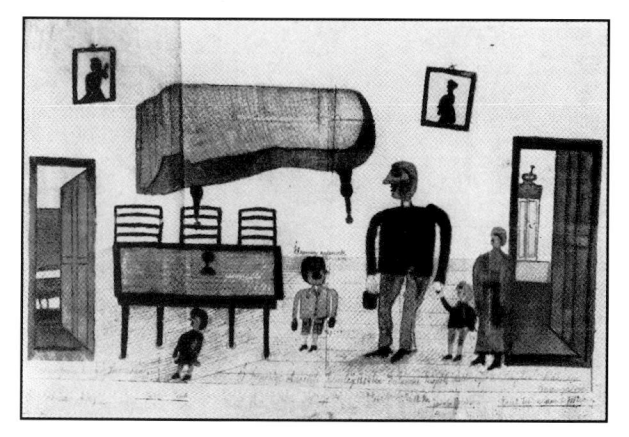

Case 5 - Fig. 62
Aquarelle. 32.5x51

Some figures populate the foreground of his drawings without perspective. The open doors without handles allow a view into other rooms.

In the pencil drawing in *Fig. 63* we see, besides an open piano, a woman placed in a "casket with mirrors". All the objects drawn are shown as if seen from above. A series of ornamental and stereotyped motifs complete this drawing.

Executed on a cardboard in colors, *Fig. 64* has a mystical air reminding us somewhat of the art work of the Middle Ages. Because of the peculiar arrangement of the figures, this painting produces a feeling of uneasiness in the spectator. The woman on the right holds a child in front of herself, while another child in front of the woman in the middle appears to be hung by his legs.

In the following passage, we are describing three aquarelle paintings of unusual dimen-

moons arranged in a line. Motifs of plants and fruits in equal number create a symmetrical arrangement of an ornamental nature on the two sides of the picture.

The patient also draws some scenes of the interior of houses. In *Fig. 62* he represents a table with three chairs and a piano as if suspended in midair between two paintings on the wall.

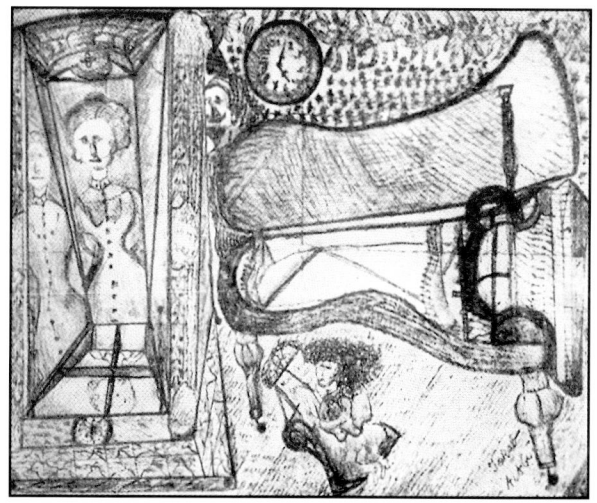

Case 5 - Fig. 63
Pencil drawing. 17x21

sions. Stereotyped motifs appear repeatedly in each painting.

*Figure 65* (31 × 108 cm) is stereotypical. The human shapes are repeated rhythmically at equal intervals.

Another aquarelle of unusual dimension is that of *Fig. 66* (33 × 105 cm), on a brown background with small green parallel lines and little green dots representing a grassy field. One can divide this picture into two different parts. The continuity among them is established by the figure of a tree, in front of which the shepherd sits on a tree stump. On the right half there are horses.

The gray horses are drawn in a stereotyped fashion, in regard to both their form and their color. In the middle of the picture, in front of two horses, a huge bird flies toward the top of the tree. On the left half of the picture the same grassy field is continued; it is populated by a herd of cows drawn in a less stereotyped way than were the horses. On the left edge of the field there is a cow standing in front of a tree. One has to note the rigidity by which the patient separates these two kinds of animals on the same "single field". The composition is characterized by the lack of coherence and by stereotypy.

An even more obvious stereotypy characterizes *Fig. 67* (33 × 163 cm). The contrast between the windows colored in red, as if they were illuminated from within, and the full daylight on the whole landscape produces a strange effect. The two human figures in this aquarelle are drawn without perspective.

*Figure 68* represents a mystical tropical scene with the inscription, "My Golden Flower". To *Fig. 69* he gives the title: "Primary School Exercise: Natural History 8. 6. 1945". The small blocks of this landscape fill the page completely like a mosaic. In the upper left part of the picture there is a little house in front of a hilly landscape topped by a line of ornamental trees.

The right side is made up of a stereotyped motif of squares. As in his other colored pictures, the sphere of the sun and half-moon formation, and the clouds form the upper margin of the picture. The proportions of human figures and of the animals are arbitrary and unreal. Their rigid expressions and the flat two-dimensional representation gives this drawing a crystallized appearance.

*Figure 70* is a symbolical work. The principal figure in this composition is the deer with silver antlers forming a bridge between two adjacent mountain peaks. The middle region of this work is made up of a mountainous landscape. In the foreground, closed on the bottom by an ornamental motif, we can see a small house and a hunter. The colors gray and silvery-green evoke the vision of a strange landscape at dawn.

In later years he was treated at the Mental Health Institute Budapest-Lipótmező. He died there. We thank the Director of the Psychiatric Neurological Institute (Hospital) of Budapest-Lipótmező, Dr. Gimes, who provided us with a copy of the medical records of this patient that we are using here.

At the hospital, in his medical record, it was noted that the patient's behavior was childish and he had several delusions. Each European state owes him an honorarium which amounts daily to a bucket of silver gulden. He complained that he did not receive this honorarium. Now each state owes him. He drew stereotyped little houses and manneristic sketches. He worked in the garden. He wrote once to the office of the diocese the following letter:

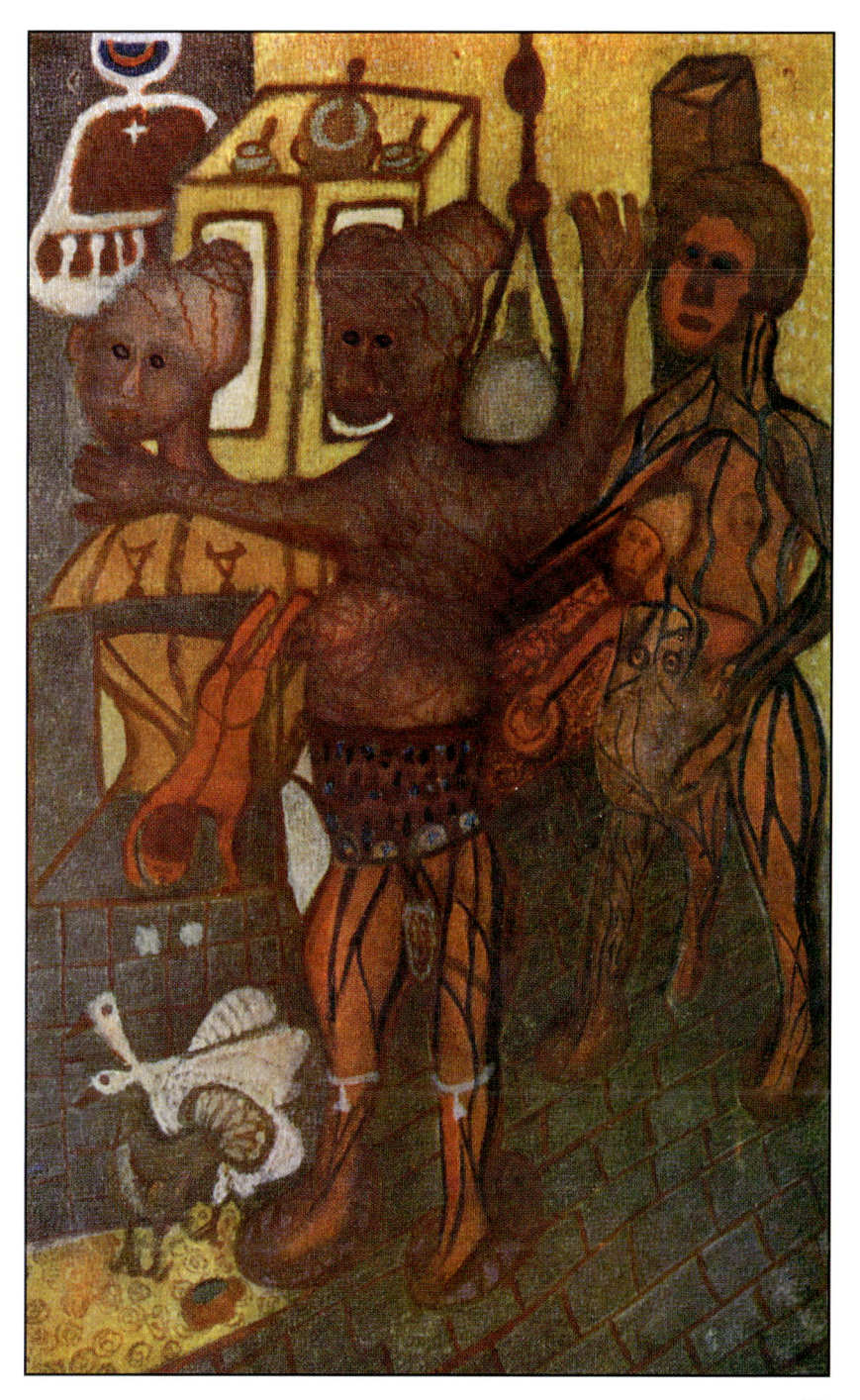

Case 5 - Fig. 64
Aquarelle. 21x13

Case 5 - Fig. 65
Aquarelle. 31x108

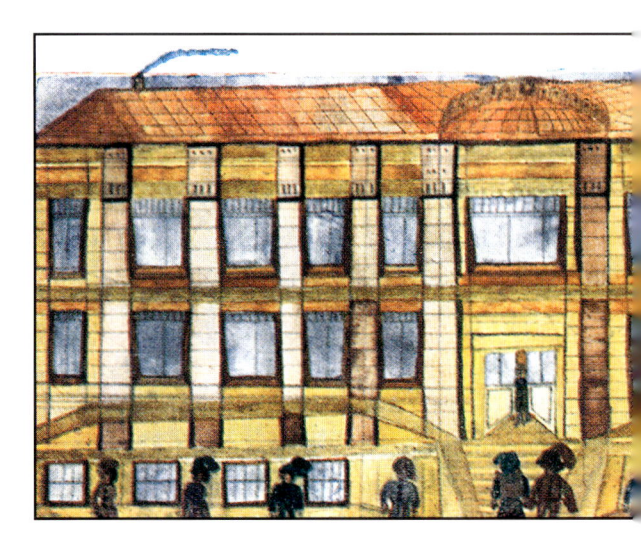

Case 5 - Fig. 66
Aquarelle. 33x105

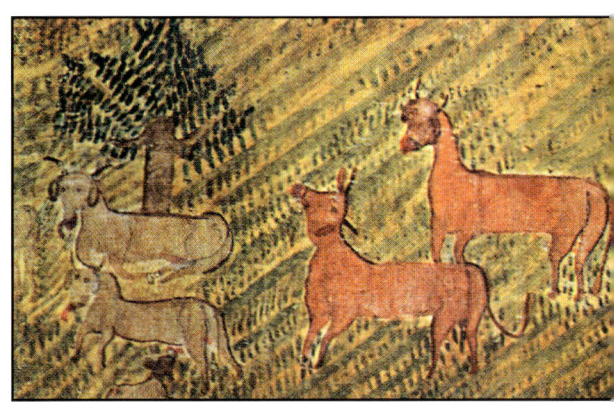

Case 5 - Fig. 67
Aquarelle. 33x163

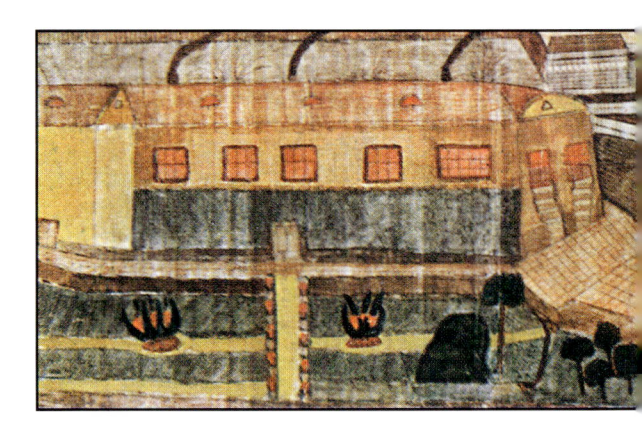

77

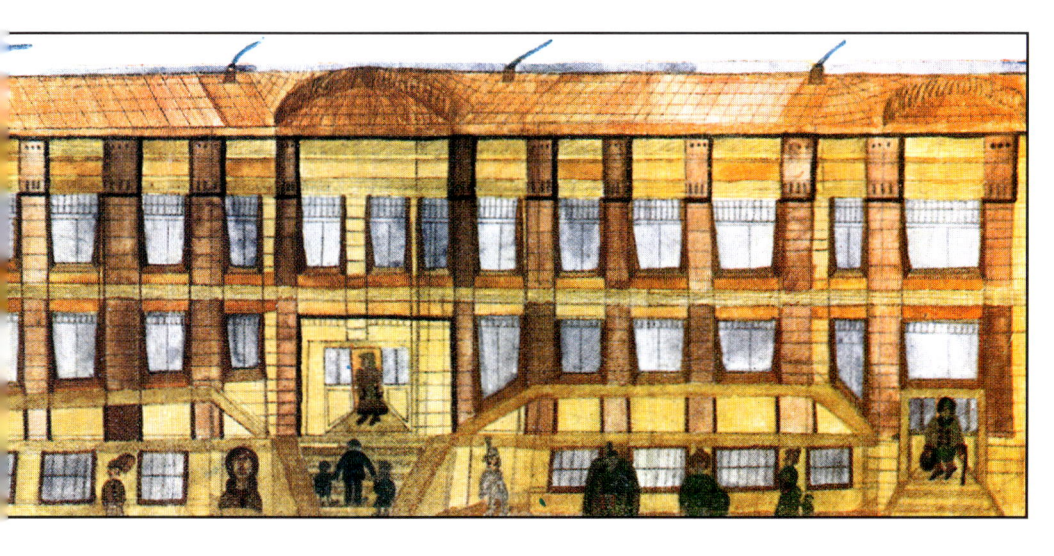

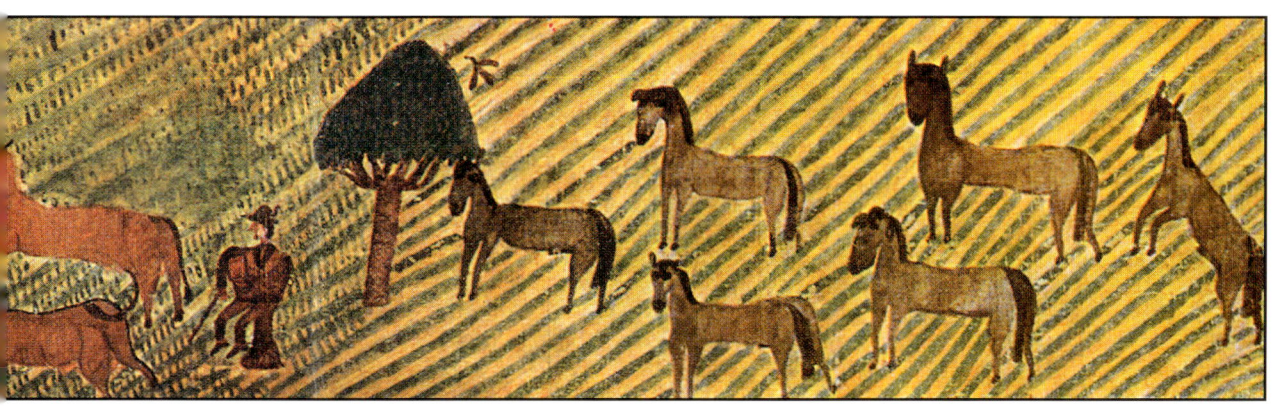

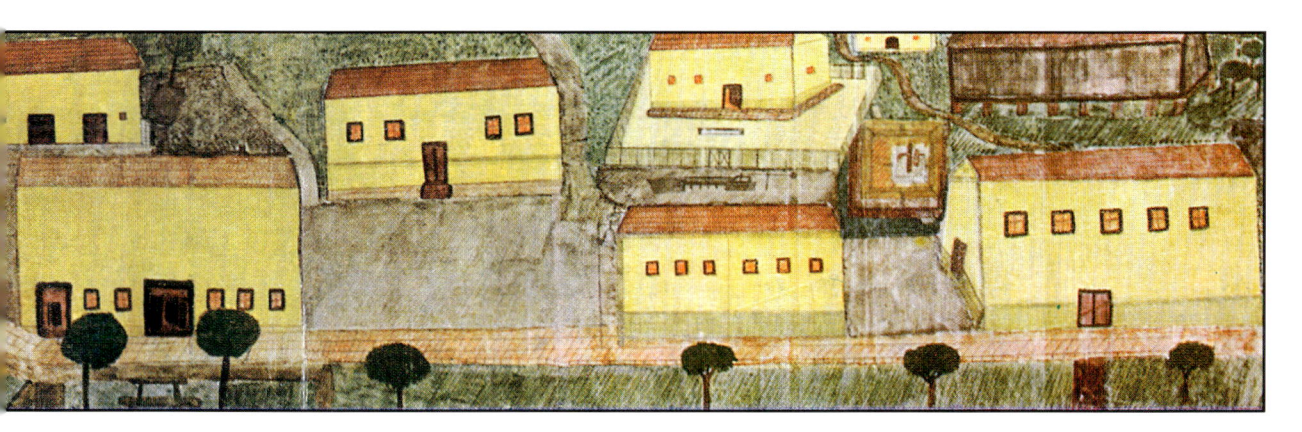

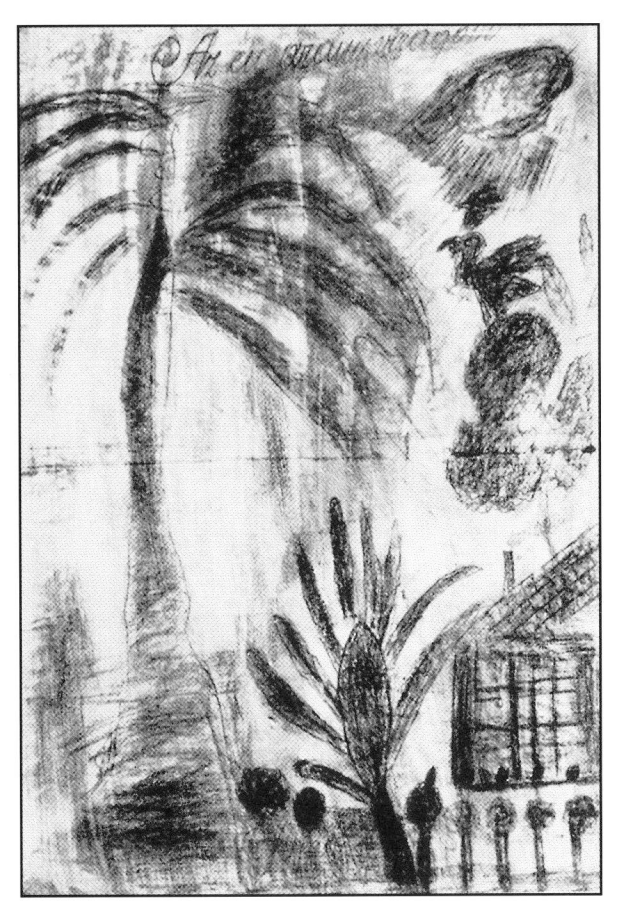

Case 5 - Fig. 68
Aquarelle. 34x21

"I am petitioning your reverency to change my name *A. J.* in the books to *A. Mester*. My name is uncomfortable. I am ashamed of it. On my name there are many rumors attached and celestial happiness. Nonetheless, it is antipathic and I have suffered with it.

And, all my works remain without honorarium. I remain by my † religion as I have been born as a Christian. I ask you humbly that you should take care of this inexpensively and to send me the certificate of baptism.

With Christian love and greetings
A. J., son of F. J. T."

From the works of his latest years, we are reproducing two pictures here. In *Fig. 71* we can see a farmyard with people and animals and a little house with windows, under which there is a ladder across the front. On the left there are ducks and a rooster. One of the ducks is sur-

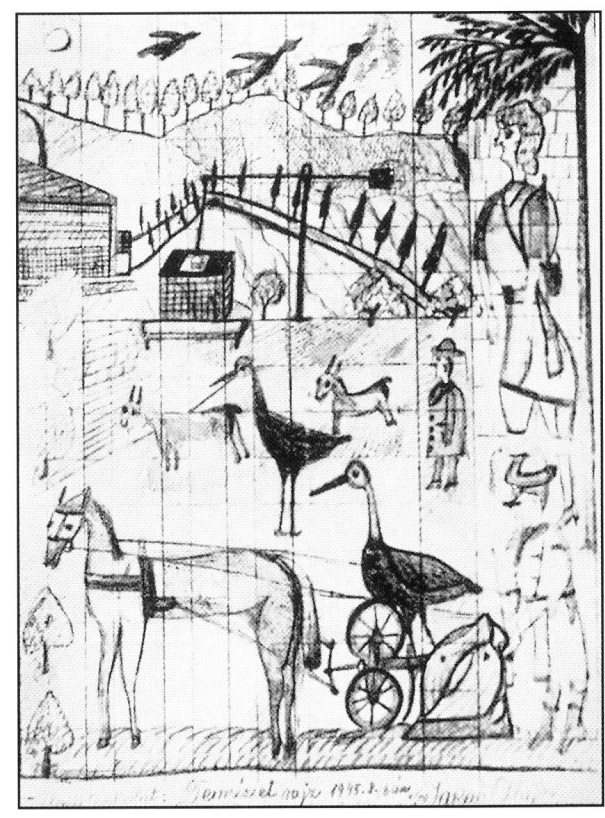

Case 5 - Fig. 69
Pencil drawing. 40x31

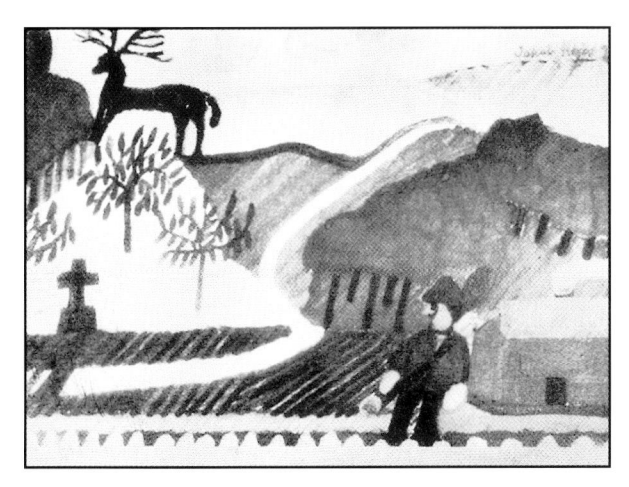

Case 5 - Fig. 70
Aquarelle. 15.5x21

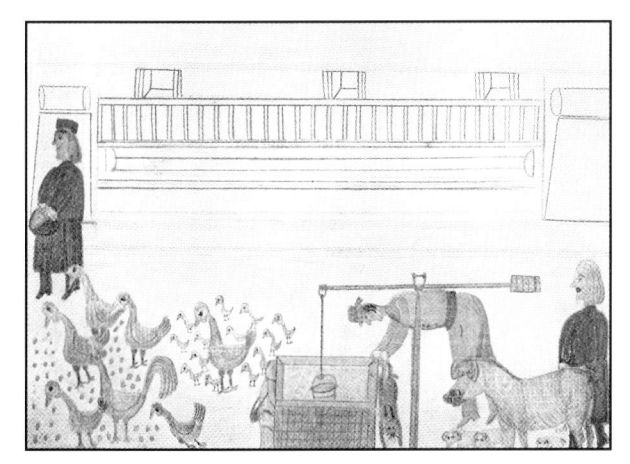

the balance beam of which is too small in comparison to the other figures. The man beside it was obviously drawn later. He is bent, in a stiff way, from the hips under the beam of the well, and holds an animal by its hind legs, which most likely is a dog. On the right side of the picture there are a woman, a pig, and piglets.

Case 5 - Fig. 71
Colored crayon. 29x41

rounded by ducklings. Otherwise, the space between the animals is painstakingly filled with grains. Probably this is corn that is dispensed by the woman drawn without perspective on the left side, in front of the animals, with a basket. In the middle of the foreground is a well,

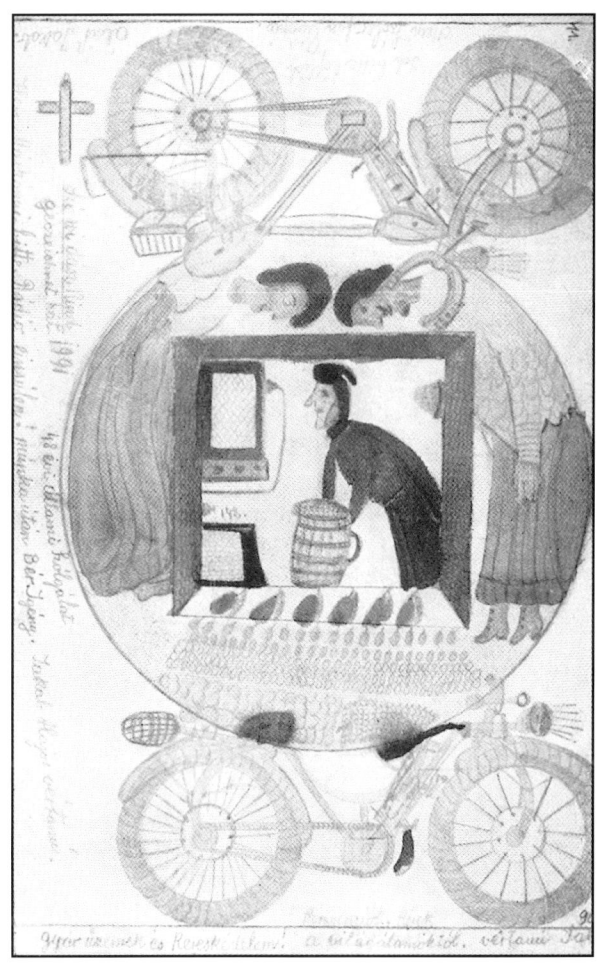

Case 5 - Fig. 72
Colored crayon. 41x27.5

79

The human and animal figures, especially the latter, are essentially similar to children's drawings. The whole picture is two-dimensional and its execution shows stereotypy in the scattering of the grains of corn and in the parallel lines on the background. The position of the man is unusual and unnatural.

*Figure 72* is a bizarre composition. The middle part of the picture is circular and encased. Inside of this circle is another space surrounded by a square frame giving the impression as if the scene painted inside of this frame would be seen through a window. A woman is bent here, without the impression of balance, over a barrel, while also leaning on it. Across from her there are two radio-like shapes. Around this frame two figures are bent, one a man with a beard and mustache but dressed as a woman on the right and a woman on the left. The back and the dress of the man is part of the circumference of the circle while the contour line of the female figure runs parallel to the circle without becoming part of it. Under and in front of the window the space is filled with stereotyped fruit arranged in minute detail. The whole middle part, in spite of its bizarre appearance, reminds the spectator of pictures of the late fifteenth century. What is very dissonant is that this picture is surrounded by two motor bicycles. A cross is on the upper left side. The text around the picture is written partly in Hungarian and partly in German.

## Case 6 — F. Cs.

*Date of birth*: 15 October 1888
*Occupation*: Teacher
*Diagnosis*: Schizophrenia

He was admitted to the Psychiatric and Neurological University Hospital of Pécs for the first time on 19 October, 1932. He died on 12 October, 1945.

*Family history*: Mother had a post-partum psychosis. Three of his brothers were mentally ill, hospitalized until their deaths which occurred in the hospitals.

*Personal history*: He finished his studies with excellent results. The patient lost one eye during World War I. He had no other injury or illness. He retired at his own request in 1923 and kept busy with small jobs in his garden. He quarreled a lot with his family members and was always impatient.

In 1932 he became increasingly nervous. One morning his speech became incoherent. He chased after everybody, and became aggressive.

*At admission* he revealed that he had been sick and that "from the moment when he first took medications all his ailments disappeared." ... "I felt at that same moment that I had been invaded by a torrential force, a stroke of lightning hit me, and I have been glorified. My beloved child who is charming and good is a double of the poet Petőfi. I have seen my dead child in the sky in a magnificent and superb celestial uniform. In that moment I died for the earth to become God, a great furious God." He explained the act of being transported to the hospital in an ambulance with the following phrase:

"An observing patrol came to me and abducted me from my room."

*Medical and neurological examination* was unremarkable. Bordet–Wassermann reaction in the blood and in the spinal fluid was negative.

*Course of illness.*The patient rests in his bed and talks incessantly: "I am God since I have been born, a horrible god and an old one whom the people had the audacity to throw in here among the dead in this abyss. Do they want to kill me? I am going to kill them! My will is the lightning and the thunder. This is not Mr. Cs, Mr. Schoolteacher who is here, this is God. I have no wife, but I do have my Alexander [his son]. I am in a different world, God, God, God, God." He beats his chest, gestures, and chases everybody. He does not observe anything that happens in his environment, but reacts to each noise. He feels being glorified and does not even find sufficiently solemn expressions or words that would be strong enough to express his feelings. He threatens the staff by his immense physical strength and power. During examination, he was asked to tell the date of today, the month, or at least the present season of the year. He gives the following answer: "In the divinity there is an eternal and infinite time! Why do you ask me such questions?"

He rests frequently with closed eyes. If someone approaches him he becomes agitated and tries to chase everyone away. Sometimes he bursts into lamentations without any exterior motives. During medical rounds, he stares with a vacant expression. At other times he catches a few words of the conversation and repeats them. He points a finger towards the people who are around him with a facial expression as if wanting to say something. Then once again he remains silent.

During the thirteen years of his illness, his family attempted to take him home several times, but because of his aggressiveness they never succeeded in keeping him longer than a few months. During his illness, periods of psychomotor restlessness and catatonic stupor alternated.

During one of his readmissions, he told the following: "I do not give references ... that you could look up in the medical history from 1932 when I have been referred by the order of the state physician H. as generally dangerous, that is because my wife was scared when I told her about my kingdom ... also my little youngster who now learns with the strength of a gorilla, who knows Mr. Professor, and who, when I was admitted in 1932, stood beside me, a little boy with blonde locks ... I consider it my holy duty to enter my son in school in Debrecen, in the same gymnasium where the muscular Hungarian ghost-of-Petőfi lives... Neither in the present nor in the past is there any law. Here is a document of my handwriting which describes Hungary as Magyarmecske (a geographical name) ... When I was here in 1932, I have seen, in a bed, my son who lived for ten days. In another bed I have seen my daughter, here beside the window is Mrs. Rozgonyi. There, near the door I saw the little King Ludwig II. And there again, Etelka Vincze. We battled with the nurses and we hit each other and threw each other on the bed ... I did not search for the origin of the predicate Cs. since I know that we have inherited the flame-soul of Alexander Petőfi and I know that we are originally from the borough Cs. ... I say nothing; my dear little son who is now in Debrecen and studies the sciences and will become a professor ... will tell it all. Do they know who I am? The promise of the future, the flam-

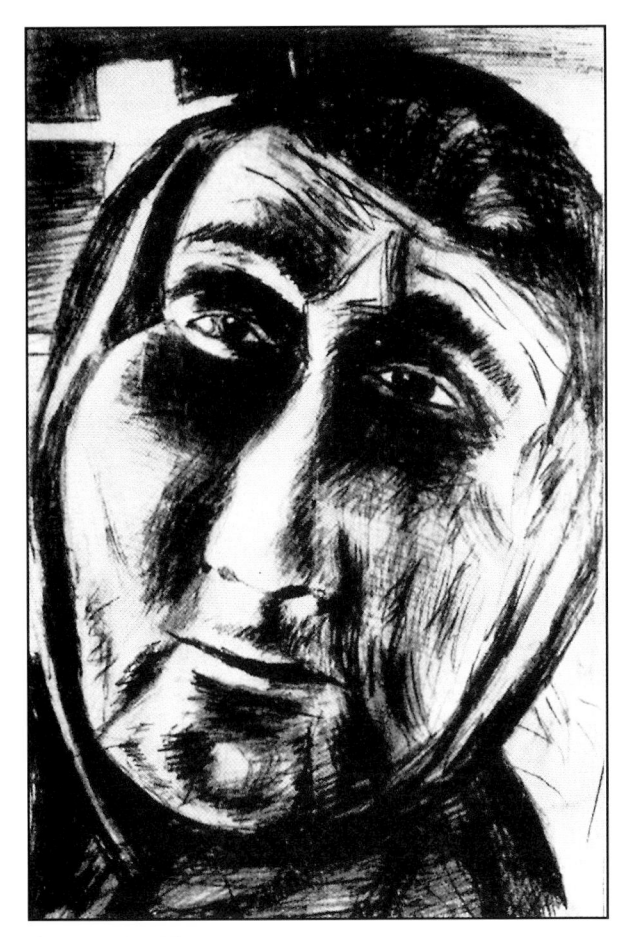

Case 6 - Fig. 73
Pencil drawing. 31x21

dust here since he was a soldier. He can only be a soldier, but he can also be a poet. I am the poet-singer of this folk. Nonetheless I cannot play on my lute. But I will be resurrected in my son who now begins to play it with his weak hands. However, he will become big so that the great spirit will revive again ... The battle from Mohács was, is it not true? in 1529, when our little king was betrayed by his army. Now the leader is not important but the troops whom

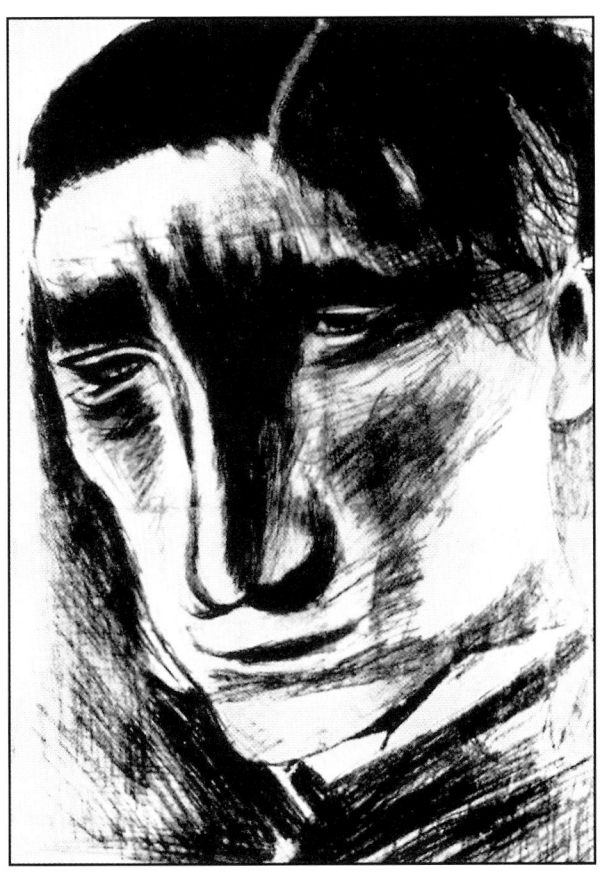

Case 6 - Fig. 74
Pencil drawing. 31x21

ing soul of Petőfi lives here with me and in thirteen years, in 1948, it will be resurrected in me again then a new land acquisition will follow, the third one ... There are namely some who believe that he died in Segesvár. There he died during the attack. There are others who believe that he died on an Asian steppe. Nonetheless, all this is not true; the truth is that Petőfi lives here with me, his flaming soul cannot become

God guides and I am fully under this in my heart, my faithful burning heart, that I am drawing, because I can draw very well. I have drawn it in coal and chalk and do you know what was on it? The head of a lion."

He started drawing only during his sixth admission to the hospital from January to March 1933. During this time he was concerned with religious problems and problems concerning painting. He is contrary and disregards the opinion of others. He discusses the different feelings that one experiences when regarding a picture from close by or from far away. He starts drawing spontaneously and brags about his work. In 1933 he drew many pictures and said: "I have gained sixty gold coins through my talent during my years of studies." Once he presented a drawing with the following words: "I am taken by dizziness, but in such a way that a drawing drops out of my head."—"I would like to break up the world, first the sun, then the moon and the stars."

He drew a madonna "to symbolize the state of the soul in time of starvation while fasting". About his other works, he said: "They will represent my life".

As suddenly as he started, he suddenly abandoned his drawing. He stated that he had lost his interest in drawing and did not find any joy in it any more.

He drew heads and busts. One can suppose that some of them are originals, while others are probably copied from portraits of famous personalities reproduced in journals.

The portrait of the woman and of the man shown in *Figs 73* and *74* reveal a disquieting and bizarre atmosphere.

The solution of the effect of light and shade is original. The relatively small and barely open eyes of the man are at a wide distance from each other; the large nose and low forehead characterize this face.

The portrait of the woman has better proportions. Nonetheless, here also the forehead is extremely low. The two sides of this portrait are drawn symmetrically and only the convergence of the eyes gives a restless character to the expression of the face.

The importance of *Fig. 75* is increased by the phrase with which he presented this drawing:

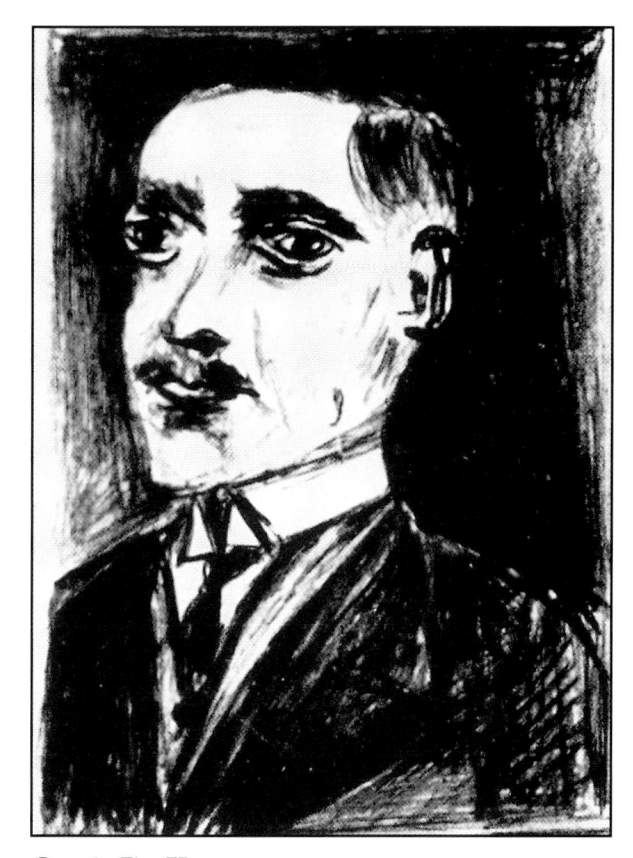

Case 6 - Fig. 75
Pencil drawing. 13x9.5

"When I drew him I felt that I was strangling his neck, and that is why his eyes are bulging". These words allow us to see the psychological act by which the patient projected his feelings into his drawings. He treated the portraits of the people in a palpable fashion, as if they were living beings.

The figures of F. Cs. are similar to the figures of L. L. (Case 2). Nonetheless, F. Cs. transposes his feelings with more dexterity and greater persuasive force and more richness. The élan and the passion of his interpretations make us forget sometimes the dilettantism and the deficiencies of his technique. An air of desperation and decay emanates from the two life-size heads of Figs 73 and 74. The characteristic traits of the portraits that he copies are generally lost. Nonetheless, one can recognize on some of the sheets the figures of Petőfi, Mac Donald, etc.

The rich scale of grays, starting with the light color of the paper to the deepest darkness of the lead pencil are characteristic of F. Cs.'s own technique. His long lines are the heaviest at the beginning and then gradually become thinner, little by little, as his hand is raised from the paper. The short lines are, in general, of the same thickness. They are not flexible. A third type of line, used only for the most difficult details to show (nostrils and eyebrows) have the characteristics of insecurity and timidity. The lines are corrected in such a way as to become overlapping.

His fashion of modeling is graphic. His traces are nervous and cross each other. His process is arbitrary. He is unable to observe attentively or to concentrate on his work. Therefore, the atmosphere of his drawings reveals the dominant role of his impulsive feelings.

## Case 7 — Mrs. J. U.

*Date of Birth*: 14 December 1905
*Occupation*: Cook
*Diagnosis*: Schizophrenia
*Hospitalized* from 9 September 1942 to 16 June 1950 at the Psychiatric and Neurological University Hospital of Pécs. In 1950 she was transferred to an asylum.

*The history* is given by the patient herself since there are no relatives and no friends to visit her at the hospital. The police requested her admission because of her bizarre behavior during a complaint made by her about the wife of her employer.

She had never been ill, except for a broken arm. She had never been hospitalized at any hospital or asylum. She had been married. Since her divorce she had been making a living by being a cook at private homes. In the recent past she had changed work every two to three months. She had the habit of presenting herself as "the daughter of the State". Frequently she had not even been hired. She made several complaints at the police station and at the Department of Justice lately because her employers had not paid her wages.

*State on admission*:
*Medical and neurological evaluation*: Negative. Underweight female. Bordet–Wasserman reaction in the blood and spinal fluid negative.

*Psychiatric evaluation*: Oriented. Attention is vigilant with a high tenacity. Thought processes formally normal. She communicates freely, but becomes suddenly enraged and threatens those around her. There is no dementia. She expresses megalomanic ideas: she claims that she is the daughter of the State. People give her favors, she is engaged to a general who is a nobleman and it is because of vengeance that she is hospitalized here. She had no insight into her illness.

Soon after her hospitalization she complained of coenesthopathic hallucinations and says that during the night weakness invades her whole body. She protests against the fact that "they take advantage of her". Sometimes she has the idea that she is being poisoned: "They put hydrochloric acid in my food to destroy my teeth".

For a time she becomes more autistic and then again becomes communicative. She calls herself "the queen" and then "the saint". "She is the proprietress of the institute." Frequently she sits in front of the radiator which is a "microphone" and holds conferences with her ministers. She requests greater privileges that others do not have. Her behavior is manneristic and her expressions are full of neophrases and neologisms.

She talks a lot about being the fiancée of a general and a count. From time to time she "amuses herself" with her fiancé. She says that he has tortured her in the evening. Therefore, he will not be a part of her kingdom. She doesn't like the generals who are not subordinated. Yesterday there was a meeting to build up the kingdom. Her fiancé spoke here and showed an attitude against the state. Anyone who has offended the state has naturally also offended the person of the queen and this she, her holiness, cannot tolerate. She had to intervene. Thus, a successor of this ex-fiancé has already been determined, a little blonde medical resident who is exactly right for reigning. She complains that the personnel doesn't show her the necessary respect. She doesn't even get as much to eat as the other patients. Actually they should give her an extra key, because she is not like the other subjects. Repeatedly, she complains about the physician and medical trainees that they are raping her during the night. At other times she complains that they don't pay enough attention to her while they are preoccupied with their own experiences of married life. She talks to the attendants who brought in another patient and asked whose subjects they are, what uniform they have, and who gave them the right to wear these uniforms. She defends herself terrified of the idea that patients "in her asylum" would be operated upon. She forbids this because it is her duty to conduct the affairs of the state. She defends herself against the present "rusty" happenings and complains that her qualities as queen are not sufficiently observed. It was also a bad state of affairs for the kings since the nurses wanted them to work, although the nurses are actually her underlings. She listened on the radio to the feast of her own sanctification and complains that she could not be there. She complains that we do not allow her sisters to come to her. She spoke with her ghost and he told her that he wants to come to her. She would like to have money to buy certain things, ten million Pengős. We show her bank notes from the time of inflation and tell her that these are not valid any more. They are worthless. After thinking it over, she said the following: "This is good money since I have not issued any other yet. After all, I am the queen of the nation."

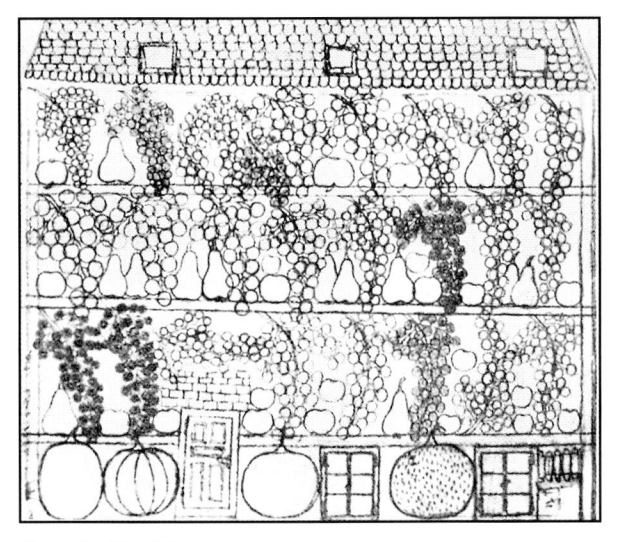

Case 7 - Fig. 76
Pencil drawing. 14.5x17

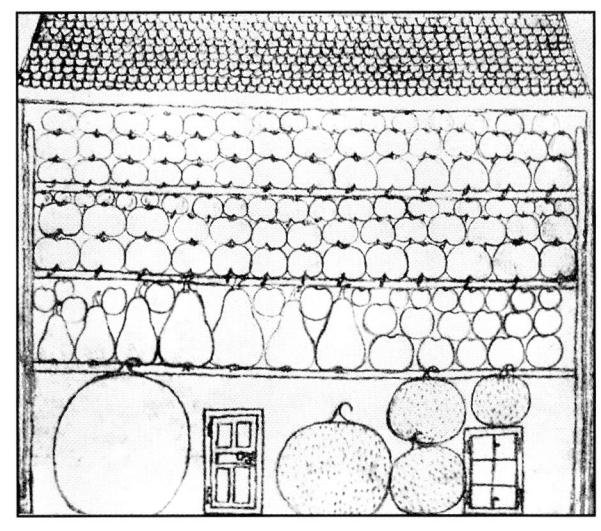

Case 7 - Fig. 77
Pencil drawing. 14.5x17

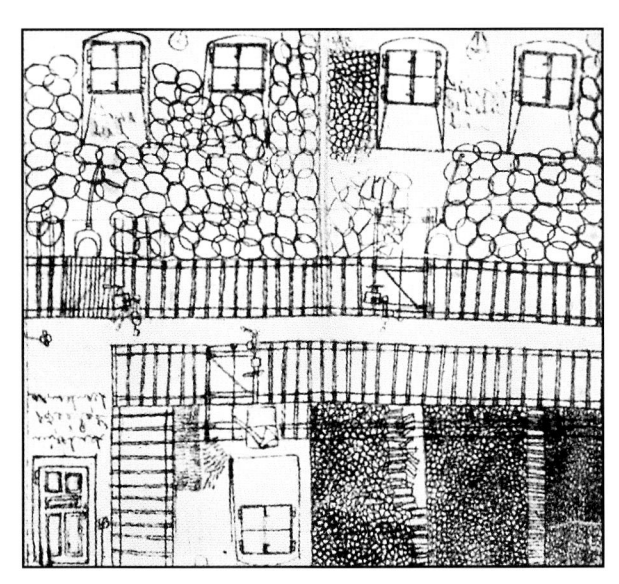

Case 7 - Fig. 78
Pencil drawing. 14.5x17

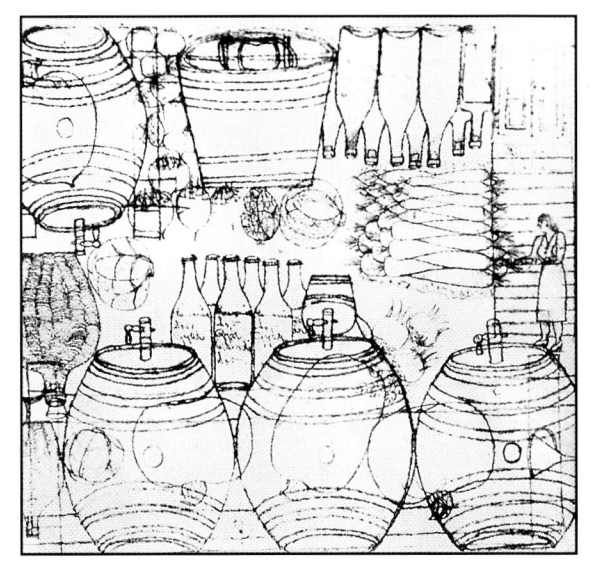

Case 7 - Fig. 79
Pencil drawing. 14.5x17

Case 7 - Fig. 80
Pencil drawing. 14.5x17

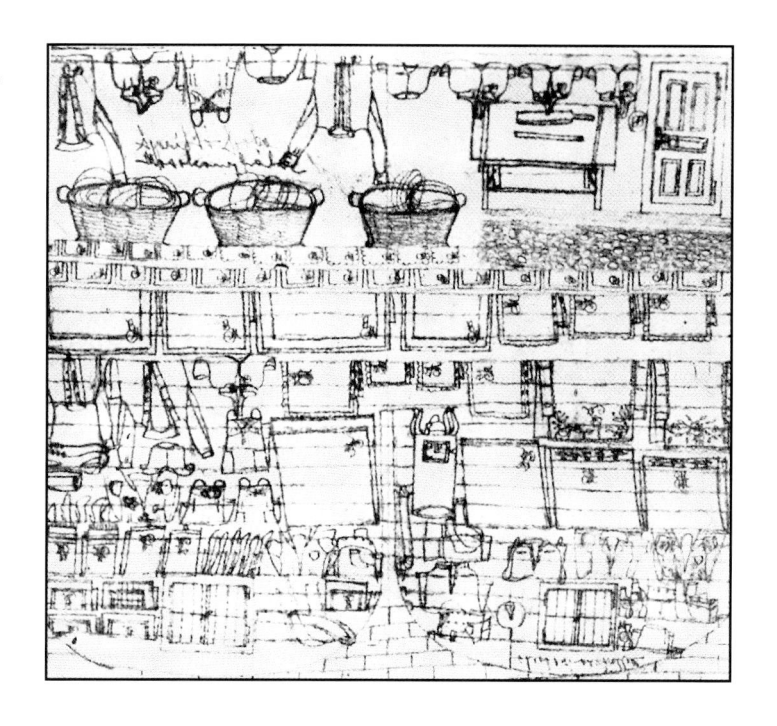

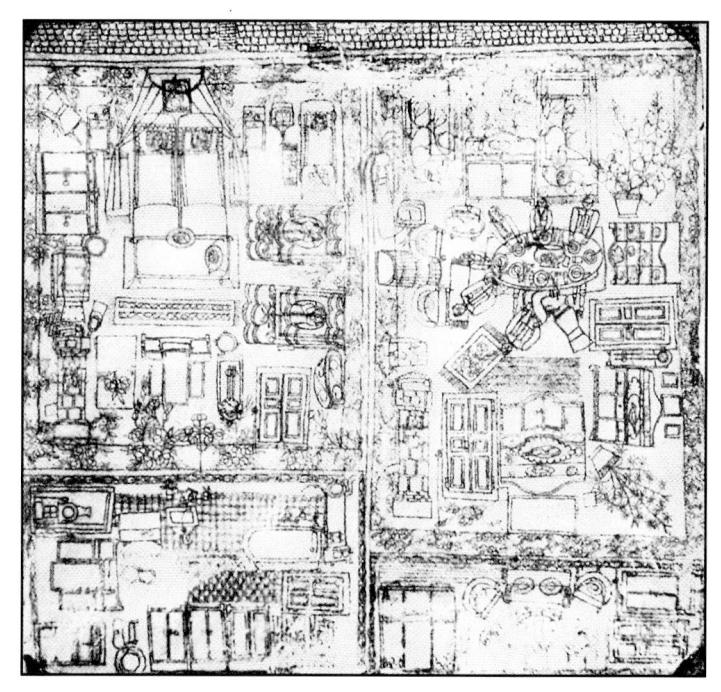

Case 7 - Fig. 81
Pencil drawing. 28x27

Case 7 - Fig. 82
Pencil drawing. 28x27

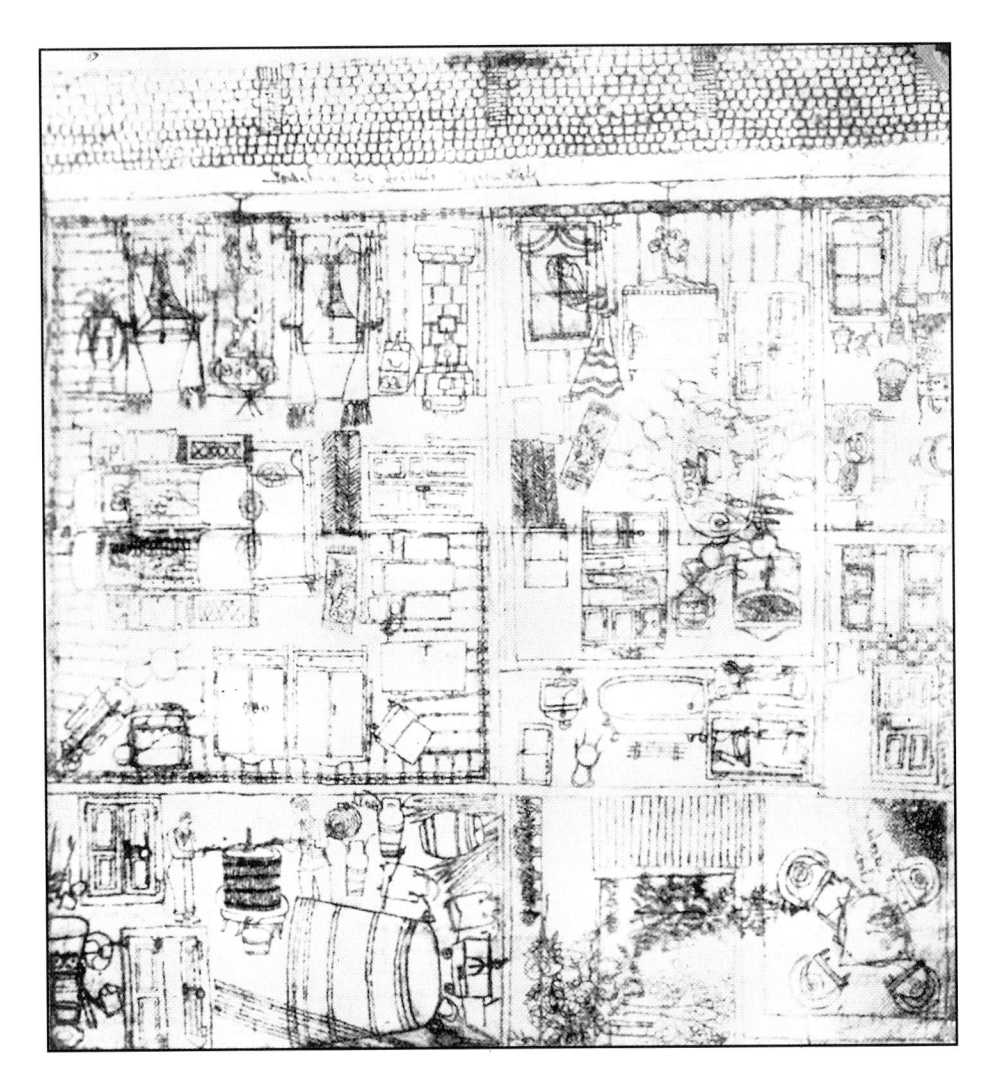

One evening after dinner she sits down and says the following without being asked: "I am the holy, the uncrowned king of the nation male as well as female, but what does the title help ...—as I came here, my holiness was recognized ... and since I bought this institute, three years have elapsed ... it is my property. Nonetheless today I only had a little milk ... Forgive me, but the institute is my property and I am the queen of the nation."

She writes letters to her fiancé in which she expresses her anger or her disgust:

"World renowned swindler!
You allow rather my beautiful picture be torn than to share with me the five years that elapsed.

Case 7 - Fig. 83
Pencil drawing. 28x27

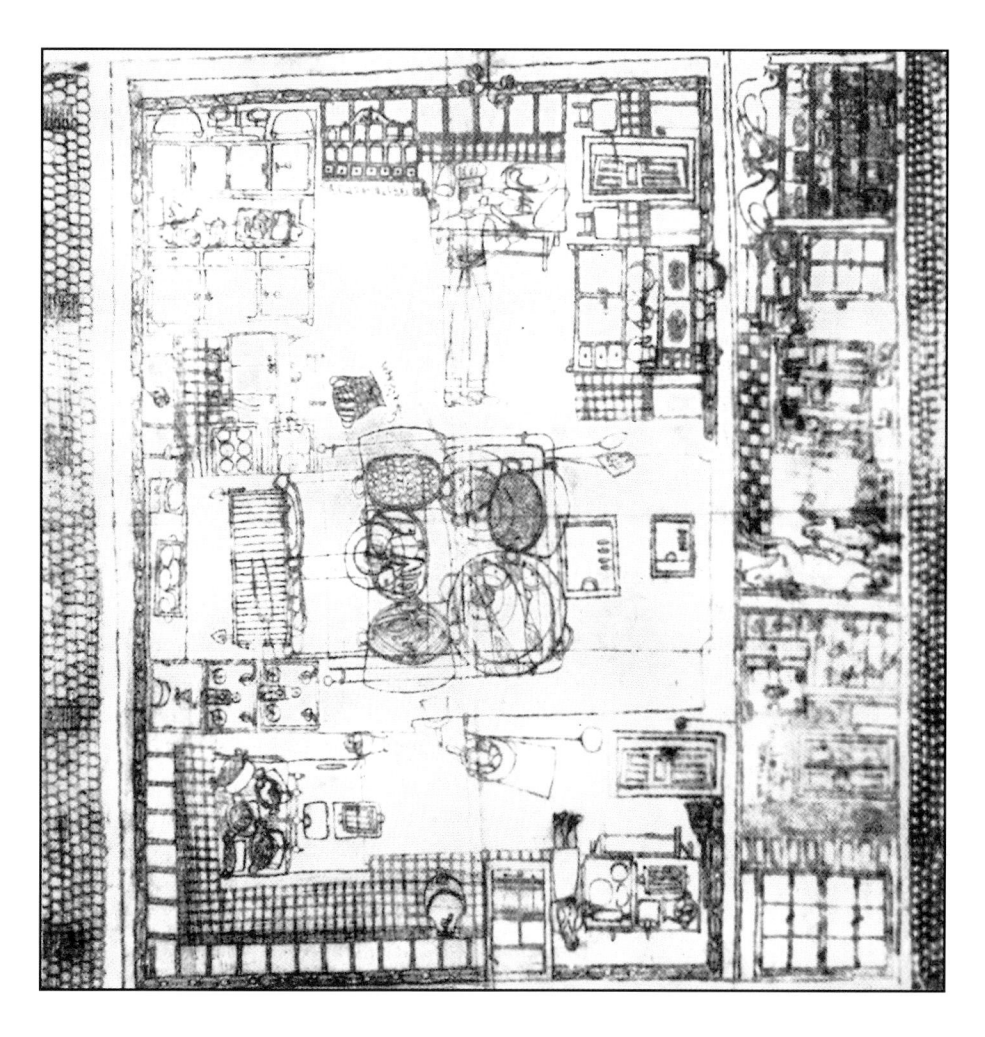

This is why you have tortured my children to death. When I ask something of you, you have broken up something and nothing remains of your holiness. This is the thanks because I have saved you from the gallows. You want to be king of Hungary. As for me, for five years I have not had even a slice of bread. You imagine that I will have enough of you when you substituted whores in my place and therefore you let me tear around with the personnel. When your unhappiness for your well-being is not fulfilled, you destroy my destiny and make my situation worse. Therefore, you allowed my children to be carried to the gallows because of your dirty ways to protect them. That you allowed them to die by starvation and in this season naked and barefoot during the night you leave. You do not accept from me the title of baron and you do not behave as if it is worthy of a gentleman. That is why you beat to death my children and allow that the nurses eat in front of me. I have considered you as king, which you do not deserve from me. I even have done that. However, I do not do it anymore while you were infinitely dirty towards me. I have no reason to bring the wrath of the kings over my head, especially when I get no answer from you to my letter. And when your dirty face does not want me close as long as I watch. Then you should not shame me of my conscience and therefore I cannot accept your military salute. You will not even shake hands with my offspring. You dirty man, for your title you should get dressed and walk around against the princes and kings and kingdoms so that it will be a success if anybody tolerates that from you. Do not tense my nerves any longer. I reject you ... I will look for a son of a king, not a physician ... but you are dirty and ask for forgiveness while nobody holds on stronger to the right of a king than yourself ..."

Electric shock treatment remains without effect. In the later years, without denying the megalomanic ideas, she becomes calmer and crochets the whole day, refusing any other work. She is clean and eats with a good appetite. Since she has started crocheting, she does not draw any more! Is this the true fashion of the manifestation of her psychological state that she has searched for in her drawings?

After several months of hospitalization, she becomes calmer and starts to draw. She draws on paper napkins. In her drawings she fills the whole surface at her disposition. She uses precise and minutious details, but totally neglects any perspective. Her drawings are not symbolical. Her figures are always represented in full view from the front or in profile, which is the characteristic trait of all her drawings. She represents most frequently the interior of a home. She prefers to repeat the pantry, the attic and basement. Her drawings are two-dimensional.

In *Fig. 76*, she drew the facade of a house divided into four stories with minute execution of the shingles on the house. On the ground floor there are a door and two windows. On all four floors pears, apples, and grapes are lined up alternating in parallel lines. These fruits are the height of a floor of the house. On the ground floor there are only four fruits of enormous size, greater than the windows, which enhances the shocking appearance of this composition.

We see similar arrangements and the same proportions on *Fig. 77* in which, on the ground floor the gigantic fruits are bigger than the door. On the first floor above the ground there is a line of pears of a size equal to the height of the floor, while the higher floors are occupied each by three rows of apples of equal size tightly arranged on top of each other. These drawings produce a strange and rigid effect due to the lack of accentuation in the identically drawn lines. *Figure 78* is a sample of her minute stereotyped drawings. This sheet is divided into two halves facing each other. The picture is filled with logs drawn apparently by turning the page around.

In the bizarre drawing *(Fig. 79)* of a wine cellar, one can see the objects arranged right and left. Some are drawn upside down. A stairway is represented two-dimensionally, by two vertical lines joined by a few horizontal lines. In the wine casks both the front and the back, as well as the bottom and the top, are visible. In this superposition, objects appear simultaneously and it is difficult to distinguish which object is in front and which is behind (transparency).

The fruits resemble pumpkins and they sometimes extend into the space between the wine casks. In this drawing the female figure standing in front of the stairs is very small in relation to the other objects. She is smaller than a beer bottle or a carrot.

In *Fig. 80* we see an attic and here the right and left sides also extend to the margins of the page. Laundry baskets and wash lines with clothing are extended meticulously at equal distances from one another indicating a strong degree of stereotypy.

Two of her drawings are very similar to each other. They represent the inside of a house *(Figs 81* and *82)*. The rooms are furnished differently. Persons sitting around the set table appear to be seen from above and as if reclining, because of the habit of this patient of turning the page in front of herself while working *(Fig. 81)*. This method of drawing is similar to the method seen in *Figs 27–28*, and *41* of PRINZHORN (1922). On both of the drawings of our patient the motif of the shingles is repeated. Also on each drawing the rooms are divided by two parallel lines ornamented in monotonous rhythm by garlands of flowers executed with minuscule obsessiveness.

On a drawing of the same size *(Fig. 82)* she represents the same interior without the people. Finally, in *Fig. 83*, we see the kitchen and the pantry drawn in a similar fashion as if folded out from the middle. Around the chef, who has a knife in his hands, there are chickens of unreal size. In front of the table of baked goods a woman is preparing the dough. The motif of the shingles can be found again on both the right and left sides of the drawing.

The patient looks at the interior of the house from above. For example, the table and the chairs around it are presented as if on a crocheted tablecloth. It is interesting that the objects having straight contour lines (for example, the window and the bed) are always seen in an identical fashion on their largest surface, while the rounded objects appear in an arbitrary perspective. This dual presentation process gives a surreal naive serenity to her works. The sizes of the objects are arbitrary and independent from each other from the point of view of proportions. They conform, rather, to the divisions of the surface. She uses equally thin lines similar to the threads used for crocheting. This reminds the spectator of a pattern drawn for crocheting laces.

The method of turning the page while drawing gives the impression of objects spread out from the middle of the page as if seen from above.

# Case 8 — Miss R. A.

*Date of birth*: 2 October 1902
*Occupation*: Primary school teacher
*Diagnosis*: Schizophrenia

She was hospitalized from 9 August 1944 to 29 November 1951 at the Psychiatric and Neurological University Hospital of Pécs. She was then transferred to an asylum.

*Past history*: She was brought to the hospital by the police. She had no domicile and had been living in caves in the area around Pécs. Occasionally when she came out of the cave she addressed "absurd words" to passersby. Earlier she had lived alone and this is the reason for the lack of an objective case history about her previous behavior.

She said that she had always been very religious. Because of her "desire for a convent" she wanted to enter a religious order, but they found her too young. She was employed in the capacity of primary school teacher for ten years in a village. After 1937, when she retired, she lived alone. She moved into a cave "to wait for her fiancé, the Pope".

*Medical and neurological examination* revealed no pathology. Bordet–Wassermann reaction in the blood and spinal fluid was negative.

*Psychiatric evaluation*: The patient is well oriented in time and space. There are no signs of dementia. Her thought processes are confused and often bizarre. The content of her thoughts is characterized by religious delusions and other associated delusions. She uses symbolism. Her behavior is conventional, but sometimes under the influence of hallucinations she becomes agitated and irritated, accusing the people around her without ever attacking anybody.

Throughout the day she keeps herself busy. She began to learn the English, French, and Russian languages. Writes "daily report" as "head nurse". She has created a neologism in Hungarian to form the word head nurse. "Head head head nurse." This patient, in her delusion, believes that she is the super head nurse of the hospital and, as such, she writes daily reports about the ward. In these reports, her delusions and hallucinations are described: "In the name of Jesus! Peace be with you! Super-head-nurse-report 17/12/42. Yesterday soldiers have taken Mrs. S. to the medical hospital and from there they brought her back. In the afternoon, she was in agony. From her closed mouth, foam came out. Her face has changed over into the face of Mrs. U. Following this it changed to the face of M. W.? Has she inhabited again, Mrs. S., and A. K.? The seamstress from Püspöknádasd P.–Schs., Sch.–F. spoke in the evening as follows: At home she was not received, therefore she was brought back. She has been shown to me in front of the bureau as Mrs. S. She was, throughout one year, the wife of this physician under the masked name B. She was teaching with B's diploma. B. is an uneducated woman with only elementary school education. K. knows her, maybe. In the mask of A. Havai and of my school diploma for A. which they transcribed as they were talked into this by Mater Valeria and Mater Anna.

Today I gave myself, as head nurse, three weeks of vacation. It is not my duty to work without being paid. I am not an inhabitant of a jail. I am entitled to vacation too."

In another of her reports, we read the following: "God's ointment is peace and quietness—not sinfulness. He creates from the greatest saints—easily. Devil—Antichrist, 666 shakes his environment. The bridegroom of the foolish virgins is the false god of 666 fallen armies of angels. Starts with a paralyzing storm. Has many victims!

I am tolerant of a child beside me, but not of an old fox with a child's face! This is a room in an institute which means that it has two beds, the Spotless who steps on the serpent cannot stay alone in the 'big biting' hole. A murderer belongs there too! Also, in H three are stuck! Many good sheep find place in a small room. For two nights the world has been searching for me through an electrical telephone. Thankful are those whom I have discharged to their home. Those to whom I have refused my consent threaten me.

The patient works on a big "educational plan". She buys paper and notebooks to write down her "concentrical educational plan".

In the writing of the theater "piece" we see how the concept of a ring will be presented in a study plan as related to different disciplines. These examples show that the patient has given concrete interpretations to abstract ideas. These interpretations are connected to her hallucinations and delusions.

"*Connections:* What are all the things related to the rings? Within which disciplines?

*Chemistry:* Fine things: Gold and silver branding! (What is branded this way belongs to the devil).

*Religion:* 'I have no gold, no silver. In the holy name of Jesus, I tell you stand up and walk'.

*Crafts:* Goldsmiths work. Wooden ring for the actors—artifacts—home-work.

*Song:* What did he take off his finger, a ring of gold and silver. (This last sentence was written by the patient in German).

*The game:* the ring goes around wandering ...

*History:* since when was the ring used for cohabitation? And what does that mean? Honored by the Antichrist? The creation is a holy thing, but nothing to imitate. Valuable things buried! ...

*Geography:* in which land it is customary to wear a ring!

*Hygiene:* for many the ring becomes too narrow and cuts off the blood circulation.

*Natural history:* the thief of the ring is the magpie.

*Concept:* why can one not heal today through miracle?

*Summary:* What did we understand today? The series of the rings. Where does it come from? What is its meaning? Why does one have to abandon it? How much cheaper is life without ring and jewelry? Who was the first who had a ring?

*Utilization:* what are the children's rings made of?

*Educational connections:* Let us forego the devilish pomp! What kind of jewelry had the bride of the Song of Songs?"

The patient composes "religious symphonies" and writes theater pieces in which several actors recite unconnected texts. In these her delusions and hallucinations are expressed by the words given to the actors. In one scene she presented herself as the Virgin Mary, she expresses also other megalomanic ideas; she is a descendent of the English royal family "in the form of Mrs. U.". She is embodied in several forms and was "artificially born" by which she understands the symbolical immaculate conception. Sometimes she abandons the fluent text and describes bizarre delusions. Then suddenly she remarks, "We have strayed away from the actual topic", and returns to her theater pieces.

Then again, within a short time she leaves the topic and describes a vision:

"On the hands of the Immaculate there were several visions of rings, God, the three different aspects of the sun which practices cohabitation with her in spiritual ways. Also, the three rings are made by her ... She was also the wife of the moon: they are many of those—666. They have put rings on her finger. Their radiation of light is gold and black: those who accept his blessings become a radiant life besides the moon. Those who are rejected by him remain in the shadows. The church cleans them from the rings of the moon. She had a vision, from her hands which were spread out for ten minutes, rays of light were emanating over the sky and from this a headless Christ has been fashioned. What does this mean? Has she projected her moon? The man of sins? She is a woman! She asks frequently to exorcise the devil but they do not listen to her because she does not rage!"

The patient makes projects for the "map of a new Vaduz".

Repeatedly she edits a newspaper with the title, "Cosmopolitan Daily Paper" and writes in this different "articles and news". Among these we find, for example, the following news: "In the psychiatry in Pécs there are about seventy women under my name. They live under my name and with my face unnecessary and they are bourgeois: they receive monthly wages of 50,000 gulden in the world on the chain of M. M. One needs a healer who heals the sick here! Not a useless Sassa! The damage to my honor and for the bodily harm in being robbed—everyone who is a chief criminal must pay milliards of dollars into the charitable funds of the people! I also need a winter coat."

The holiday number of her newspaper "Eternal Spring" shows the following lead article: "Will the holy ones in heaven become old? When there is no radiating radium horseshoe—in lime water and dusted with the fruit of the tree of life, then it becomes difficult to lie and the angel will fall to destiny... His natural history. In heaven there are many beautiful roses. The biggest one, which is better than the La France the red velvet rose was fragrant: gold rose—with shades of light and bronze gold—not as dark as the roof of the St. Paul church, but like my star crown, the queen of the roses on my immaculate sack. From this kind—from the Benedictine Monks' castle: from the castle, from Astric, I brought a young bud of tea rose to Rome to Pius the XIth who, following his death in my sublet apartment of the Hungarian internal ministry: our electric clock and in my electrical flame burned—while the Lord Jesus and the Devil Jesus were my guests in the night: I have been anointed as a priestess and the crocheted forget-me-nots from my tablecloth have risen for a few seconds. I have gotten three tea roses from this giant rose—as a vision in that bed in which I have the wonder bronze? The gold? I have kept them as a throne on the floor. I have given it over! Some vision bent over me in this bed with a forehead of rainbows? Who?"

In the same newspaper we read under another title "New Kitchens": "What we eat we will smell of it. In the evening we take rose tea. Let us rose tree have rose oil. Roses cooked in pancakes. A golden rose is very delicate, distill it in water with honey. A little wine doesn't hurt for improving."

She writes a theater play and composes "religious symphonies". She wears robes sewn by herself ornamented with blue ribbons when she

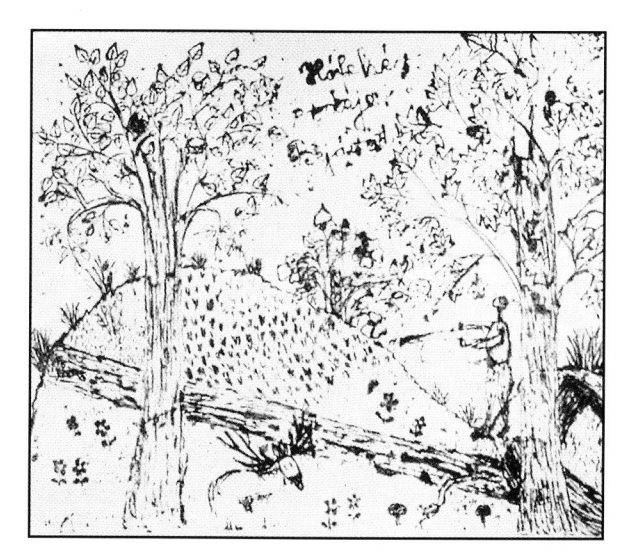

Case 8 - Fig. 84
Ink drawing. 28x35

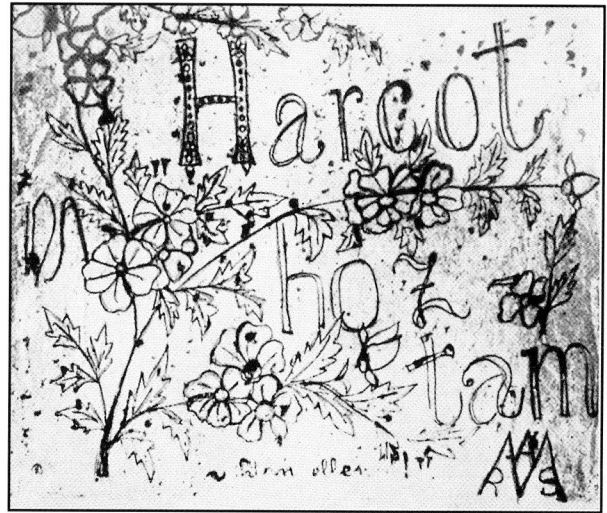

Case 8 - Fig. 85
Ink drawing. 28x35

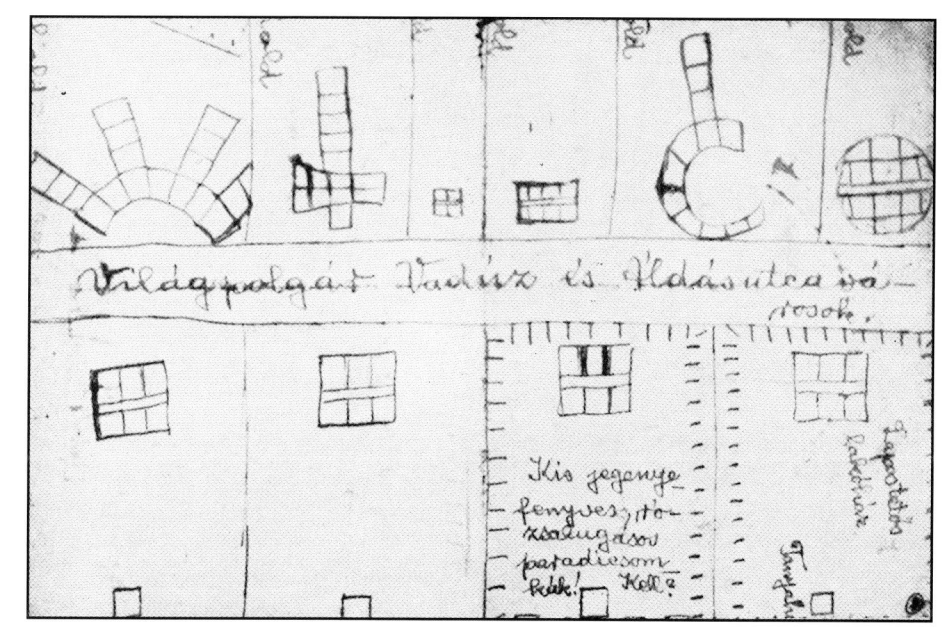

Case 8 - Fig. 86
Ink drawing. 20x29.5

declares her identity to be that of the Virgin. She participates in various tasks at the hospital. Nonetheless, she requests an exceptional position among the patients because of her being "head nurse".

She was hospitalized for several years at the same time as the patient of Case 7 (Mrs. *J. U.*) who has been "her Majesty and Sanctity, the proprietress of the institute". They had sometimes quarreled about "the question of power". One morning, under the influence of her hallucination, Miss R.A. complained that they mutilated her during the night when she was subjected to "extraordinary operations" (castration).

She sees her face on several individuals who are walking around "impersonating" her and at the same time "they are assuming her body". The persons in her environment present themselves as "incarnations each time in the form of a different body and under the appearance of another person".

From time to time she makes additions to her writings and drawings. Her "programs" are also illustrated by drawings. Sometimes she draws on large sheets of wrapping paper her "celestial reports"; "a celestial rose" and "a rainbow".

She explains minutely to the other patients the symbolical meaning of her drawings. The title of one of her drawings is "The Map of the New Jerusalem with Twelve Gates and the Houses of Pilgrimage".

*Figure 84* is a landscape drawn in ink in a primitive fashion without perspective, done on wrapping paper. The hills are covered with flowers and mushrooms. A hunter holds a gun pointed forward and held tightly against his chest. His look is fixed upwards and in a very different direction from where the gun is pointed. In the foreground there is an antlered animal (deer?). The text written on top is the following: "The Forest of Snow White, Entrance".

On the bottom part of the same sheet we find the drawing of an ornamental flowering branch ("celestial rose") and around that the following sentence is written with an ornamented initial: "I have brought the war against Satan" *(Fig. 85)*.

Her technique is monotone. No parts of her drawings are especially accentuated. The landscape has no balance.

*Figure 86* is a schematic map. The maps are constructed of geometric figures. They represent houses, streets of the cities, and imaginary countries created by the patient. This is a primitive symbolical drawing. The patient's autistic concept of the world is reflected in these symbolical drawings, which are incomprehensible unless they are explained by the patient. Her way of representing objects is that of a five-to-six-year old child (maybe she had been accustomed to drawing in this fashion so that she would be better understood by her little students). Her capacity to represent is severely restricted. She populates the surfaces with motifs of plants of simple shape, executed in the fashion of embroidery. As she draws with ink on paper of inferior quality (absorbent) her lines are washed out. Nonetheless, one can see that the traces are formed by short interrupted lines of equal length.

The incoherency of the composition and of the surfaces show the instinctive and irrational fashion of her work: for example, the solution of the theme of the straight road on the surface of the hill on *Fig. 84*.

# Case 9 — I. J.

*Date of birth*: 15 June 1905
*Occupation*: Dairy worker
*Diagnosis*: Paraphrenia
He was hospitalized from 2 June 1954 to 26 July 1954 at the Psychiatric and Neurological University Hospital of Pécs.
*Family history*: No illness. One brother is a sculptor whose statues grace some places in his native city.
*Personal history*: The patient was hospitalized in a hospital for the mentally ill during the years 1951 and 1952. He suffered hallucinations and visual and acoustic illusions which were very vivid and to which he attached delusional ideas later. His behavior was aggressive to the point of attacking the members of his family.
*Medical and neurological examination* reveals no pathology. Bordet–Wassermann reaction in the blood and spinal fluid was negative.

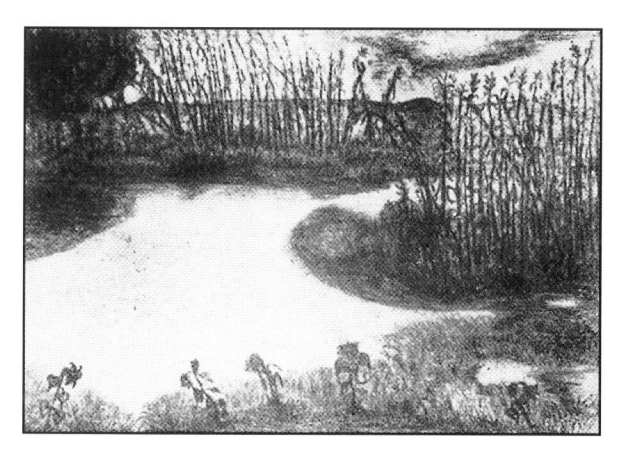

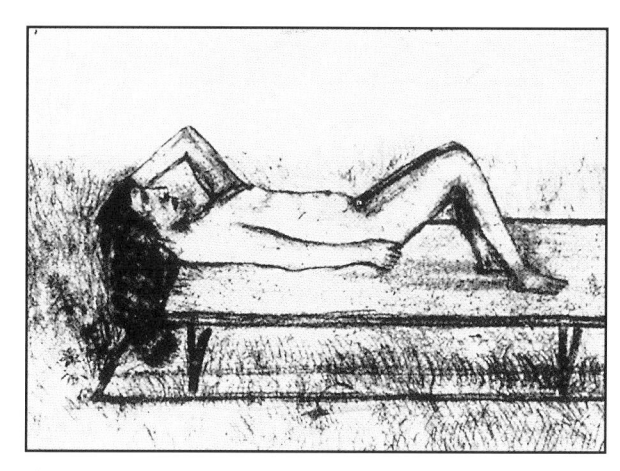

Case 9 - Fig. 88
Pencil drawing. 16.5x23

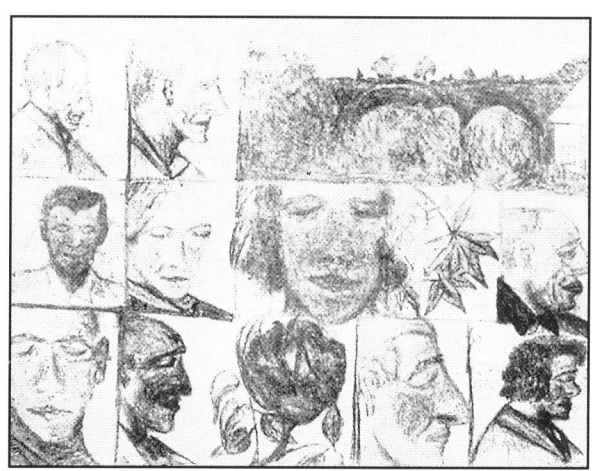

Case 9 - Fig. 89
Pencil drawing. 16.5x23

Case 9 - Fig. 87
Pencil drawing. 16.5x23

*Psychiatric evaluation*: His thought processes are incoherent. He expresses delusional ideas, for example: having been robbed, he is imprisoned for a reason unknown to him and does not feel mentally ill. The world has changed around him and he finds the behavior of peo-

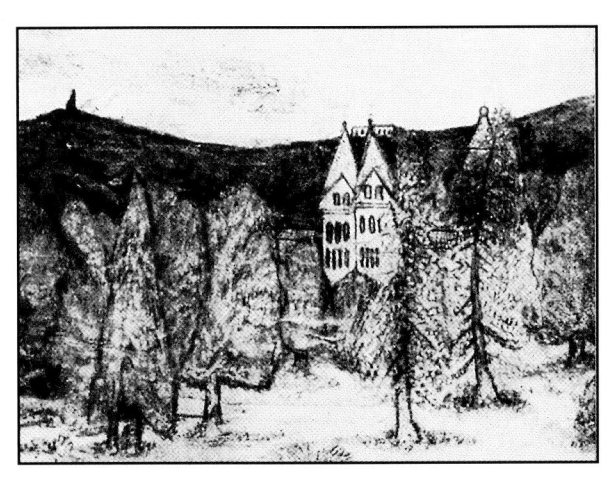

Case 9 - Fig. 90
Pencil drawing. 16.5x23

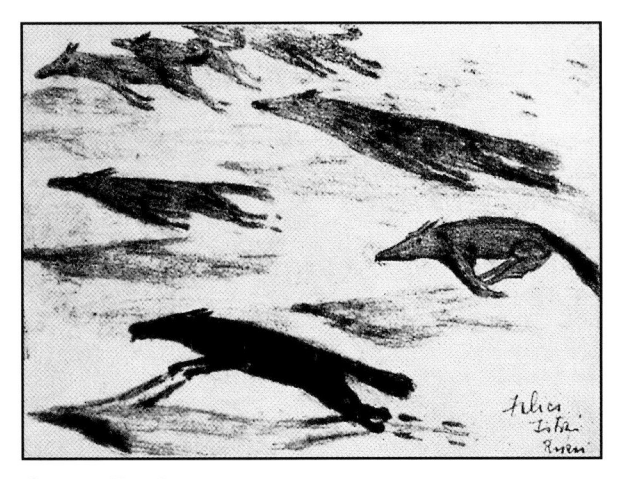

Case 9 - Fig. 91
Pencil drawing. 24x32.5

ple around him strange. His behavior is generally withdrawn; if one addresses him, he answers quickly in a superior tone of voice. He tries to deny his hallucinations.

Following a series of electric shock treatments and a cure of Sakel (insulin shock treatment—translator's note), his state has not improved.

He draws a lot, in a special sketch book. He also draws on the margins of journals (newspapers) where he repeats the same profiles, one underneath the other at equal distances. These portraits are sometimes replaced by flowers and geometric figures. We find a series of repeated motifs also in his landscapes. For example, one of his last works is framed by a series of animals all alike. He draws statues and flower vases ornamented delicately with decorations.

The perspective of the vases is incorrect. When he represents human figures in movement, he shows a complete lack of knowledge of the anatomical relationship and of the dynamics of the movements. He invites the patients and the physicians to pose as models for him. He draws them in profile, but the likeness to the model can be found only in the accidental details, for example, the hairstyle, the mustache, the eyeglasses, the striped cape. The faces are similar in all his drawings.

Before leaving the hospital he destroyed his best drawings.

On *Fig. 87*, according to his explanations, he drew a swampy landscape that he had seen in the past. This pencil drawing gives the impression of appropriate depth, while, in the foreground, there are large flowers represented two-dimensionally.

His leaden gray surfaces are worked over by unskilled black lines, making the atmosphere more somber and creating an even more menacing landscape.

*Figure 88* shows a reclining nude who has no shoulders; the right arm is a continuation of the neck. The construction of this picture is primitive. The proportions are not realistic. The head and the trunk are too big in relation to the legs.

*Figure 89* is composed of ten profiles in rectangular frames. Among these ten portraits drawn from nature, only one resembles the model. The patient drew in the spaces between the heads some flower motifs, and in the top right corner he sketched a small, strange silhouette-like landscape.

*Figure 90* shows a view of a landscape seen from the window of the hospital. It is an unskilled, unclean pencil drawing. Behind the trees of the garden of the hospital we can see two towers of the cathedral and the tourist hotel on top of the hill—in reality the towers are at a much greater distance —while they appear here as if rising up between the trees of the garden.

On the day of his discharge he completed, in a few minutes, the "running wolves" of *Fig. 91*. These animals are put out on the surface and give the impression of unusual postures rather than movement. The shadows and footprints convey the fact that he wanted to represent running animals.

The pictures attest to the fact that I. J. had no artistic training. The surfaces are completely filled out and only the horizontal and vertical lines are meaningful. Through this, his work becomes monotonous and motionless. The scale of his colors is poor and the gray colors are monotonous.

## Case 10 — T. S.

*Diagnosis*: Schizophrenia
*The medical record of this patient was lost during World War II.*

Professor Reuter (who collected the drawings and paintings at the Psychiatric and Neurological University Hospital of Pécs) remembered this patient who was hospitalized at the end of World War I in which he participated as a simple soldier.

The patient signed his paintings as "the Commandant Painter and Author of Projects, Sallay". In our collections we have three similar paintings by this patient; they represent "the assault of the castle" and they have an unusual effect. Above each of these castles there are bizarre images. In *Fig. 92* three gigantic cats form "the reconnaissance patrol", and stylized airplanes are flying over them. In *Fig. 93* on top of the castle is a human figure, "the observer", whose dimensions attain half the height of one of the towers of the castle. Finally, in *Fig. 94*, above one of the towers a nude figure with wings and with a frizzy hairstyle holds in his hands a large red heart.

The cannons as compared to other objects are extremely big in all three paintings. The one in the middle of *Fig. 93* is larger than the ship in the foreground and it is being fired. Aside from the bizarreness, we must admit that the colors of these pictures produce a lively and surprisingly agreeable effect. *Figures 95* and *96* represent a map of a military operation. The patient explains, on the margin, the significance of the colors (green: his own army, red: the enemy). In *Fig. 97* the landscape on the banks of a river is entitled "the assault on Belgrade, 25th November 1920". From different parts of the city flames rise, surrounded by circles sprinkled with red spots, which indicate probably the ex-

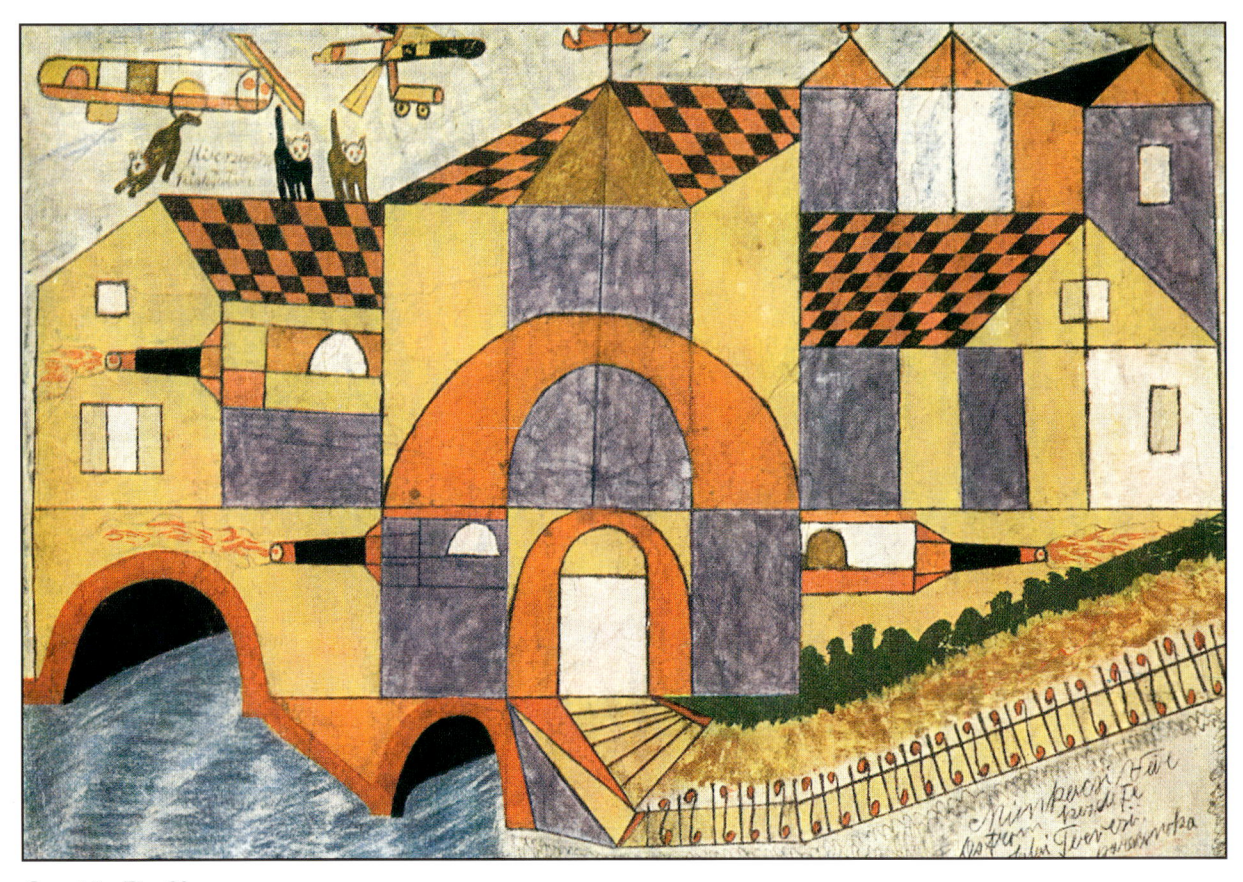

Case 10 - Fig. 92
Aquarelle. 31x45

plosion of the shell. This painting is more primitive than *Figs 92, 93* and *94*.

The paintings in *Figs 98* and *99* represent human figures. The dynamism and the colors of *Fig. 98* are surprising. The man with an astonished facial expression is represented up to his knees and is leaning somewhat backwards. His hairstyle is a kind of wig which is continuous with his beard, leaving only his ear out. The man holds in his right hand a small dog by its tail. The rigidity of this tail extended horizontally is unnatural and in contrast to the dog's limp body. The foreground of this picture is a green band of uncertain nature which could represent water as well as grass. The human figure emerges from this band in front of a rosy-colored background (hills?) and a cobalt blue sky. The sky has a disquieting effect due to the deep blue clouds in movement over a blue-gray background.

Case 10 - Fig. 93
Aquarelle. 40x53

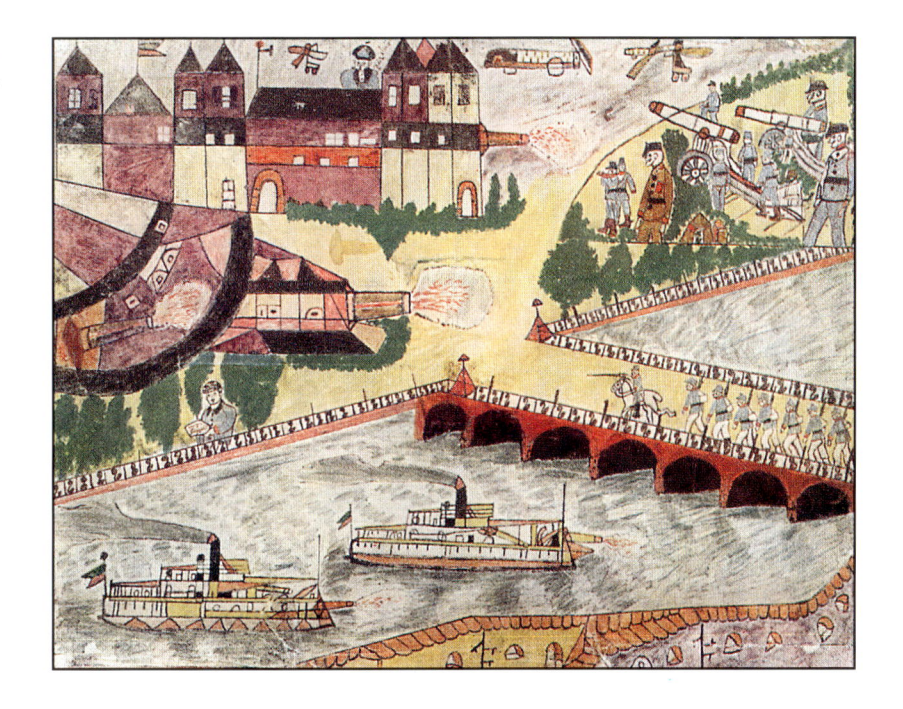

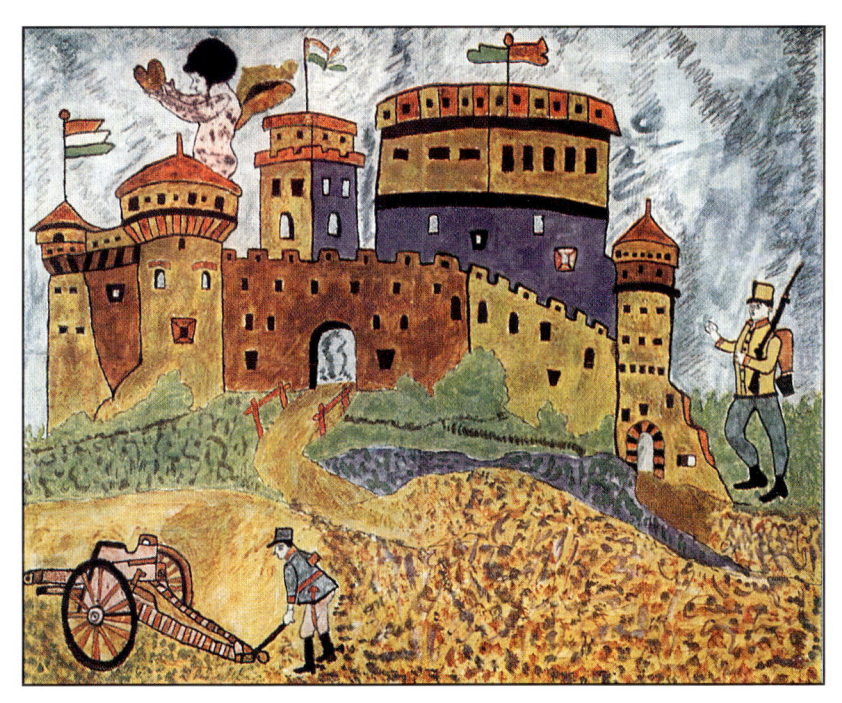

Case 10 - Fig. 94
Aquarelle. 34x41.5

101

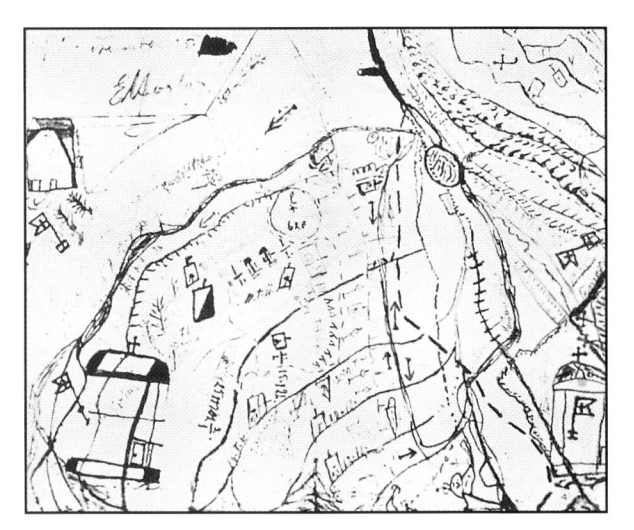

Case 10 - Fig. 95
Aquarelle. 34x42

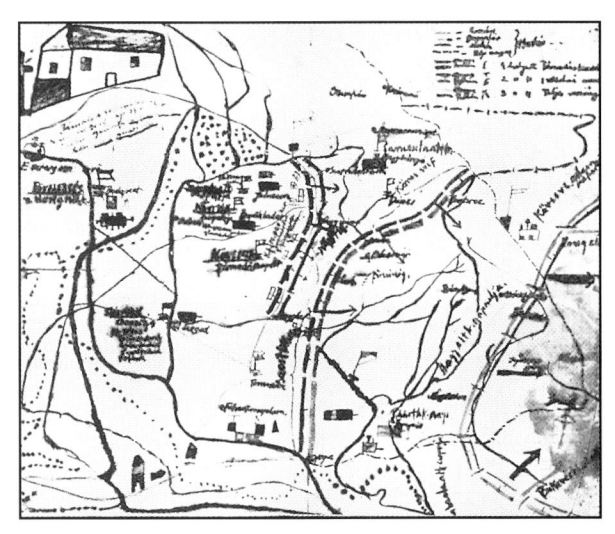

Case 10 - Fig. 96
Aquarelle. 34x42

In *Fig. 99* the man on horseback has a similar facial expression. The artist called him "the Archduke Joseph". The sky, with dark clouds in movement gives the same dynamic effect as the sky in the previous picture. This picture has, nonetheless, a more indifferent atmosphere. Flowers are used as ornamentation.

*Figure 100* is an ink drawing on brown background. Here, among other figures, we see once more the known face. The hands of this figure hold sheets of paper with the inscription: "Lecture, secret communications". The other figures, of varying sizes, are independent from one another and all are in movement.

There is a certain analogy between the art works of this patient and *A. J.* (Case 5). They both produce, on one hand, drawings of constructions and, on the other hand, large pictures of strong and striking decorative aspect vigorously conceived.

Neither of them had had an artistic education. They did not even know the most simple elements of painting. They had no idea of per-

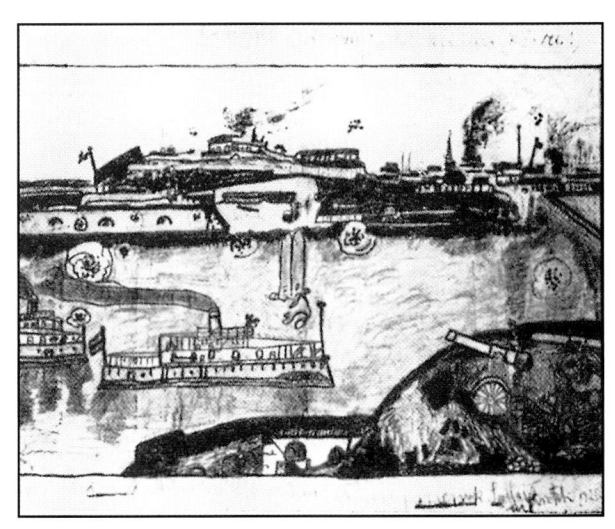

Case 10 - Fig. 97
Aquarelle. 31x43

spective or of the anatomy, and had not even learned from the simple observation of objects around them.

The harmony of colors, the principles of composition, and even the most simple techniques are unknown to them. Their lack of skill surpasses even that of the Sunday painters. Their works are characterized by the expressive power and the perseverance of their creativity. They totally lack the meticulousness and the inhibitions of the dilettantes. The dilettante, the child and the folk artist express subjects in a logical fashion and spontaneously delineate the limits of their representations. On the other hand, our two patients, *A. J.* and *T. S.* assembled unconnected motifs on a previously determined subject. This logical and visual incoherence is truly striking.

The art works may, nonetheless—although we reserve judgment on this—be compared to the paintings of Sienna of the twelfth and thirteenth centuries. They may also be compared to those of modern artists (Paul Klee and Salvador Dalí). This comparison is based on the char-

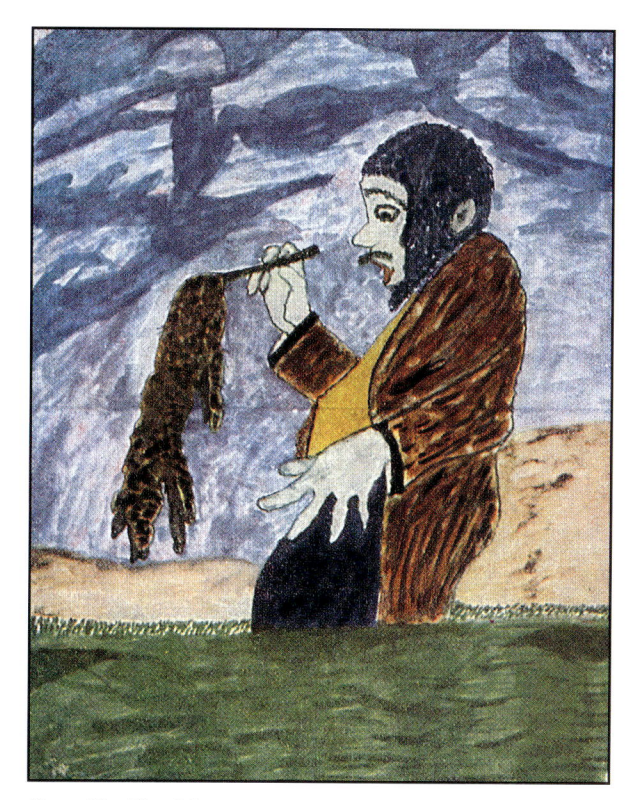

Case 10 - Fig. 98
Aquarelle. 21x17

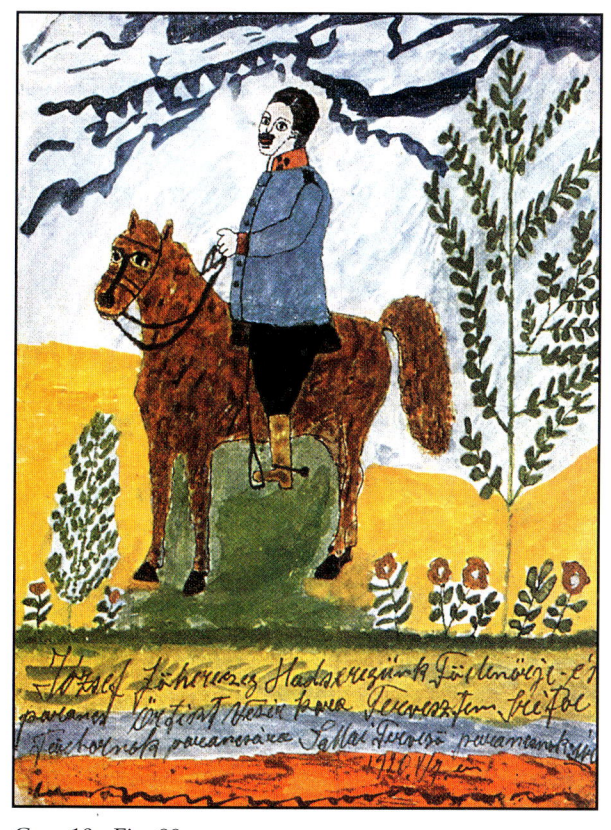

Case 10 - Fig. 99
Aquarelle. 23x17.5

Case 10 - Fig. 100
Aquarelle. 20x23

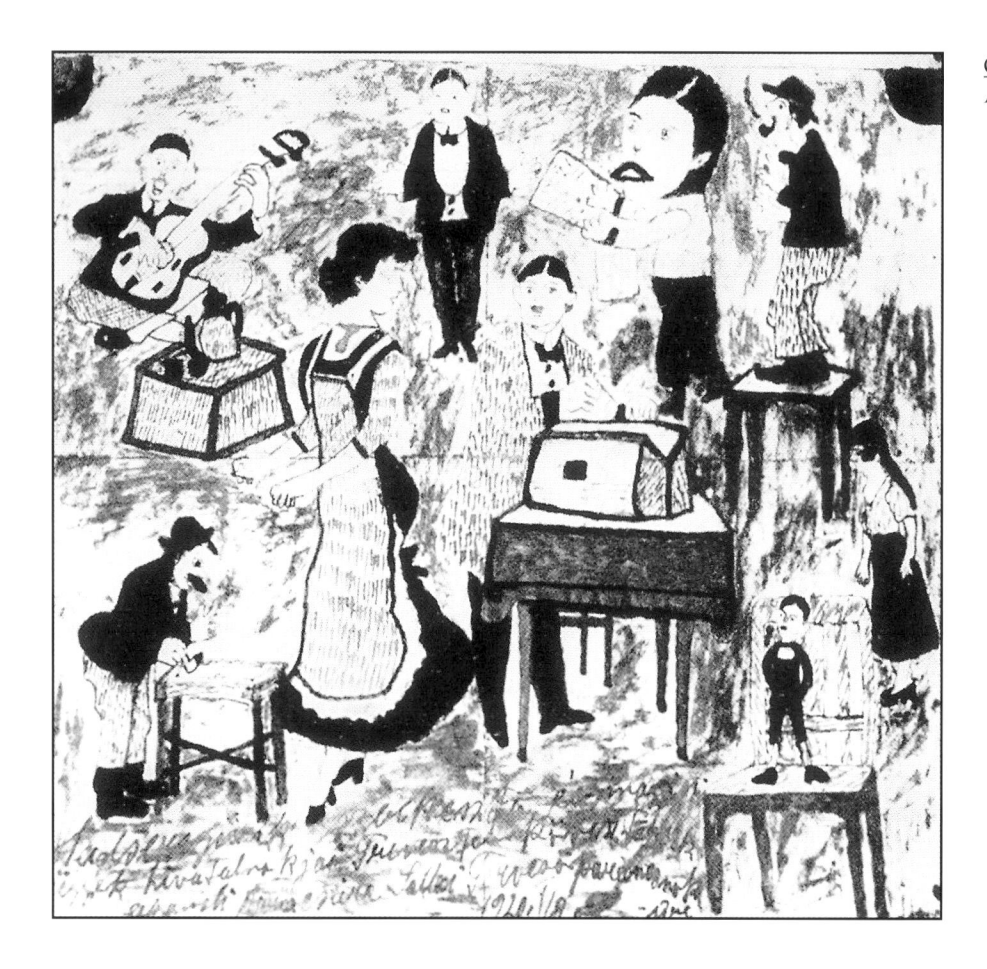

acteristic interpretation of the affective content rather than on the shaping of forms.

The difference between the modes of expression of our two patients is that *T. S.* first makes a sketch with expressive lines, although unskilled, which he leaves in the painting. *A. J.* also makes sketches in crayon, but finishes his work by going over these lines with color. Nonetheless, it occurs to *A. J.* to trace crayon lines (sometimes even with a ruler) over the completed painting. This method serves as rich ornamentation of the surfaces.

Both patients represent scenes. The constructions of *T. S.* are massive. *A. J.* cannot order the surfaces and his figures are frequently crowded at the margin of the page *(Fig. 61)*.

Their lines are unskilled, interrupted, and of the same width regardless of whether they are at the beginning, in the middle, or at the end of the traced line.

We may wonder what kind of works these two painters would have produced if they had had artistic instruction in painting. Would the artistic instruction have strengthened or, on the contrary, weakened the expressive force of their works? This is an unsolvable problem which applies to the majority of our patients.

We may also ask what was their goal when drawing, and what was the event that they wanted to express in their works. Without doubt, the events of the war left profound imprints on the affective life of *T. S.*

The lines traced by brush by *A. J.* and those in crayon by *T. S.* have the same effect. From the point of view of the colors, *A. J.* is more picturesque and sometimes shows a surprising harmony. The pictures of *T. S.*, based frequently on the contrast of colors, are crude decorative items.

## Case 11 — *S. F.*

*Date of birth*: 1886
*Diagnosis*: Schizophrenia

The patient was hospitalized from 17 January 1932 to 2 May 1932 at the Psychiatric and Neurological University Hospital of Pécs. His medical record has been lost.

Several of his drawings have been preserved. On the back of the drawings the patient wrote text. In part, he describes the hallucinations he has just drawn. Other times, he describes in writing some of his hallucinations of which there is no graphic representation.

An example is the following:
"Heavenly appearance which showed itself in the bathroom of the Hospital for Psychiatric and Nervous Diseases in Pécs.
On the tenth of February 1933 I had to take a bath after I got a strong injection. As I stepped into the bathtub I saw that the water was murky bluish. I was very scared and became aware that there is a sin on my soul for which I made no penance. Crying with teary eyes, I have asked the powerful and much suffering Christ and the Holy Virgin Mary to forgive me if I have done something wrong to them, following which immediately I started hearing in my ears a heavenly godly music of thousands and thousands of bells. I heard from this music the words of God: Your water is not dirty but blue as the sky and look up to me; your parents who came to me a long time ago are happy in the lap of the angels that their child also became the son of God, just like their ancestors who have been resting for 3000 years and whose mummies are also godly and possess the body and the jewels of the pharaohs which will belong to you later. My dear parents to whom I have never spoken anything in my life that was not true smiled at me from the lap of the angels and reached with their hands with several little angels. I took to my heart this feverish vision so much so that on the following day I heard on the radio of the clinic the high mass of the dome during the late lunchtime and I prayed on my knees in the unfriendly corridor of the clinic. I thank you dear God for your good deeds.
S. F. von Kapos Szentjakab Fieldmarshal."

Finally, he wrote his testament which informs us of his bizarre megolamanic ideas.

"Testament.

In the name of the creating God. The undersigned assigns through this testament belongings which are my real estate and cash money of 39 0000000 and also 1400 dollars as well as my pension as an invalid which is about 45 million Pengő, in addition the Diadem of the original Pharaohs and about 50 00000 the factory Zsolnai and the brick fabric 1 700000 Pengő

| | |
|---|---|
| Total | 390 00000 |
| Dollar | 1 96000 |
| Retirement Income | 450 00000000000 |
| The Pharaoh's Wealth | 500000000000 |
| Zsolnai | 170000000000000 |

The end amount of the testament 600 million 500 thousand Pengő. This should be given to my wife my relatives and other charities in the name of God.

S. F. Fieldmarshal m. p."

He produced drawings with colored crayons. On one of his drawings he represents his family home *(Fig. 101)*. The transparent curtains float outside of the windows and give a dynamic and unsettling effect to this otherwise quite rigid painting. It is interesting that on one side of the front door is the portrait of the patient himself—a man with mustache, eyeglasses, dressed in a checkered suit. Under the window on the facade of the house he writes little verses (quite banal) similar to the little verses that used to be written in "memory books". In the right corner the half moon emerges with rays; a childish and conventional representation.

*Figure 102* is fashioned like a greeting card for Easter, surrounded by a border of flowers. The picture is composed of two different parts. On the left side are a man and a woman, half naked, whose heads are surrounded by a halo. They stand in front of an animal similar to a donkey. Their clothing is barely sketched by rough lines. The extremities are very small. The inscription underneath is the following: "God and the Virgin Mary and a deer wish you Happy Easter". The right third of this picture is separated from the rest by a tree with a very tall trunk. Its crown is formed only by a few branches. This third of the composition is filled by the bust of a man with his face in profile and with small deformed hands. The inscription is the following: "The bishop of the diocese". This drawing is executed on a cardboard like the one used by bakeries, as suggested by the folds of the cardboard. The patient has drawn on the upper left corner of the cardboard an arm with sleeves folded at the elbow.

*Figure 103* is the portrait of a woman with a deformed face, done in colored crayon. Her pear-shaped left hand (or shoulder?) is only sketched. The misconception of the anatomy, the very large almond-shaped converging eyes, and the arbitrary changes in the proportions of the face give a disquieting air to this portrait. The distance between the tip of the nose and the chin is much bigger than that between the nose and the hairline on the forehead.

*Figures 104* and *105* represent the two sides of a postal card. On one side there is the address (to the woman doctor who treats him) and the portrait of a man with eyeglasses surrounded by garlands of flowers (self-portrait). On the other side of this "postcard" we find Easter greetings illustrated by a big bird standing on a bed. This is perhaps a symbolical drawing. The patient frames his ink drawings with colored crayon.

*Figure 106* is the representation of a hallucination. This is evident from the text written on the back side. After having scribbled over the paper with ink, he has drawn, in pencil, over this dark background, the crucifix and some landscape motifs. Only the drops of "blood" are red. He describes the meaning of this sinister picture in the following words:

"My fever dream has taken me to the hills of the Calvary of Pécs where, among a few leafless trees, I have seen the recently crucified body of Christ with drops of blood, all fresh on the cross. While I was looking at him, the crucified Christ

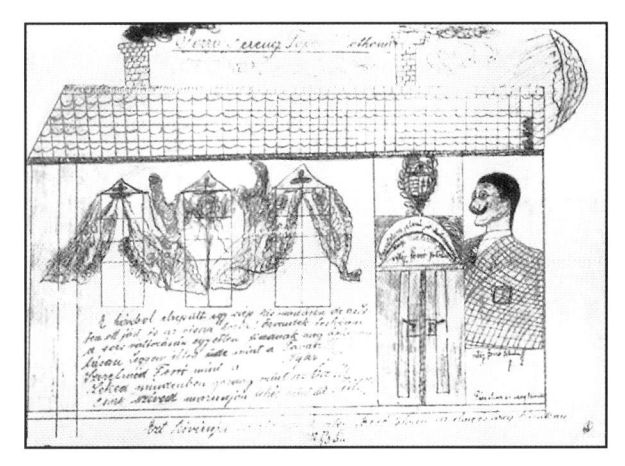

Case 11 - Fig. 101
Aquarelle and pencil. 21x34

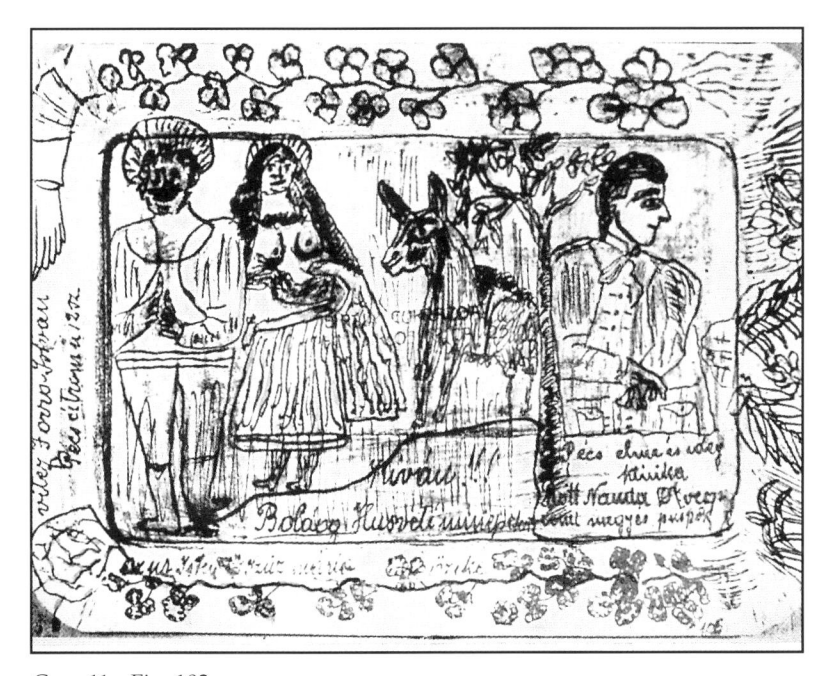

Case 11 - Fig. 102
Pencil drawing. 13x20

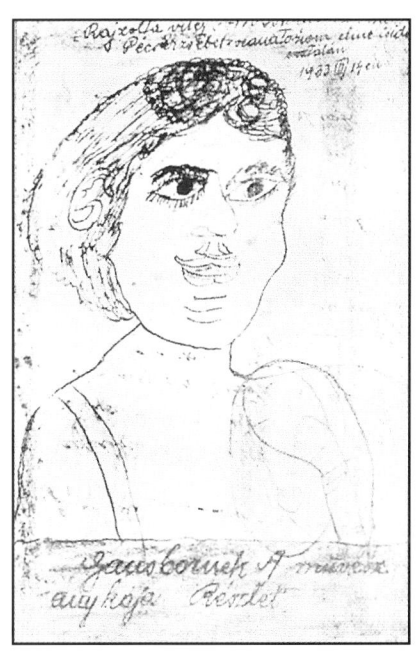

Case 11 - Fig. 103
Colored crayon 17x11

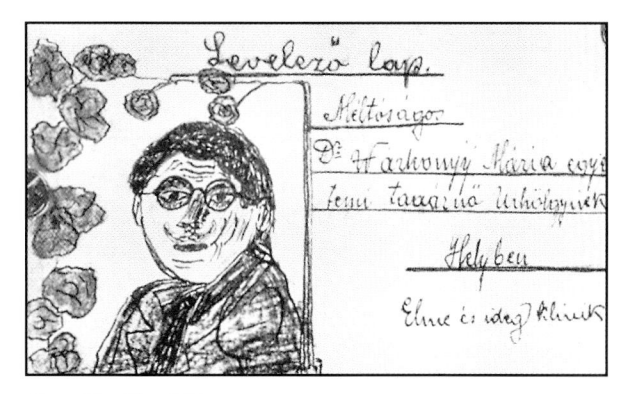

Case 11 - Fig. 104
Pencil drawing. 10x16

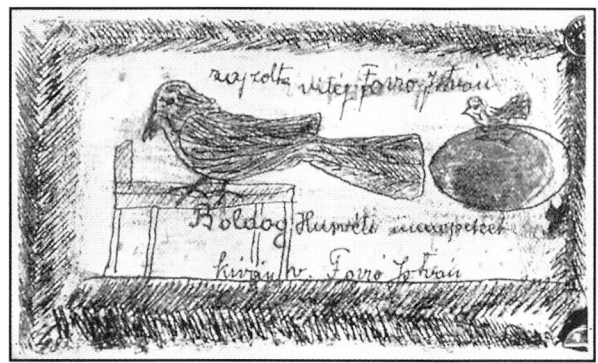

Case 11 - Fig. 105
Pencil drawing. 10x16

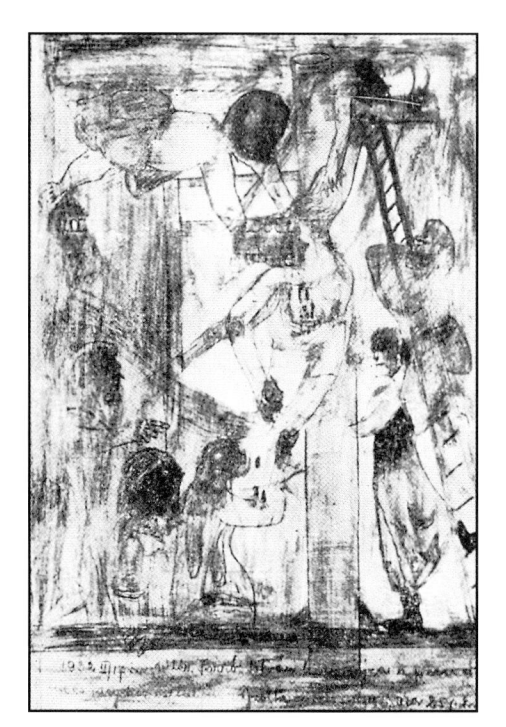

Case 11 - Fig. 106
Ink and pencil. 34x21

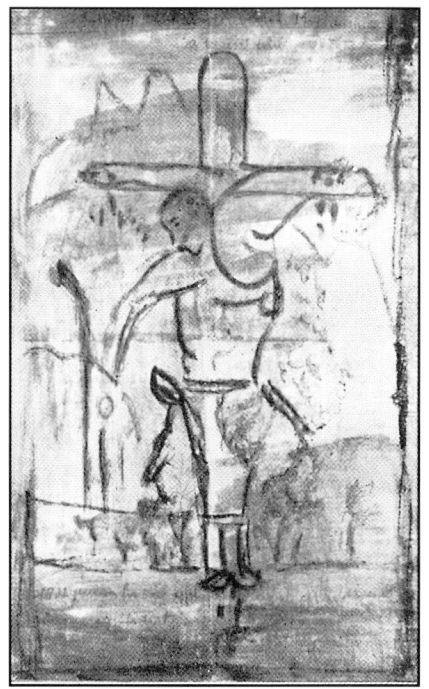

Case 11 - Fig. 107
Ink and pencil. 34x21

108

moved and came off the cross. He detached his hands and legs from the nails with great heads, called nails of Christ, He came towards me with these words: 'My son, what color is this glass?' The glass in his hand was snow-white; I answered that it was white as snow, upon which I received the answer that 'only one of its sides is white, while the other is black'. The Son of God told me then: 'You are right, my son, it is white as is your soul; stay with your family as you have up to now; you will be my faithful child.' He then took a few steps towards me and three drops of blood were pearled on his forehead. I wanted to wipe them off, but I received this order from him: 'Don't bloody your hands because that is a sin. Nonetheless, I shall forgive you.' and he wiped them off himself and then went up onto the cross again, where he first put the nails through his feet and then through the left hand with the right and then with his right hand he made a sign to me: "Come nearer, I want to tell you something: 'Your charitable director at the state factory of air and electricity has judged your illness and wanted to give you three hundred Pengős (Hungarian monetary unit from 1927 to 1946), so that neither you nor your family would be deprived of recreation; his good heart has become even better and he has given to your family the help of, not only three hundred, but five hundred, and this has already been done.'"

*Figure 107,* which represents by its more vivid colors and more assured lines the descent from the cross, was probably suggested by reproductions of ancient pictures.

## Case 12 — S. K.

*Date of birth*: 28 October 1912
*Occupation*: Artist, painter
*Diagnosis*: Paranoid schizophrenia
He was hospitalized from 18 August 1954 to 31 December 1954 at the Psychiatric and Neurological University Hospital of Pécs after having been hospitalized earlier from 1953 to August 1954 in an asylum.
*Family history*: One brother was epileptic and alcoholic. One sister is paranoid.
*Personal history*: No previous illness. He finished eight grades of normal school and then the College of Applied Arts. After having finished his studies, he worked as an artist painter. He decorated churches with frescoes and also painted pictures that he sold up until 1951. Since then he kept his art works and only rarely gave away a few as gifts to people "who understand these paintings of a very particular significance". He married a primary school teacher in 1936. In the last years his wife was the breadwinner.
*Admission*: Medical and neurological evaluation was negative. Bordet–Wassermann reaction in the blood and spinal fluid was negative.
*Psychiatric evaluation*: The patient's affect is labile; his mood is mostly depressed. His behavior is manneristic. The associations are dominated by paranoid ideas. He does not have real hallucinations. His intellectual ability corresponds to his level of education.

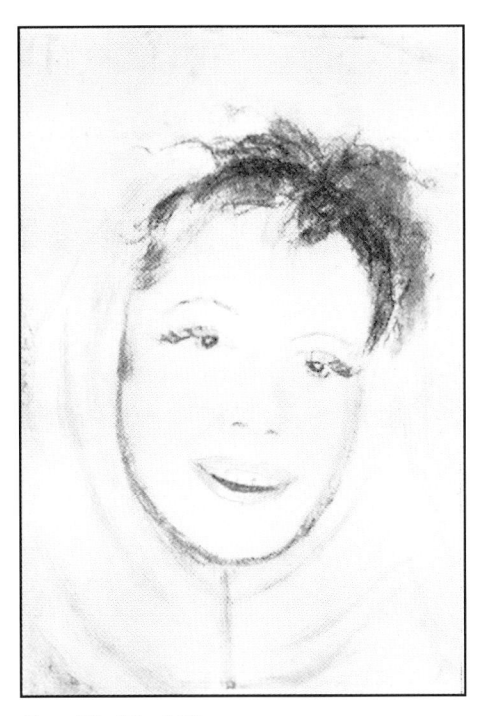

Case 12 - Fig. 108
Colored crayon. 29x21

According to his wife his behavior has changed in the last three years. He has become very jealous. Sometimes he talks to himself. He has delusions. He is afraid that he is surrounded by spies; "Men turn around after me to observe me and to spy on me." He attacked his wife twice, accusing her of having "divulged" his thoughts. He is afraid of being betrayed by his wife who is going to give away his secrets. He distrusts everybody. He has locked up "his secrets" (that means his drawings and paintings) in an armoire. He does not go out into the street anymore because "the whole world observes me. They are interested even in the weight in grams of my excrements".

He wants to exterminate the whole world, including himself, or at least wants to commit a crime in order to be condemned. One night he ignites several boxes of matches "to burn everything". He assumes that when they repainted the walls of his room they mixed with the paint a certain material which can reabsorb sounds and transmit them to his neighbors who are equipped with a radio transmitter and receiver through which they supervise all his actions and listen to his words. "I have unveiled in Paris, in America, and in India, men who were stationed by Monquar (a name probably invented by the patient). I have observed those men for several years although I cannot follow their traces in a direct way, but I observe every step of their society." Furthermore, the patient confides in us as follows: "My environment has changed in the last three years".

He has discovered that his wife reveals his thoughts (secrets) mostly to teachers who are her co-workers. He is always the subject of their observation. They try to penetrate his secrets—through his words. They register his words through a microphone on a tape. They steal from him.

He talks to himself, asks questions, and answers them. He listens to foreign radio stations and is in conversation with them. This brings it about that people are jealous of him, and these people have destroyed his sending machine in vengeance.

He has frequently found a little thread in his food that his mother-in-law has put there: (in Hungarian "ugye Rácné, cérna, zöld, öld"). (Translation: "isn't it true Mrs. Rác, sewing thread, green, kill them." (The first two words Rácné–cérna are anagrams and the two last words rhyme: zöld, öld).

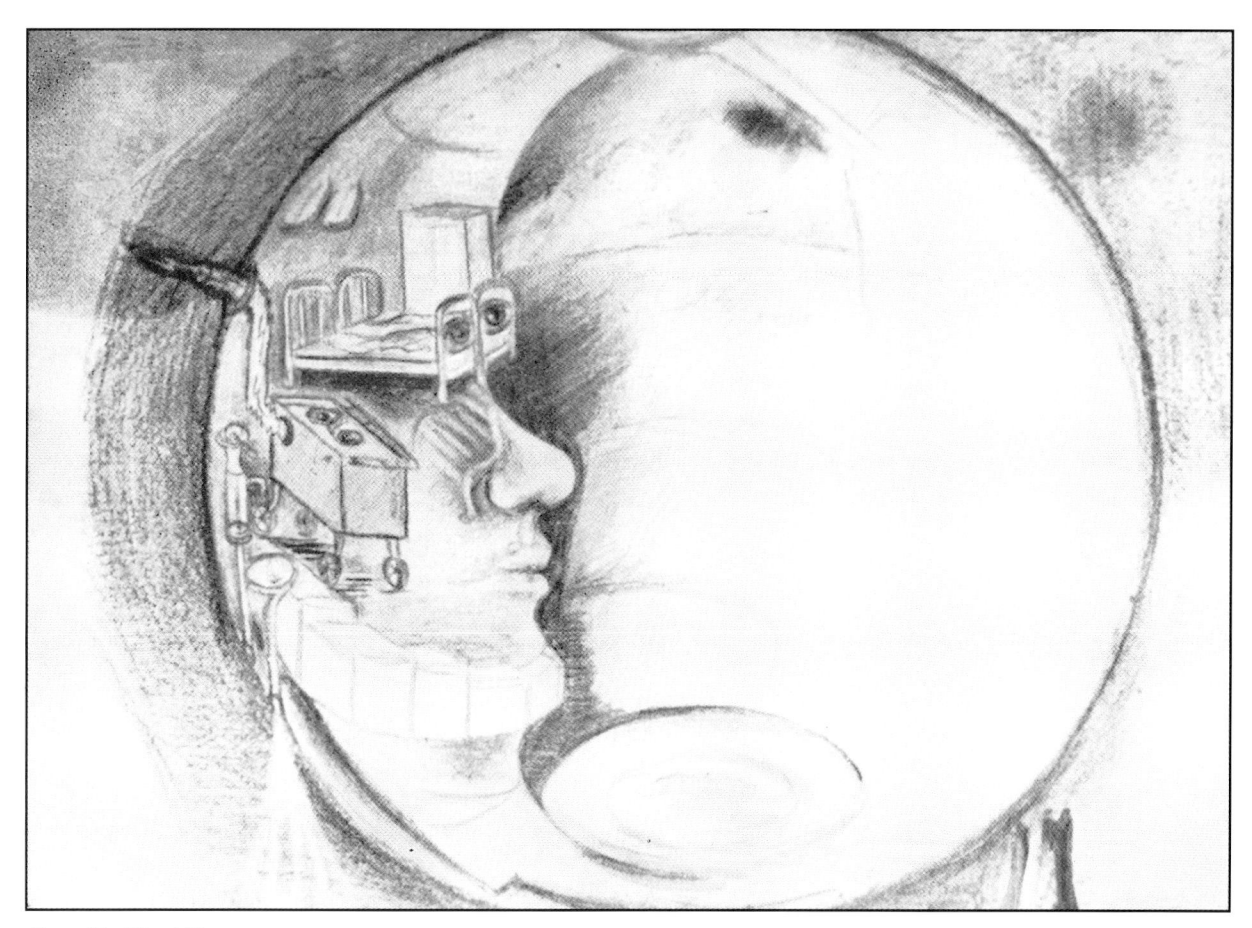

Case 12 - Fig. 109
Pencil drawing. 30.5x43

He has found in his bed a red thread "because the name of my wife's friend is Piroska". (Translation: Piroska is a feminine first name which has no correspondent in English and has the meaning of Little Red Riding Hood. "Piros" means red; Piroska means Little Red.) "They are always confusing me. They throw knives at me and put rods across in front of my legs."

*Course of illness at the hospital*: At first he is distrustful and withdrawn. He is afraid of being robbed. "The patients want to steal my secrets." He gives special meanings to words and letters, which he replaces by numbers. "Each letter corresponds to a special number: b = 6, and its reverse is the p. v = –7; g = 9, its reverse is the k."—"We add the numbers and then we decompose them again, we add the letters which are missing and the text develops." He

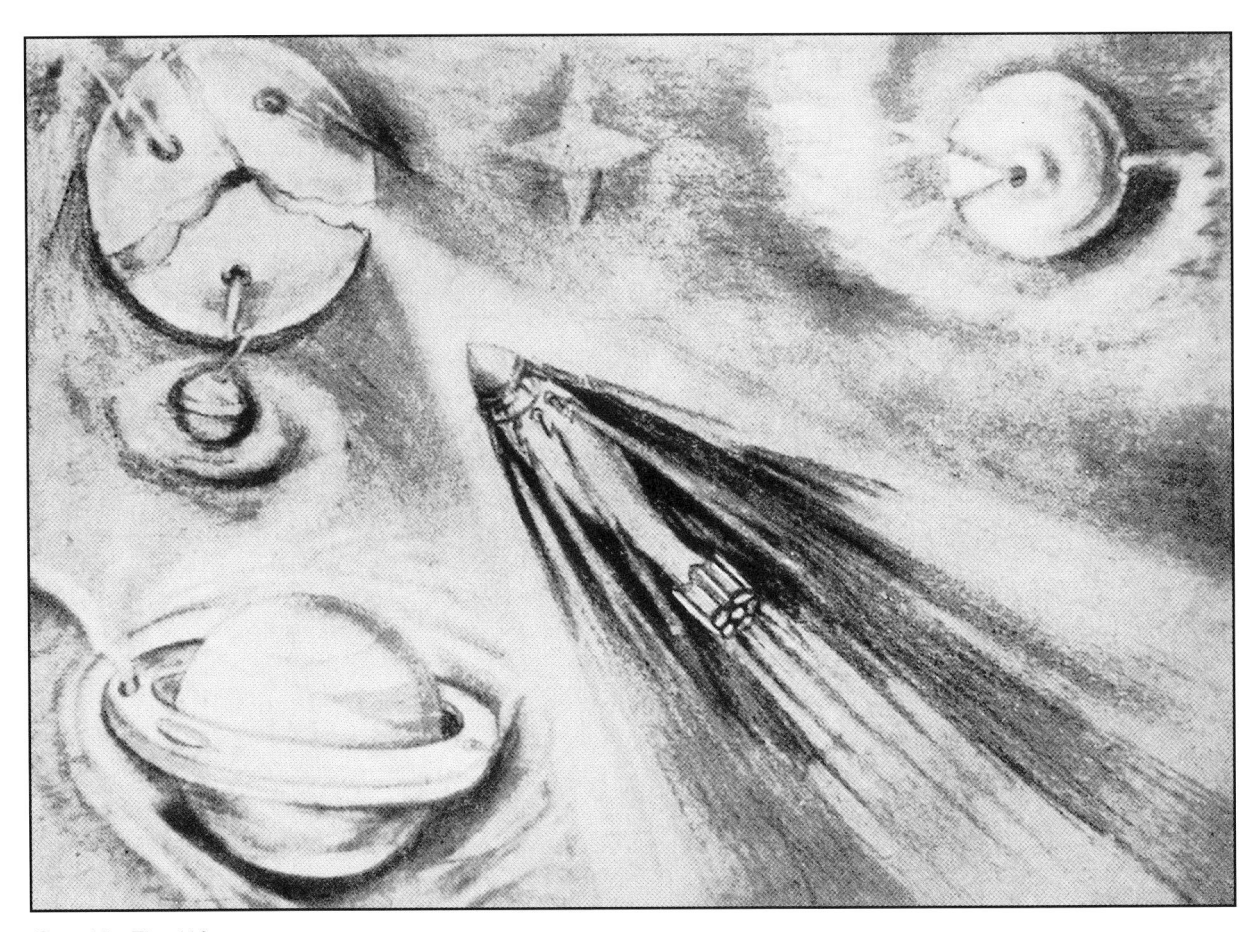

Case 12 - Fig. 110
Pencil drawing. 30.5x43

has the habit of isolating certain words in a text, 'to decipher them' because the letters have additional meanings.

The numbers have remarkable properties: "20, 40, and 60 cut and hit". 20 = the huszárs [20 in Hungarian is pronounced Housse. It is a word which produces an alliteration with the word huszár (pronunciation: houssar). This is an association by homophony followed by a sophism.] (cavalry) who cut with the sabre, 40 is the double of this one, and thus they kill twice as many." He replaces, by numbers, the letters of the last names and first names of his parents and of his friends. At other times he produces anagrams by transposition of the letters.

He states that he has made "the industrial map of the whole world; that it contains all the localities, all the factories, and all the people".

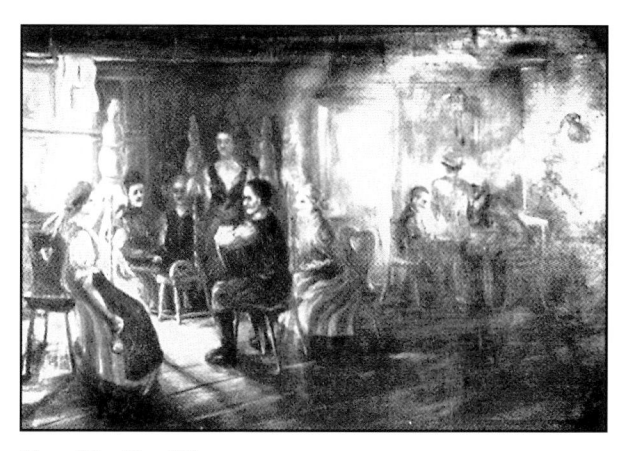

Case 12 - Fig. 111
Oil on canvas. 60x84

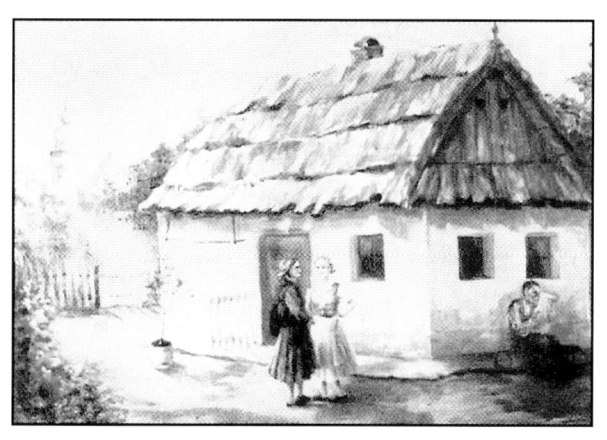

Case 12 - Fig. 112
Oil on canvas. 62.5x84

He guards these documents, well locked up. He tells us that his wife cheats on him and questions whether that is a symptom of an illness of his wife. "Maybe this idea has gone to her head?" He would like to do anything to heal his wife.

He talks about his visual hallucinations: he has seen radiations in his room, in the mirror and in the garden. These radiations may cause him bad moods.

All the figures in his pictures "have a specific meaning, and all are members of a group of spies.—In the last three years, my painting has changed. I use different colors. One could write books about each of my paintings, I express so much in them." Lately, he never finishes his paintings, "in order that nobody could see them". "I have secrets, strange secrets"—he says—"with me the red is different than that of other painters."

According to his wife, before his illness, he always worked from memory, except once, when he attempted to paint a landscape from nature. Then he was much disturbed by the curious people who stood around his canvas while he was working. Nonetheless, he made some portraits in pastel from models.

About abstract paintings, the patient declares: "This is a sick tendency, neither the form nor the content are aesthetical and it is incomprehensible without the help of explanations". Immediately after this statement, he says that he can paint musical notes. He will draw tree leaves in different colors, flying in an undulating line. All colors will have their significance, each will represent another sound. These will be musical notes. When questioned about the reason for the change in the style of his works, he refuses to explain.

He never makes sketches, but starts with a minute detail with the brush and develops the painting successively, detail by detail. Asked about this method, he gave the following explanation: "If I should start by sketching a picture, the whole world would guess what I intend to do and they would talk about it."

Case 12 - Fig. 113
Oil on canvas. 60x84

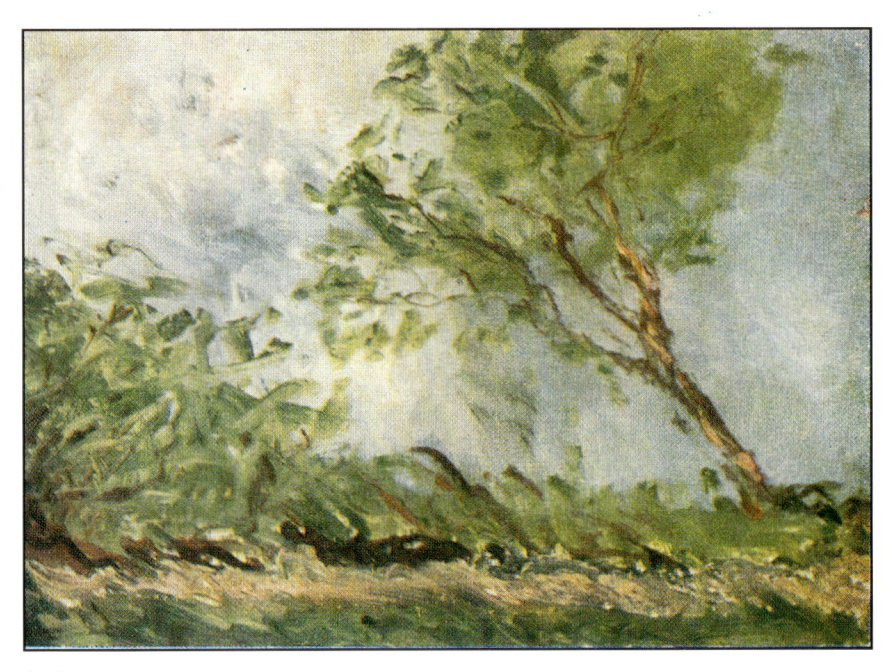

Case 12 - Fig. 114
Oil on cardboard. 26x35

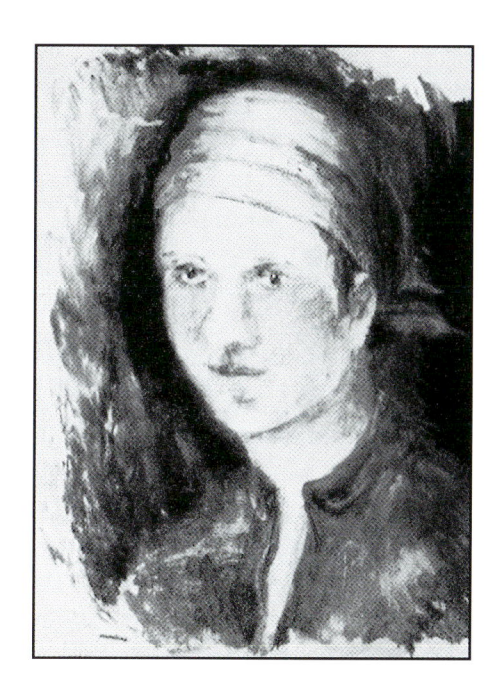

Case 12 - Fig. 115
Oil on cardboard. 36x26

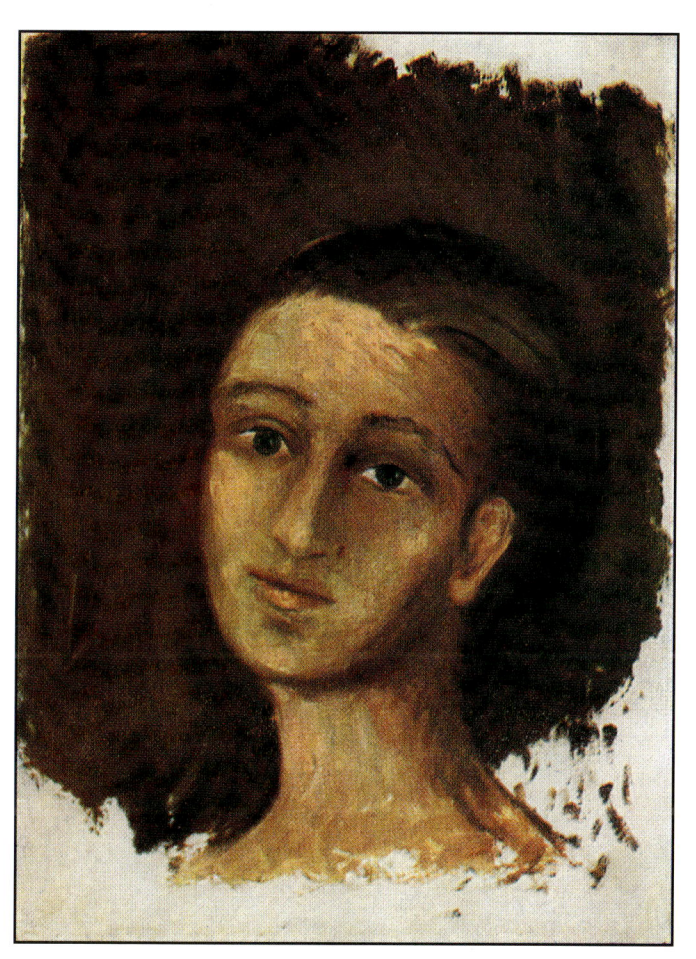

Case 12 - Fig. 116
Oil on cardboard. 36x26.5

115

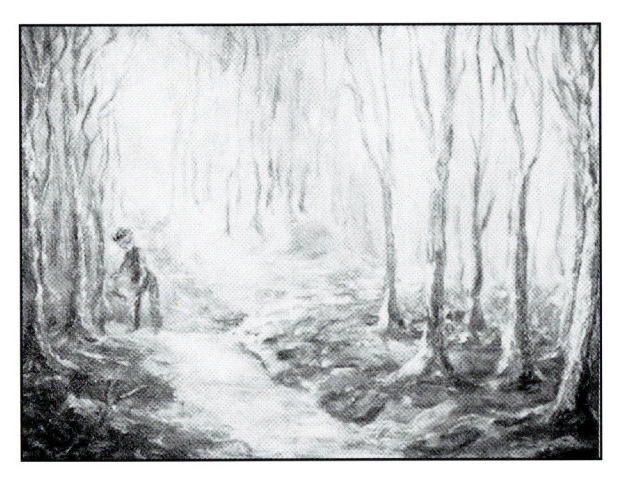

Case 12 - Fig. 117
Oil on cardboard. 26.5x37.5

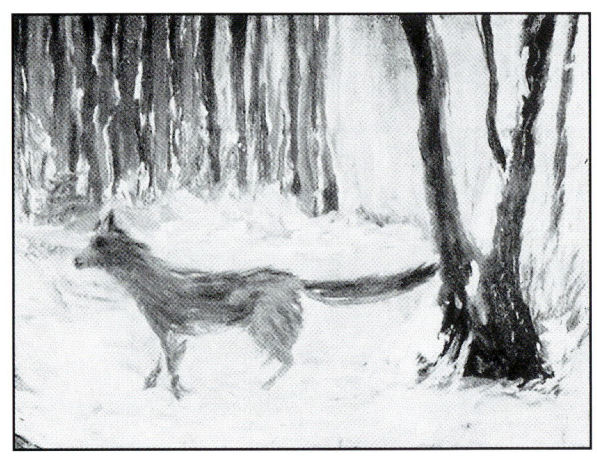

Case 12 - Fig. 118
Oil on cardboard. 26.5x36

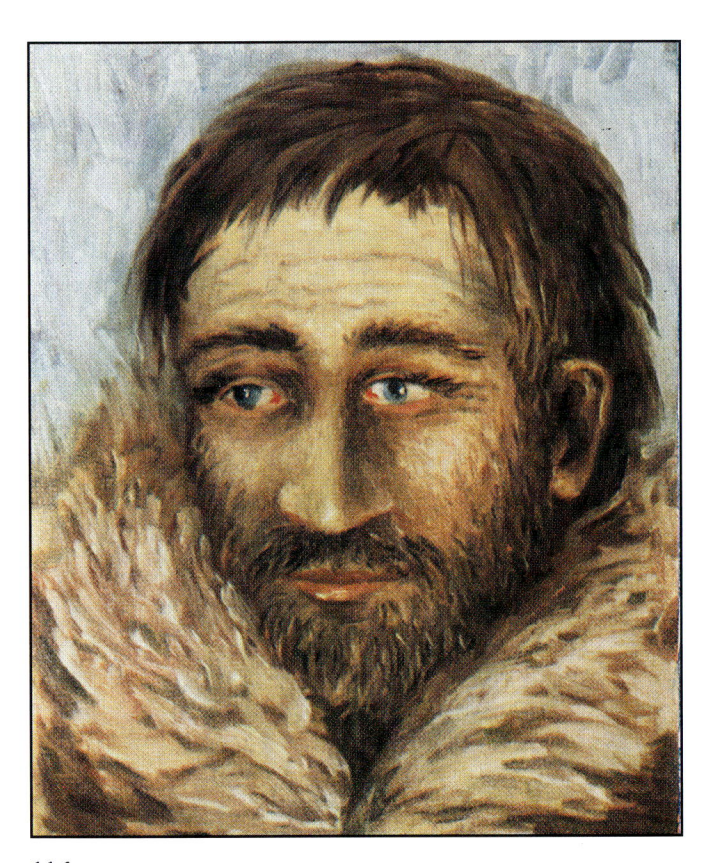

Case 12 - Fig. 119
Oil on cardboard. 34x21

He has started, for example, *Fig. 112* by the head of the woman placed essentially in the middle of the blank canvas. Once the head has been meticulously worked out and completed, he painted the whole figure the same way, and he continued to develop the rest of the picture in an identical fashion.

Occasionally, it occurred to him to start a new subject on a painting already completed as if he had a blank canvas in front of him. He starts painting the new picture by a small detail without being disturbed by the previous painting which is on the canvas.

Following electric shock treatment, his status has improved. He is less withdrawn. He pursues his paintings with pleasure. However, after the twentieth shock treatment, he complains of memory deficiency. The two pictures produced during this period, "are very primitive"—the patient says—"as if they had not even been painted by me".

At the time of his discharge, he denies paranoid ideas: "If I had known the number of factories in the world, and if I had made that map in the possession of such a great science, I would not be here". He does not remember his assumption (which he had previously adamantly voiced) that his mother-in-law wanted to poison him. He recalls the history of the sewing thread found in his food and he says: "That would have been stupid, if I had thought about such a thing". He decided to work at home and sell his paintings.

*We can divide the works of this patient into two categories* with two very different styles.

*The first group* consists of pictures produced during the most severe state of his illness, before treatment. These are symbolical pencil drawings, understandable only by the patient's own explanations.

*The second group* of his works is made up of pictures which have been produced before his illness and by those he has painted during his convalescence. These are canvases painted in the naturalistic style. The portrait of the young woman in *Fig. 108*, done in pastel at the beginning of his illness, although it remained incomplete, has a certain strength of expression.

He drew *Fig. 109* during the most severe phase of his illness. The superposition of several unrelated motifs over the portrait of the man produces an extraordinary effect.

In this profile, the patient has put in the place of the ear, an "electric shock machine which is, at the same time, a kitchen stove". Near this "stove" is a faucet with water spouting from it—an association purely mechanical. The eyes of the portrait are above the nose in the footboards of two beds. One side of the nose is modeled like a "garden bench".

*Figure 110* represents a rocket and planets. The patient gave the following explanation: "The picture represents the medical staff of the hospital of Kaposvár. In the upper left corner the doctor is the head of service of internal medicine and his assistant is represented as a satellite. The other planets are also physicians, heads of services. The rocket in the middle is the head of psychiatry, full of electricity."

Already during the electric shock treatment, the patient started painting in oil. *Figure 111* represents a scene in a room with looms and weavers. This scene is lit from two different sources which gives the whole painting a golden tone. The woman at the left side of the painting appears to be sitting on the edge of the chair. The other figures are done with better skill, nonetheless, the whole composition is banal. *Figure 112* is an even more primitive representation of a house in a village. On *Fig. 113*, the patient paints an autumn scene in a forest with his preferred warm colors. He has worked for a long time on this painting. As usual, he finished each tree with minute detail and only then would he start another one. Because of his training he was able to give depth to this landscape. However, the picture of the forest with an animal produced two weeks later *(Fig. 118)* has no perspective. It is to be noted that this later painting *(Fig. 118)* was produced during his period of amnesia caused by the electric shock treatment. He completed *Fig. 115* before *Fig. 118*. This is a study of the portrait of "My Roman woman". *Figures 116* and *119* are also studies of heads in oil on cardboard. One represents "a sinning woman" *(Fig. 116)*, the other is "a polar explorer" *(Fig. 119)*. He produced the picture in *Fig. 117* soon after *Fig. 118* at the end of his period of amnesia.

Before his discharge the patient painted, with rapid gestures, in less than an hour, his last picture in oil on cardboard *(Fig. 114)*. This sketch, dynamic in effect, is lively and reminds one of a painting by J. F. Millet, entitled "The Oak and The Reeds".

## MANIC DEPRESSION

### Case 13 — *L. V.*

*Date of birth*: 30 May 1912
*Occupation*: Primary school teacher
*Diagnosis*: Manic depressive psychosis
Hospitalized from 13 January 1932 to 1 September 1932 at the Psychiatric and Neurological University Hospital of Pécs.
*Family history*: Unremarkable.
*Personal history*: No organic illness. At the end of his studies, "at the time of his last exams, he felt so ill that he could not even answer the questions". He received his diploma, nonetheless, because he had been "an excellent student until then". During the five months during which he was preparing for his examination, he cut off all contact with those around him. He did not even speak, and if anyone spoke to him, he only answered briefly. He spent all day doing nothing. He stated that "he was love sick". After this, his mood changed suddenly and he engaged in megalomanic projects. He had fantastic plans and became aggressive toward the members of his family. On the street he attacked several men and tried to kiss young women and girls.

*The medical and neurological examination* was unremarkable. Bordet–Wassermann reaction in the blood was negative.

*Psychiatric evaluation*: At his admission he set three conditions: "(1) That I should wear the uniform of the Hussars; (2) that I should be with my dear fiancée the whole day; (3) that I may

Case 13 - Fig. 120
Colored crayon.
34x21

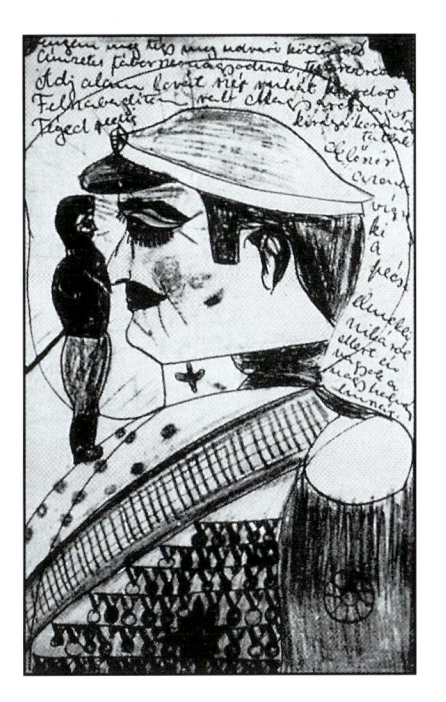

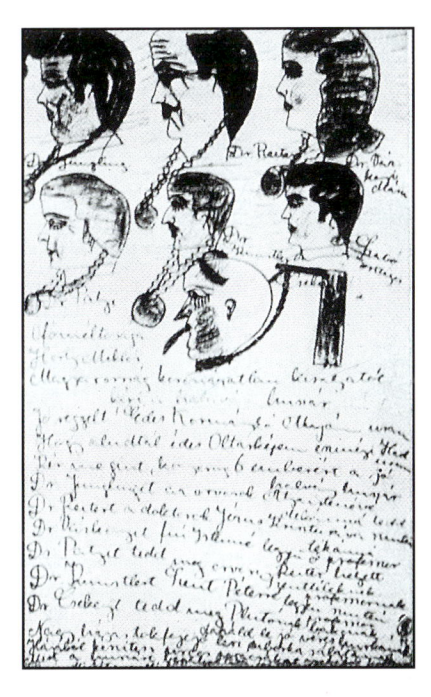

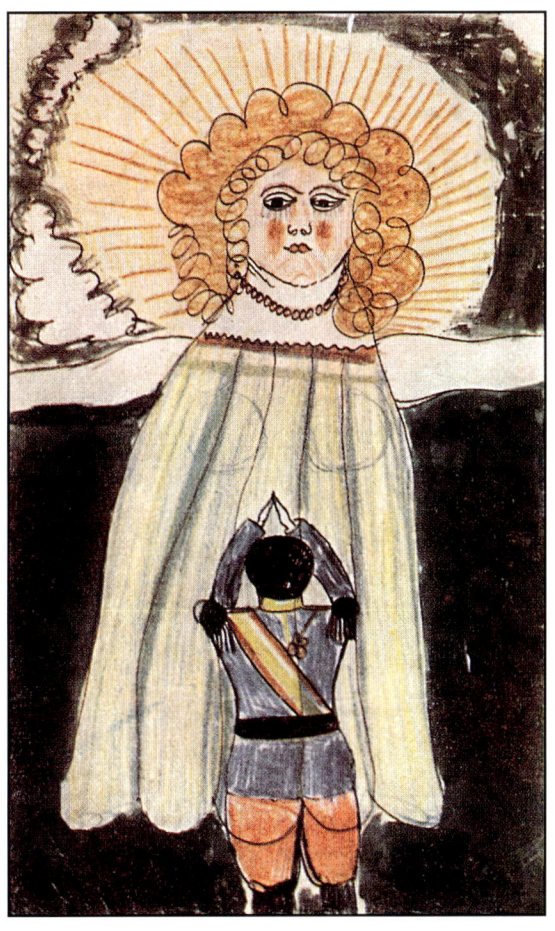

Case 13 - Fig. 121
Colored crayon and ink. 34x21

Case 13 - Fig. 122
Colored crayon.
34x21

sleep at your home, Mr. Doctor, during the night because I become crazy among these mentally ill patients."

*Course of illness*: During his hospitalization he was sometimes very agitated, ripped his shirt into shreds and made megalomanic statements. His language was obscene.

Once he stated that he was a murderer, having killed his friend with a hatchet and buried him in a 30 centimeter deep hole dug with his fingernails. He wanted to do penance for his act. He frequently "provoked his physicians to an American duel". "We have to choose which one of the two of us is going to die." He wrote poems and scenes for the theater where the principal actor is "the pale Hussar" (himself).

One month after his hospitalization, he began spontaneously to illustrate his poems with primitive drawings. He bragged about his talent as a poet and called himself "the pale Hussar", "the master poet". He collected postal cards and illustrated journals, stating that his works were published in them. He drew people kissing each other. Once, during the medical rounds, he spread all his drawings on the floor to show them. He made plans to escape and requested the help of the physician, inviting him at the same time to a gala dinner, with wine and champagne, and promised him "I will make a great man of you in Italy if you come with me". Later, he became calmer. He drew a lot and wrote little verses. He drew portraits. He asked his physician to send his works to the editors of journals. One day he decided to compose "a musical drama" and requested different musical instruments.

He illustrated his letters addressed to actresses of his time. Sometimes he drew only parts of a body (eyes, arms, feet). After a certain time, his productivity increased. He drew more and more and decorated even his envelopes with drawings.

His megalomaniac ideas had, for subject, his marriage with a star of the theater to whom he addressed his poems. Occasionally he called himself the Czar of Russia or the Emperor of China. At other times he stated that he was the supreme general of the Japanese army. One day he declared himself to be a movie star who had played great roles. On another day he "was the son of a professor". He was a "specialist renowned in the treatment of pulmonary diseases". He walked in the corridor with long strides and with a cape over his shoulder. The pockets of this cape were filled with illustrated post cards. He also drew geographical maps and boasted about his competence in that field.

His mood was still elevated and his intense drive for activity was present, even on the day of his discharge.

In his drawings, the patient uses vivid colors. The perspective is completely missing, but he fills the total surface in a raw primitive way with ornamental elements.

He represents homage to an honorable personage by the disproportionate size of the figures. In *Fig. 120*, in which he represents himself in military uniform with many medals, we see also a small figure in military uniform saluting "the general". This soldier is smaller than the head of the principal figure, which indicates that in face of such a glorious person, a simple soldier is very small and is frozen in a position of saluting. This drawing is surrounded by text in which he glorifies himself.

*Figure 121* represents a big female figure resembling an idol with a halo around her head, in front of whom a small man in uniform ex-

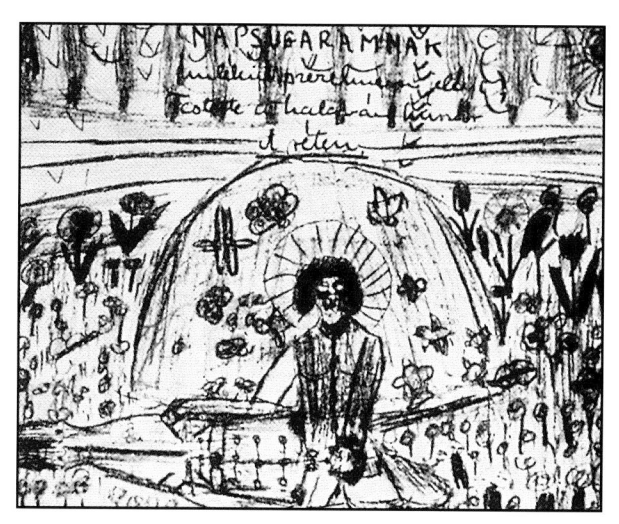

Case 13 - Fig. 123
Colored crayon. 17x21

presses his adoration with joined hands, as in prayer. The style of the woman's hair—drawn in a single trace—resembles the hairstyle of ornamental character of *Fig. 46* in PRINZHORN's book. On the dress, with a two-dimensional effect, the patient has drawn two circles at the level of the breasts. He traces in ink the contours of the dress and the margins of the folds; these lines remain visible across the figure of the man in the foreground. Obviously, he has drawn the figure of the woman and only after having completed it, has he placed in front of her the small soldier (a self-portrait made on a rare occasion when he shows his smallness in front of the adored woman). He filled in the rest of the paper with ink, most likely fingerpainting it.

The subject of *Fig. 122* is based on the reality of his everyday life. On a sheet he draws seven profiles, all similar, except for their different hairstyles. He writes underneath these heads the names of the doctors in the hospital. The seventh head is horned and his large tongue is protruding (this is the head of a hanged man attached to a small symbolical hanging post). In the text underneath this page the patient requested the head of government to give the doctors different decorations and medals and to name them to high positions (Dean, God, Christ, etc.). Only the seventh must be condemned to hell, and he should be destroyed by the most terrible tortures.

*Figure 123* is an idyllic scene. A young woman is sitting in front of a haystack. She has a halo around her head. The head of the "pale Hussar" rests in her lap. The flowers and butterflies and the haystack are roughly sketched and disproportionate. This picture reveals how scattered his attention was. In the background there is a road surrounded by trees in the form of a garland. The representation of the sun is similar to children's drawings. He dedicates this picture to his love.

# Case 14 — F. B.

*Date of birth*: 5 May 1902
*Occupation*: Locksmith
*Diagnosis*: Manic depressive psychosis (manic state)

He has been hospitalized twice in the time span between 1919 to 1954 at the Psychiatric and Neurological University Hospital of Pécs.

*Family history*: Unremarkable.

*Personal history*: A few weeks before his first hospitalization his mood became elevated. He made projects to travel to Fiume, Italy, as a "violinist virtuoso".

*Medical and neurological* findings were normal. Bordet–Wassermann reaction in the blood and spinal fluid is negative.

*Psychiatric evaluation*: He is oriented in all spheres. His attention is very short, he is vigilant, but the tenacity of his attention is practically zero. His mood is continuously elevated. He believes himself to be a great actor and a great artist. His associations are accelerated (flight of ideas). His thoughts are jumbled, his behavior is agitated and his judgment is poor.

The patient has always been hypomanic. During psychotic exacerbations he expressed megalomanic ideas. Sometimes he was the king and a general, at other times a "violinist virtuoso". The manic episodes of his illness have generally lasted for about two years. During that interval he often continues his work, but changes employment several times.

His latest hospitalization became necessary because of agitated and aggressive behavior.

During his hospitalizations he draws a lot. He draws and scribbles on any little piece of paper that he can put his hands on. He never makes original compositions, but copies illustrations from journals. Mostly, his human figures are grossly caricatured. He adds inscriptions—frequently obscene—around his drawings. He prefers to copy illustrations from comic papers. His preferred subjects are the automobile and the motorcycle. He works on these drawings very minutiously for several days. His

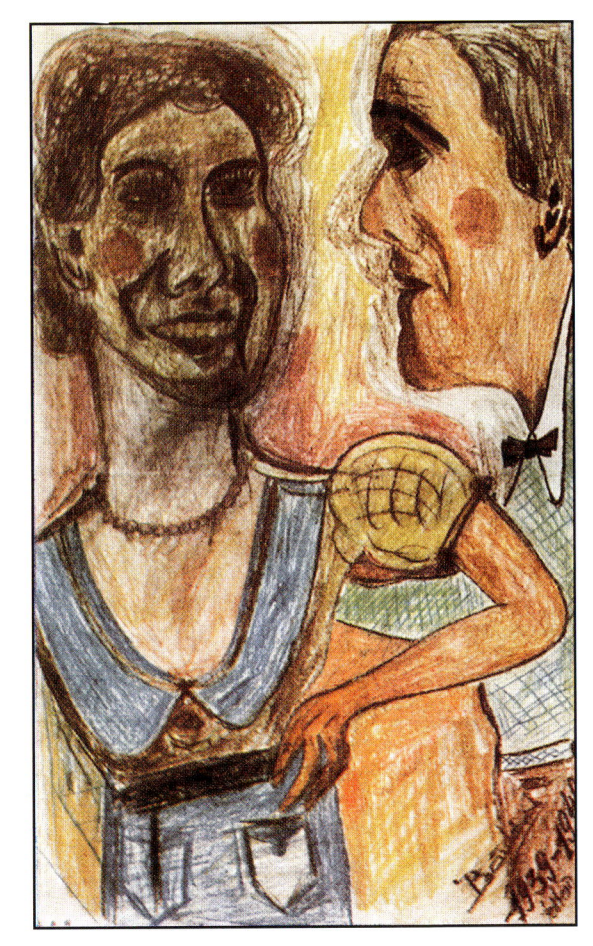

Case 14 - Fig. 124
Colored crayon. 34x21

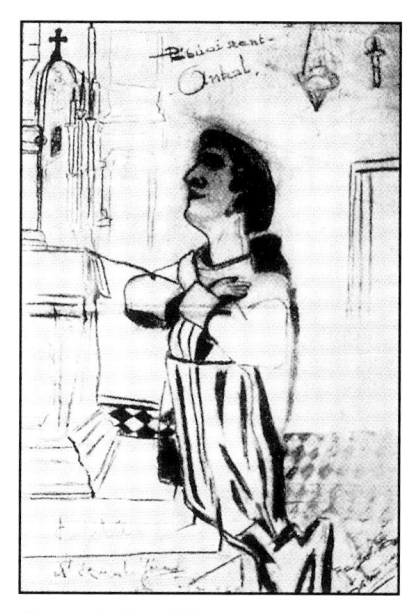

Case 14 - Fig. 125
Pencil drawing. 43.5x30.5

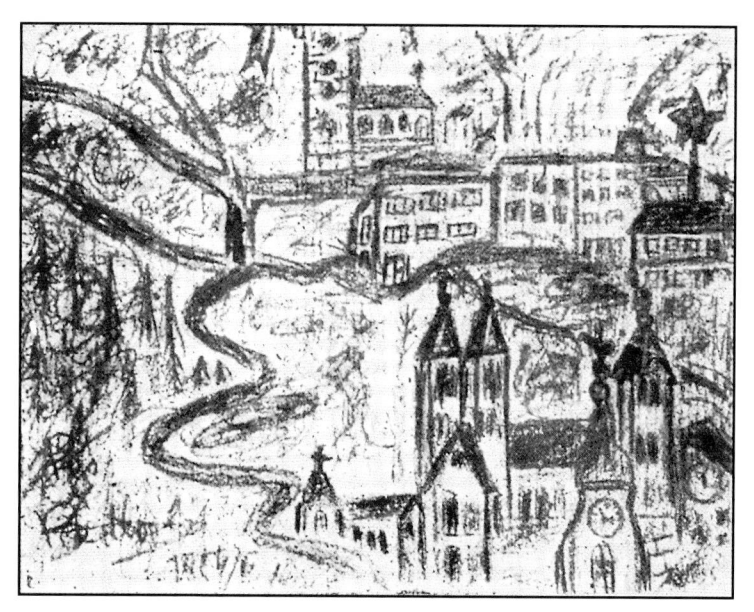

Case 14 - Fig. 126
Colored crayon. 15.5x21

way of working is unique. At first he makes sketches which reveal a certain aptitude for drawing. Nonetheless, because of his habit of going over the same lines innumerable times, his drawings become more and more scribbled over and dirty until they become almost unrecognizable.

Sometimes he works with colored crayons. He brags about his talent. Occasionally he adds his signature to other patients' drawings done at the same time. He paints personalities from the political life and writes obscene words around these pictures.

*Figure 124* represents a female figure in three-quarter profile and a man in profile who look at each other. Their bodies are disproportionate, too small in relation to the heads. The light and shadow in this picture are incorrect. This drawing—made in an unskilled manner in colored crayon—exaggerates the brutal traits of the woman.

In *Fig. 125* he represents Saint Anthony of Padua, the head and extremities are disproportionate. The lines were done rapidly, sometimes repeatedly drawn over and strongly accented. The background is only sketched by a few uncertain lines. The mosaic of the floor design shows that he worked fast in a superficial way and drew with quick gestures. This way of working is in contrast to the usual precious and minutely obsessional work of schizophrenic patients (for example, the precise work of the floor design in *Figs 29* and *30* of Mrs. *A. P.*, or the shingles by Mrs. *J. U.* on *Figs 76, 77, 82* and *83*. In general, the drawings of *F. B.* are unskilled, scribbled and confused.

*Figure 126* represents a view of the city of Pécs in several superimposed levels, drawn in red and black crayon. The lines are crudely done, the details are not in the same visual plan but ordered on different vertical levels. He drew from memory the public buildings of different boroughs of the city, one near the other, independently of their actual place. A serpentine road borders the left side of the picture. On this side one can guess at a few skeletons of trees. One can assume that this inadequate sketching represents the mountain of Mecsek. The objects in this picture are generally linear, but sometimes they are modeled, which gives an unsettling atmosphere to the composition.

## ALCOHOLIC HALLUCINOSIS

### Case 15 — N. N.

This patient's medical record has been lost. He was treated during World War I.

According to Professor Reuter, who remembered this case, the patient was diagnosed as suffering from alcoholic hallucinosis. He was an employee of the railroad company.

The patient drew monsters which he saw during his hallucinations in alcoholic delirium. These monsters frequently have a human head and the body of an animal. Another figure frequently repeated by the patient is that of an animal with four small legs and from which several snake-heads arise. The serpent is one of his preferred motifs.

In *Fig. 127* we see a real crowd of these monstrous figures in a kind of nebulous veil from which an eye, as well as certain human faces and stars, are emerging. Some contours of the human faces are at the same time the borders of monster figures in this "veil". The monsters, frequently with horns, have iron forks or an axe in their hands *(Figs 127–129)*. Next to them the patient fills all the negative spaces (free space) with other monsters. For example, in *Fig. 128*, under the abdomen and in the space between the back and the elevated tail of the monster with four legs there are small animals and heads of serpents which populate the entire surface. In the same composition we see a bizarre figure with its arms ending in animal heads, which grow out of a bird standing on top of the central monster.

These works are truly surprising and of a disquieting effect.

His ink drawings are done in two dimensions.

*Figure 129* is an almost grotesque scene. In this drawing facing a monster with antlers like horns and with a human face there is a little figure, hard to define, which sticks out his tongue. This last one stands on the large duck tail of another horned monster.

*Figure 130* shows a kind of turtle whose head is decorated with antlers. From the convexity of its shell, small serpents arise, among which the one in the middle has its head decorated by a cross. Above the principal figure there is a clock from which little flags arise in the same directions as the heads of the serpents. At the top center of the clock there is a cross. Finally, underneath the principal figure we find some kind of a tent, also surrounded by flags with a cross on its top. One can assume that the principal monster has arisen from an illusion based on the perception of a clock which next changed to the vision of the tent underneath.

One can get an idea about the nature of these hallucinated figures through the text surrounding some of the monsters.

On *Fig. 131a*, one can read: "This one comes to me every night. He is going to treat you in the other world, I have already talked with him, because you have not been faithful to me +++...."

On *Fig. 131b* the text is the following: "My wife, I know, this man comes to you every night."

In *Fig. 131c* he draws besides the monster with serpent heads, two small hearts and he also adds the word "heart". Around the border of this sheet, he writes: "I greet you and send my kisses to the children and to my brother. They have nothing to fear; this one will help me and the children. Kisses from your Papa". Related to the horned monster *(Fig. 131d)* with frightening teeth he makes the following threat: "This one will destroy you in the other world; I have already seen him and I talked with him".

*Figure 132* is not composed of such monsters. In the upper part there are six small coffins with a cross on top of each and in the middle of the sheet there are three larger ones also with crosses. From the coffins human figures arise with very small bodies and large heads, except for two of them on which birds are standing. Underneath the top line of coffins one can find arabic numbers in four digits (dates of death?), while beside the three large coffins in the middle there are numbers composed of three arabic digits. Serpents climb over two crosses.

The subjects of *Figs 133* to *135* evoke the idols of primitive people.

It is evident from the marginal text written by the patient on some of his drawings, that the monsters have different meanings. There are idols of good will to whose patronage he recommends his children, and there are other gruesome monsters with which he menaces his "unfaithful" wife.

This patient is the author of the most disquieting drawings in our collection. His figures, lacking in perspective, are placed side by side. A certain tendency to produce a composition may be deduced from his "desire for order" and the fact that he fills the whole pictorial surface. His monsters have a horrible head with frightening teeth and stuck-out tongue. They have a massive trunk and their raised tails beat in the air. They are created by the fusion of human and animal figures such as birds and other animals, which gives these drawings a strange character of being at the same time both ridiculous and frightening.

These figures are similar to those used in carnivals, but their menacing infernal atmosphere is beyond the humorous and mocking aspect of the carnival figures. They remind the spectator—with respect to quality—of the pictures of Hieronymus Bosch. SULLY (1909) mentions that children's animal drawings often have a human-like head.

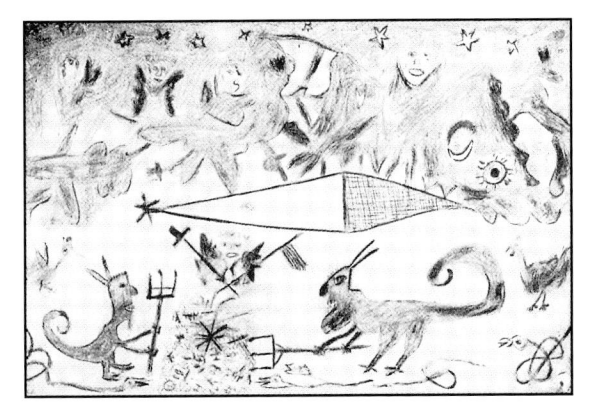

Case 15 - Fig. 127
Ink drawing. 21x34

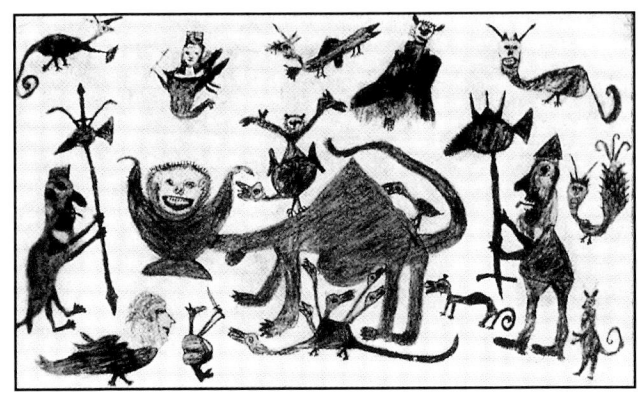

Case 15 - Fig. 128
Ink drawing. 21x34

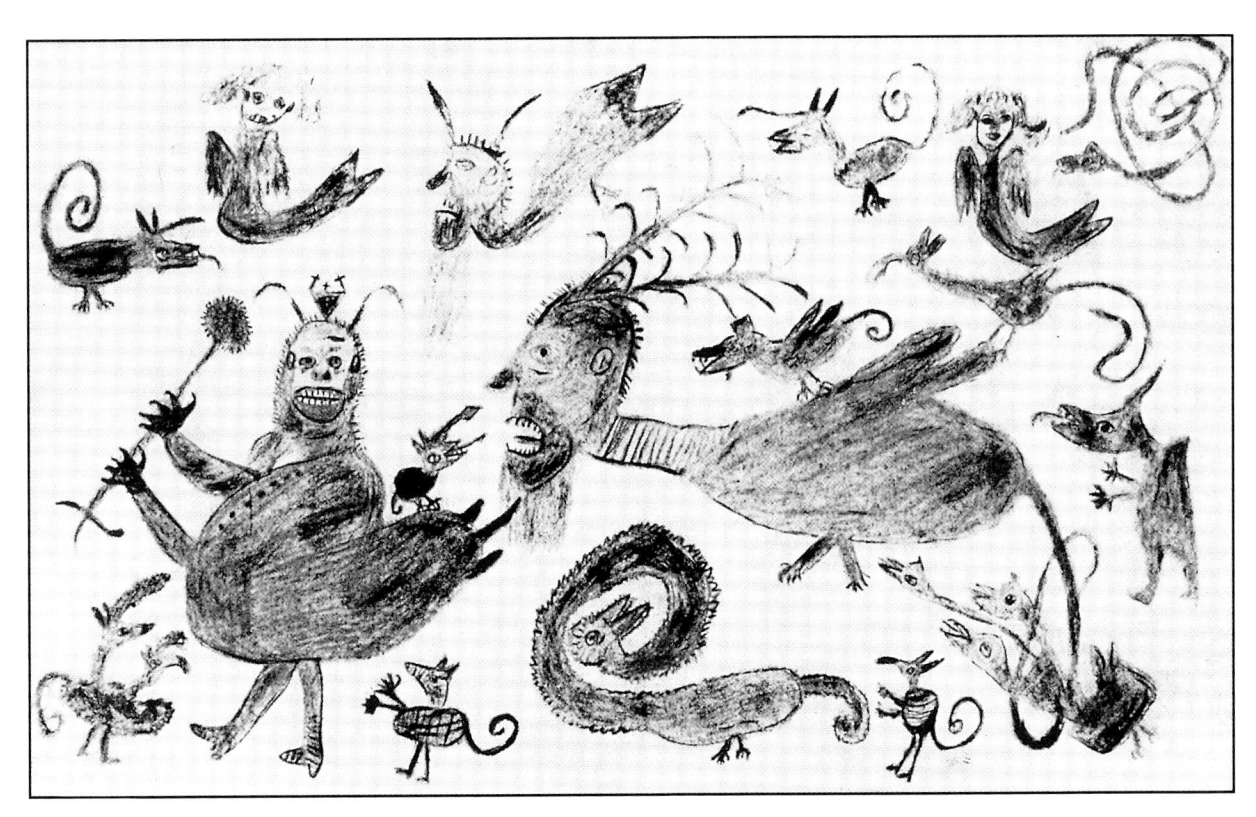

Case 15 - Fig. 129
Ink drawing. 21x34

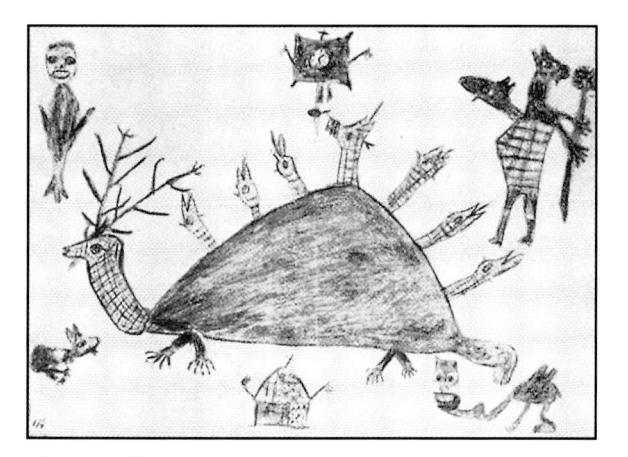

Case 15 - Fig. 130
Ink drawing. 16x24

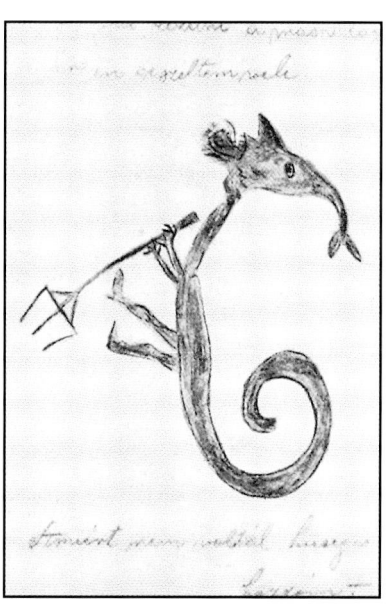

Case 15 - Fig. 131a
Ink drawing. 20x12

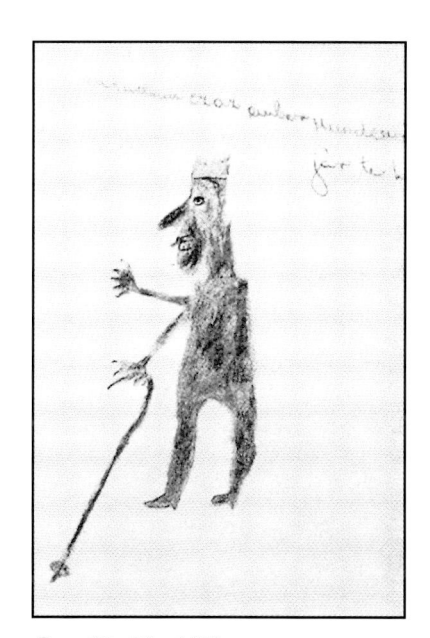

Case 15 - Fig. 131b
Ink drawing. 20x12

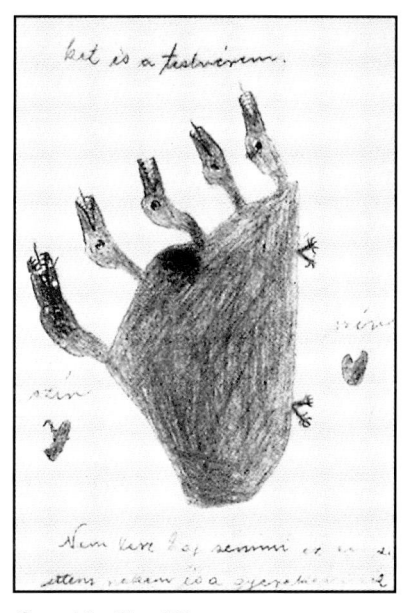

Case 15 - Fig. 131c
Ink drawing. 20x12

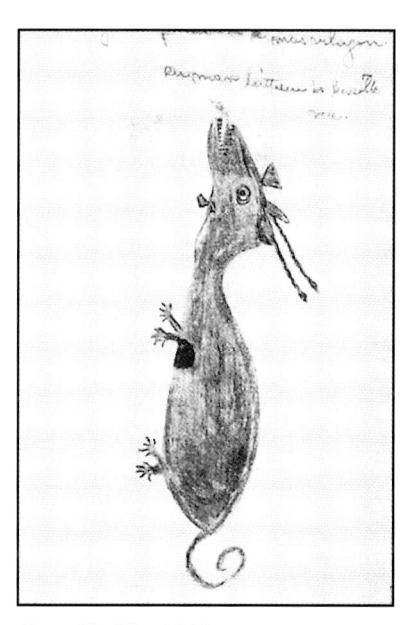

Case 15 - Fig. 131d
Ink drawing. 20x12

127

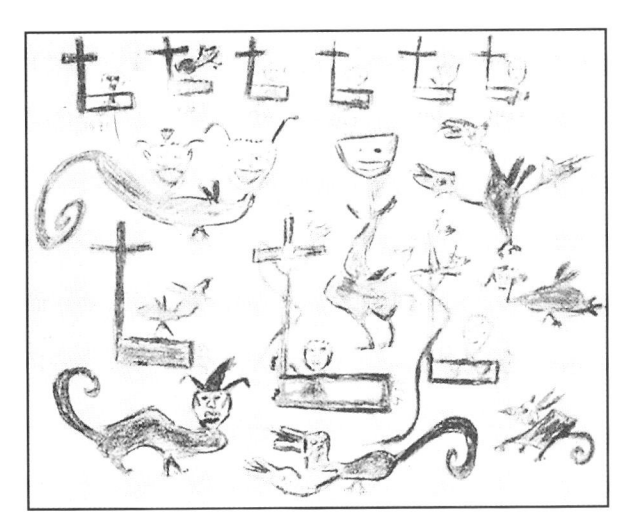

Case 15 - Fig. 132
Ink drawing. 16.5x21

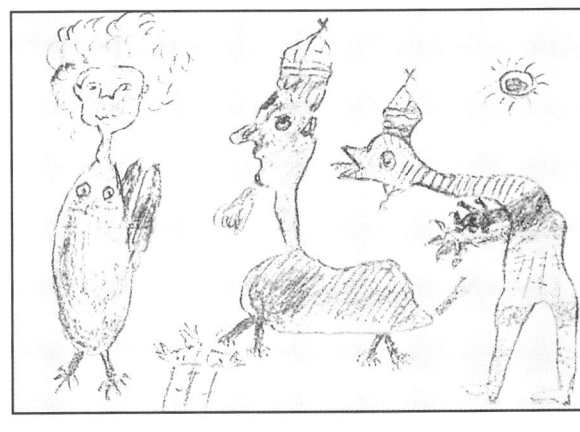

Case 15 - Fig. 134
Ink drawing. 8x11.5

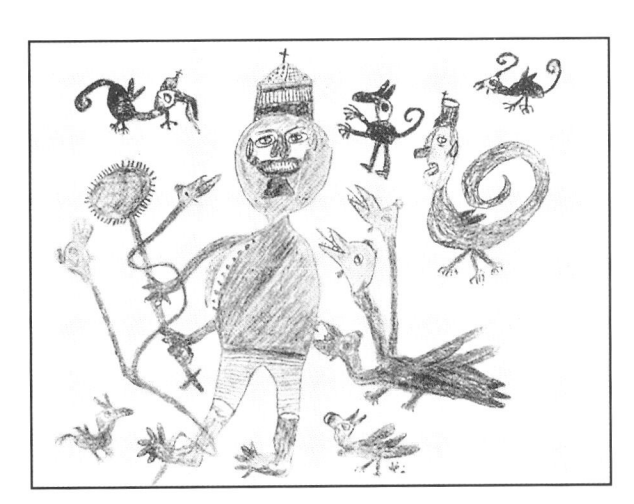

Case 15 - Fig. 133
Ink drawing. 8x11.5

Case 15 - Fig. 135
Ink drawing. 21x17

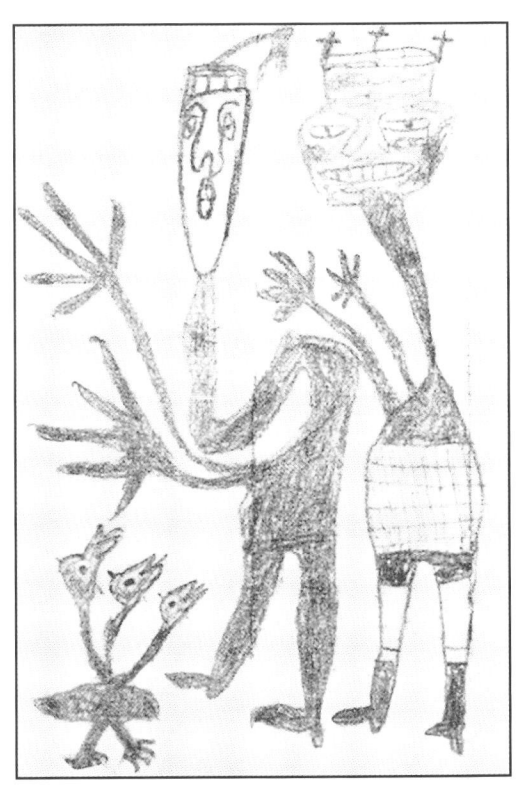

The works of our patient are rich in forms. His subjects are original. The interpretation is primitive, although uniform and consistent. The painter is unskilled, but nonetheless he shows a remarkable expressive strength. A certain tormented agitation emanates from these drawings with the extremities extended in all directions.

This patient lacks all knowledge of the artistic notion of space. He presents his figures in shadow-like silhouettes and in two dimensions. They have mostly a pictorial rather than a graphic effect.

# NEW CASE WITH LONG-TERM FOLLOW-UP ON OUTPATIENT BASIS

## Case 16 — Zs. H.

*Date of birth*: 29 January 1943
*Occupation*: High-school student
*Diagnosis*: Schizophrenia
*Date of hospitalization*: hospitalized from 7 January 1959 to 28 March 1959 at the Psychiatric and Neurological University Hospital of Pécs.

This case has a special interest for the study of the psychopathology of expression because of the opportunity to follow the development of this patient from a young age when he was first hospitalized through adulthood. He now lives in the home of his mother and has become a professional painter. The follow-up covers a thirty-five year time period. The case history of his first admission was published by this author in the *Medizinische Bild* (JAKAB 1960).

The description of this case is based both on this article and on the patient's medical record, which is updated to the present with follow-up progress notes of later readmissions as well as on the records at the outpatient clinic which provides ongoing psychiatric support and the monitoring of his medications.

Zs. H. was a student at the middle school for artistically talented children. He was admitted at the Psychiatric and Neurological University Hospital of Pécs on 7 January 1959 for the first time. He was released on 28 March 1959.

*Family history*: The father was an architect. The houses built by him are still favorite homes in the city. One brother (B. H.) is also architect, and his son is studying law. The mother is a home-maker, she is in good health and it is in her home that the patient lives. Grandmother on the father's side was mentally ill. One of the younger sisters of the father was also treated in a hospital for a nervous breakdown after she attempted suicide following the birth of her child. This was obviously a postpartum depression. Otherwise the family history reveals no further pathology.

*Personal history*: Birth and early development was normal. The patient is right-handed. At the end of the eighth grade of school he was very nervous, felt weak and tired. Therefore, in the last month he did not attend school. However, he received his final report because he was a good student up to then. He was talented in painting at a young age.

Already in his early childhood he was rather withdrawn. He had no friends and spent his free time reading and drawing. In the summer of 1958, he frequently said that art is not good because all artists will end up in mental hospitals. *He did not want to become an artist painter because he did not want to be mentally ill.* During this whole summer he did not draw or paint. In the fall he returned to the middle school for artistically talented children in Budapest. Nonetheless he had to be brought home again because he became very fearful. He believed that the people wanted to kill him and that they were coming at him with opened knives. He himself felt such a strength that whomever he looked at became mute. At home he read the Bible constantly and talked about hearing voices which were calling him.

When he was admitted to the hospital, he said the following: "There are four blacksmiths, my two parents, and my two brothers. They are hammering all the time and they will change the world because they have such strength in them. They pull atoms through the electrical wire and the whole world will be switched over."

He skipped and sang and whistled and danced around restlessly in his room. He carried on conversations with non-existent persons. He told his father not to come near him because the father is Satan and the patient will fight Satan. He did not accept any medication and stated that one wanted to poison him and that in his drinking glass there is fire.

*Medical and neurological evaluation* was within normal limits. Bordet–Wassermann reaction in blood and spinal fluid was negative.

*Psychiatric evaluation*: At the time of his admission he showed a high degree of psychomotor restlessness, and dissociated thought processes. His attention span was short. He talked about hallucinations and delusions.

We asked his name: "My name is nothing, I am the anonymous ... Now comes the crucifying, but what is that for me. I descend from the cross ... doctor. You are the anonymous, we are both ... I love mankind, the whole mankind is for me cha cha cha ... You don't believe it? This one serves me (patient points to one of the nurses), and you also, all of you are my servants."

At the question of where he is presently, he gave the following answer: "Aha you are coming now with the Mars. I like this kind of gossip. You say that we are in Naples and you want to bend for me the tree of wisdom, ha ha ha, only a passing cloud she goes as she has come. If I had a name then the tree of knowledge would be by me the one from which Eve plucked the apple. You are bringing an invisible enemy upon me. The atomic war. A human child has also a need for you stupid peasants. Do you want to kill me, isn't it so? I don't need any poison, you should drink that. My father also offered me poison but I knocked it out of his hand."

"This one here is Elijah and that one is Moses (he points to two attendants) and I have the power to destroy everything because my father is Satan ... With the soul I kill people, but there will be no more deaths because I am already dead. I simply kill. I have a few friends, Leonardo and the Michelangelo. I love one goal? I am a new school. I have three paintings. Actually these have already withstood the atomic explosion."

When he was requested to draw one of his visions that was a crucified body, he said, "but without the cross".

At the hospital he received electric shock treatment and gradually became calmer. After the sixth treatment he complained of memory problems. These persisted throughout his hospitalization. He received a total of eighteen shock treatments. Gradually his hallucinations decreased and disappeared. He said that he did not remember them, but if he had felt such things that was "caused by his illness".

One month after his discharge he returned for follow-up in the company of his mother. The mother reported that the patient behaved well at home although he was very withdrawn. If he was asked to do some household chores, he willingly participated. He was reading a lot and did not draw spontaneously.

Before his illness he drew and painted portraits which, according to his professors, showed good talent. The oil portrait of his mother and his self-portrait *(Figs 136, 137)* were painted before his illness when he was only fourteen and a half years old. Regardless of the depressive expression of his self-portrait, these pictures show good composition, balance and good color combinations.

During his hospitalization he drew a lot, partially spontaneously and in part when he was asked to draw. But he was never requested to draw a specific topic. At the beginning he drew his visions. Later during the amnestic period after the electric shock treatment he produced primitive scribblings, paintings and drawings without any composition. In the next phase he drew sexual themes, some symbolical, others with coarse pornographic expressions. Finally, during the improvement after the electric shock treatment he produced portraits of the people in his environment. At first he used very bizarre colors. Later he worked essentially with crayon. His models were well recognizable from his drawings.

In the following we are describing his works during the production of the drawings and paintings which are reproduced. We report verbatim his verbal comments during his activity of drawing or painting:

*Figure 138.* The patient draws his first vision. "A chest as if made of stone under a cross on which it was nailed. But one could not feel it. This figure has just appeared as if he was very heavy and his flesh as if made of stone and not touchable. Then he disappeared. He was a shimmering mass." He completed the picture by first drawing a chest and the arms. It was similar to the head of an ox and he said, "Yes, it has that meaning also". He drew the head and the extremities after this.

*Figure 139.* As he started, he said: "This is Adamuk—a frightening and complicated being because it is a molecule that returns into itself." He started on the left corner of the paper with circles and little appendices. Next he composed the form, a star in which he incorporated one side of the previous drawing. The other sides were three interlocked curves. He redrew the whole figure three times, one after the other. He decorated the star with ornaments between the curves that intersected. From one corner of the star he drew an oblique line to the middle of the paper. "This is part of the head", said the patient, and requested a little pause to rest. Then he stated: "The important thing is that in Harlem everything is in order. I draw it from my knowledge. I think it out." Then he continued to draw detail after detail, one beside the other in geometrical forms. Over this he drew a female head which he then scribbled over with black lines. "Since this is a woman whom one has to rescue from the Black Sea—not only one, but many! This must be rescued, cha cha cha." We gave the patient a new sheet of paper to

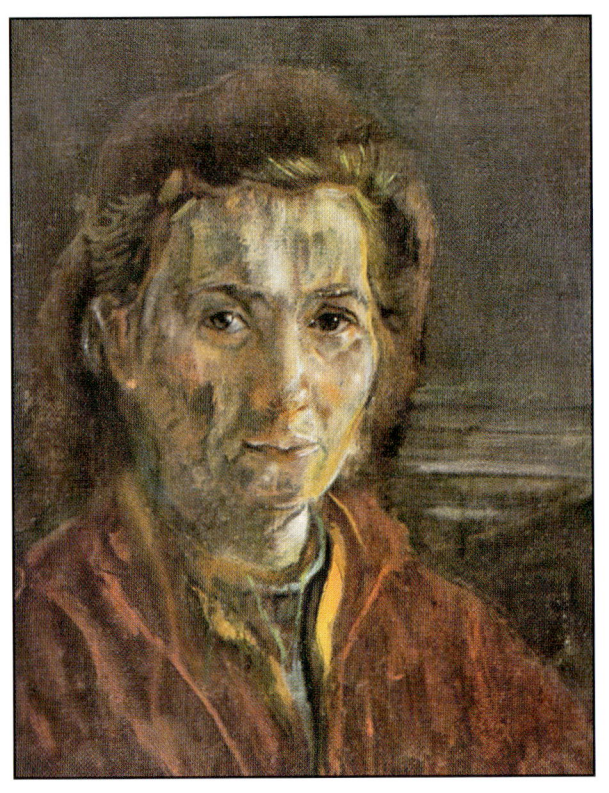

Case 16 - Fig. 136
Oil on canvas. 45x30

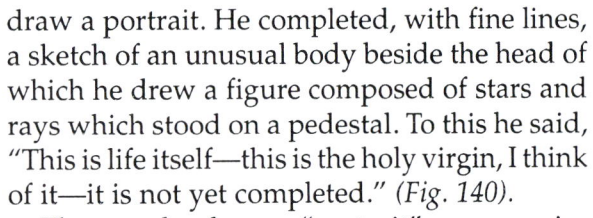

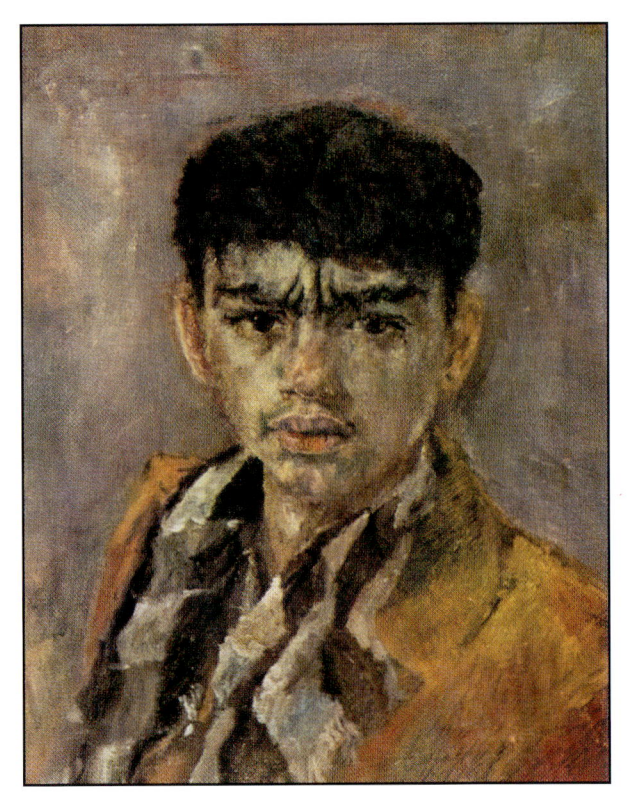

Case 16 - Fig. 137
Oil on canvas. 45x30

draw a portrait. He completed, with fine lines, a sketch of an unusual body beside the head of which he drew a figure composed of stars and rays which stood on a pedestal. To this he said, "This is life itself—this is the holy virgin, I think of it—it is not yet completed." *(Fig. 140).*

The way he drew a "portrait" was very interesting. He started sketching a head and the body, but had no more space for the shoulders and therefore he attached another sheet of paper and started anew. On this he continued to draw and sketched a new head with one shoulder which overlapped with the previous gestalt.

It again extended beyond the paper. Therefore, he attached a third sheet of paper on the right side. While the patient drew he said: "This smells very strongly of oil." (He drew with pencil.) We asked if these were two different figures. Of the first figure, he said: "I don't know what this is." Again, he asked to go for a little walk. After a few minutes he returned and continued to draw. He drew lines over the papers and extended them even onto the table. "This is the Gordian knot." "Please write this for the jury and it will live."

We asked him whom does this represent?

"This is the Mona Lisa as Mona Lisa—a decent man does not break glasses." (Indeed, beside the patient a glass was dropped and broken.) "The oppressed heroic polital (?) has stood up, cha cha cha." The patient began to sing and thump with his feet. Then he started in the middle of the drawing paper again. He sketched circles. "Is it here? ... No, maybe here? Down straight there is no Gordian knot. It is a life." Now the patient has scribbled over the gestalt, "This will be the earth, maybe it is a little bit indented. Maybe the sun? But then mankind has so much energy it is like the sun. Then the sun cannot burn him." On the right side of the drawing paper he drew lines on the table and said: "This is destiny". We suggested that the patient continue and complete this drawing.

"Oh I understand it. If I had completed it, then I would be in love with death." (He indicated the pages of the medical record.) Next he attached another paper to the right side of his previous three papers and said that he drew a rocket *(Figs 141a–d)*.

He continued his associations and said the following: "There was once a half bent, not completely bent line. This had a meaning, not only one but a million. Maybe a straight line was even God and something similar and, from a socket of an eye, something is missing, that he is only this little. But on the drawings it is also a little knowledge while it is maybe a whole a total. The knowledge. You are Caesar."

During his treatment at the hospital he said once about his visions: "I saw a crucified body,

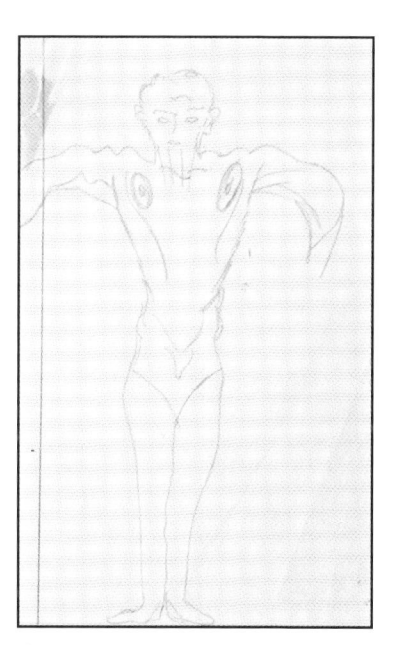

Case 16 - Fig. 138
Pencil drawing. 42x30

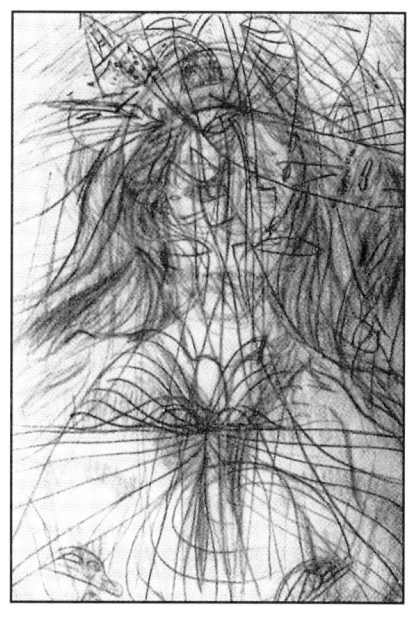

Case 16 - Fig. 139
Pencil drawing. 42x30

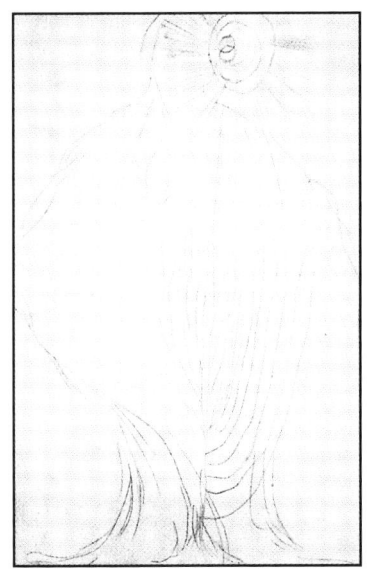

Case 16 - Fig. 140
Pencil drawing. 42x30

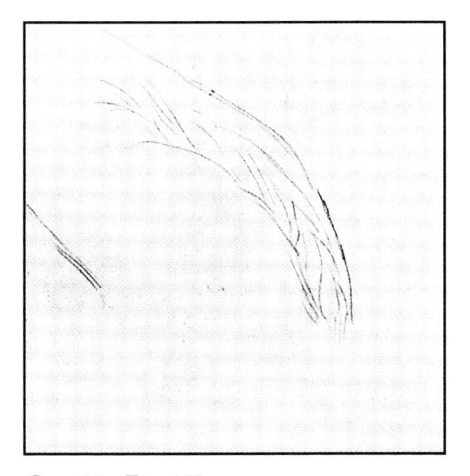

Case 16 - Fig. 141a
Pencil drawing. 42x30

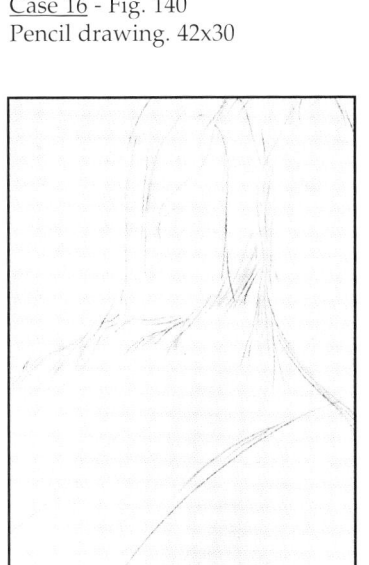

Case 16 - Fig. 141b
Pencil drawing. 42x30

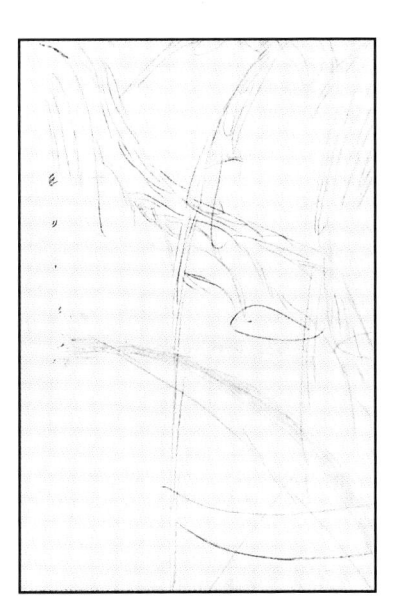

Case 16 - Fig. 141c
Pencil drawing. 42x30

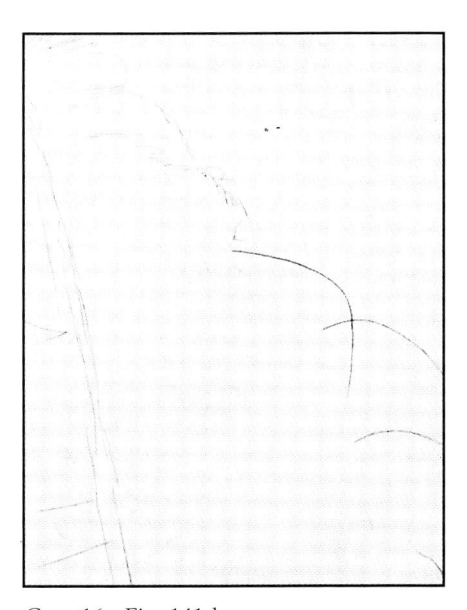

Case 16 - Fig. 141d
Pencil drawing. 42x30

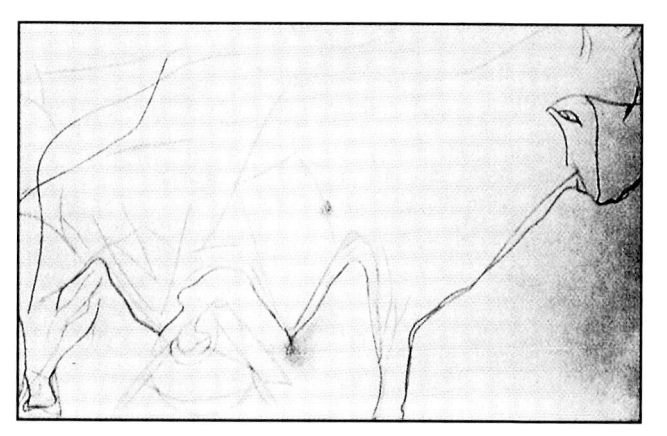

Case 16 - Fig. 142
Pencil drawing. 30x42

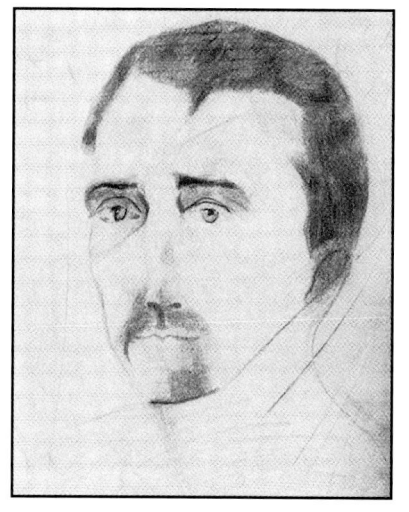

Case 16 - Fig. 143b
Colored crayon. 42x30

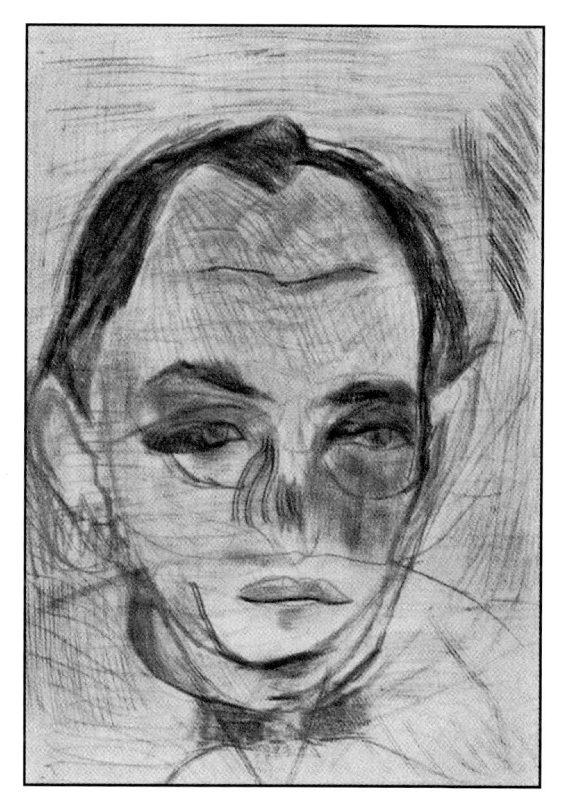

Case 16 - Fig. 143a
Colored crayon. 42x30

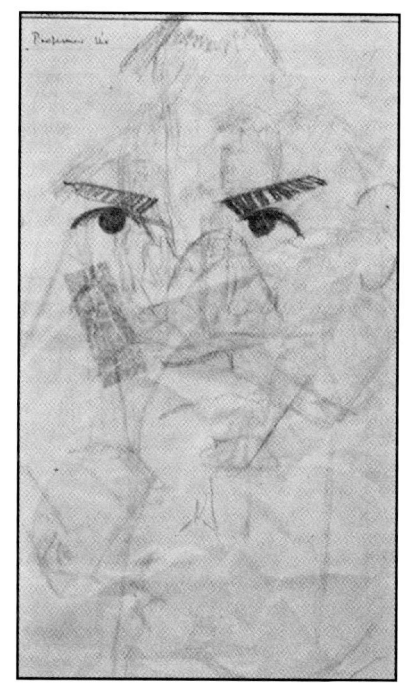

Case 16 - Fig. 144
Pencil drawing. 20x15

but without the cross; first, from the front, then from behind. I have also seen some burning forms and around their head there was light as it came. I talked mutely with him. It was St. Peter. In his hand he had a kind of whip and a lock. I thought that he had nothing in his other hand. Yet, maybe it was some kind of heart-shaped wreath of flowers, which gets destroyed, and under his feet there were flowers."

"During the summer I pushed a cart through the door and beside me I felt another being, a feeling form who just like me pushed a little cart. As I wanted to see better, I couldn't see. Actually, she didn't even exist at that time. This creature had the ability of sensory weight, which can be transferred through the sensory organs. That time I could not fall asleep for a long time." We asked the patient what does this "sensory weight" mean in this context. He gave the following answer: "Sensory weight can be for instance a cart loaded with bricks like the one that appeared to me. However, the bricks made me by so many kilograms lighter as heavy they were and this made the work always heavier.— In that form there was no intention because she was no human. I couldn't talk with her, although on the surface she had the form of a human, it could have been one, but I felt such lightness in her. She appeared and disappeared and after that I felt myself lighter."

*During the first few days of the electric shock treatment the patient did not draw. Then, after the fifth treatment, he complained that he felt as if his surroundings were from his childhood years and "that is very unusual and depressing". During this period his drawings actually had quite a regressive character. They were primitive and schematic, similar to children's drawings.*

In *Fig. 142* he drew with colored crayons, as a sketch of few lines. It is an animal of an unusual form. During the follow-up visit, he stated that he did not remember having done this picture. The patient believed that it might be the representation of an ox or a bull. *Figure 143a* was drawn during the period of amnesia and in a state of anxiety. It has no composition.

For the first time during his treatment, the patient attempted to draw a portrait. The picture is abstract and has unusual colors. The face is yellow with green, violet, and blue lines which give it an unusual frame. On the nose and on the forehead he wrote with different colored crayons his name and a few incomprehensible words. Following this first completely abstract portrait he attempted to draw a more naturalistic one but the colors and some details were still quite bizarre. This figure has green hair and green eyelids.

After completing the previously mentioned two portraits, the patient drew several more, but now he used people in his environment as models. For instance, *Fig. 143b* is the portrait of an attendant. The model can be recognized well, but the colors are still not natural. The hair is violet and on the face green, yellow, and blue colors dominate. At this time he also produced a pencil sketch representing the chairman of the department of psychiatry "The Prof" (*Fig. 144*).

On *Fig. 145a* he drew the portrait of a patient with colored crayon. This was done shortly before his discharge. The represented person is easily recognizable and the colors are more natural. The whole picture is quite realistic. It is similar in technique to *Figs 145b, 145c* which were drawn by the patient before his illness, representing classmates of his.

If we look through the series of drawings of this patient, we can establish that his work during the schizophrenic process was very different both in style and in content from his drawings made before his illness, as well as from those made during recovery.

In the most severe phase of his illness, he drew bizarre symbolical figures without any composition. As a consequence of the electric shock treatment, his drawings became schematic, primitive, and similar to children's drawings. During this regressive phase and at the beginning of the transition to recovery, he again drew some bizarre abstract portraits, but they had better composition; though they were still of unusual colors.

Later he drew more and more naturalistic pictures. On the portraits that he drew, the lines became gradually less unsettling. The colors were also becoming more natural. His last pictures were similar in technique to the ones he had painted before his illness. He drew landscapes seen from the windows of the hospital. These are naturalistic representations with excellent composition and the colors also correspond to the scene.

In viewing this patient's pictures, we can follow not only the course of the illness, but also the transitory influence of the electric shock treatment. This manifested itself clinically in amnesia and the resurfacing of childhood memories and, at the same time, his drawings showed regression and childlike style.

This patient showed a change in style at the beginning of his illness, then during the electric shock treatment and, again, his style changed during recovery, achieving the same quality of works as before his illness.

Following the first hospitalization this young patient completed high school and took courses in painting at the Academy of Fine Arts.

He continued to live in his mother's home, remained withdrawn and drew and painted almost all day. He continued this quiet lifestyle up to adulthood. He is now a middle-aged man who identifies himself as an artist painter and is a member of the artist painters association in Pécs. He had a successful one-man exhibit in a local art gallery.

Throughout the years he had to be hospitalized a few times for short periods, when he became delusional and voiced paranoid ideas. In the structured environment of the hospital he improved with psychotropic medication. He developed a trusting relationship with his physician at the hospital and accepted treatment readily.

During some of these hospitalizations he drew and painted pictures which reflected his exalted religious experiences. *Figure 146a* represents himself as "Christ crucified without the cross"; *Fig. 146b* is "Christ (himself) ascending to Heaven"; *Fig. 146c* is "An Angel (himself) with baby Jesus being adored by a woman"; *Fig. 146d* is a "Vision of extraordinary brilliance".

During another hospitalization he had a phase when he drew pornographic pictures. *Figure 147* is a surrealistic composition representing a woman in a provocative pose and attire, surrounded by unrelated details such as a detached arm and hand holding some flowers, other bizarre flower and tree shapes and geometrical figures.

Follow-up care is provided on an outpatient basis at a mental health clinic. He continues to take antipsychotic medication and reports regularly to the clinic where he is encouraged to continue painting. It was with the support of the clinic staff that Mr. Zs. H. prepared for the exhibit of his paintings. Nonetheless, the antici-

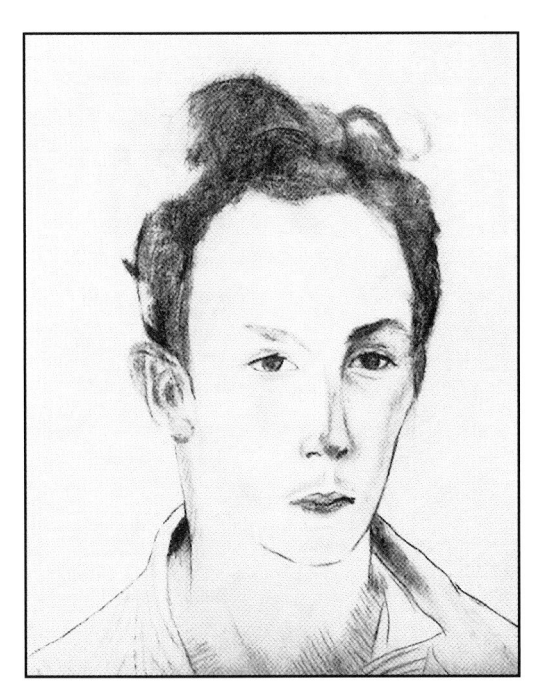

Case 16 - Fig. 145a
Colored crayon. 42x30

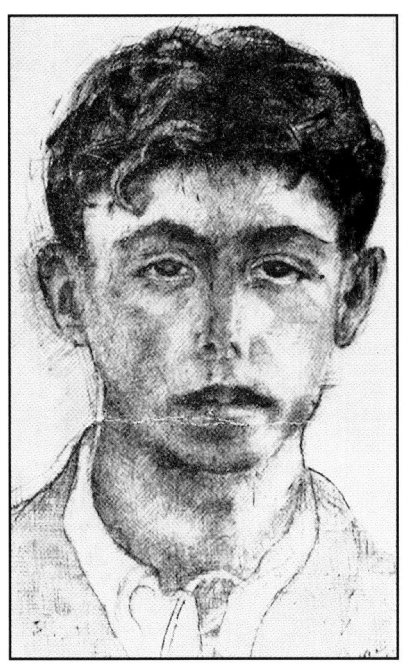

Case 16 - Fig. 145b
Pencil drawing. 42x30

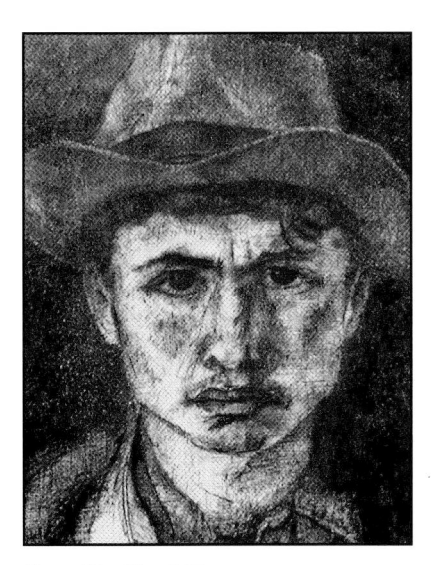

Case 16 - Fig. 145c
Pencil drawing. 42x30

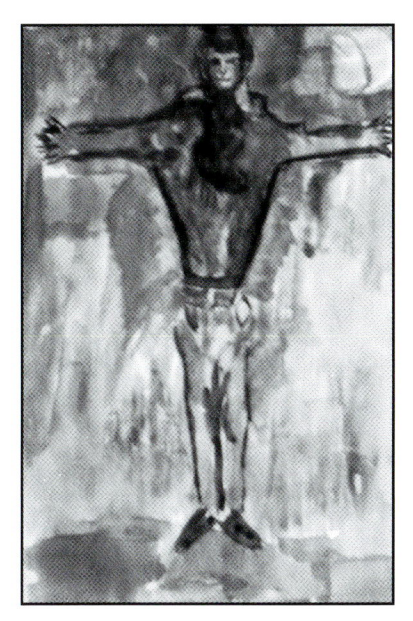

Case 16 - Fig. 146a
Tempera on cardboard. 42x30

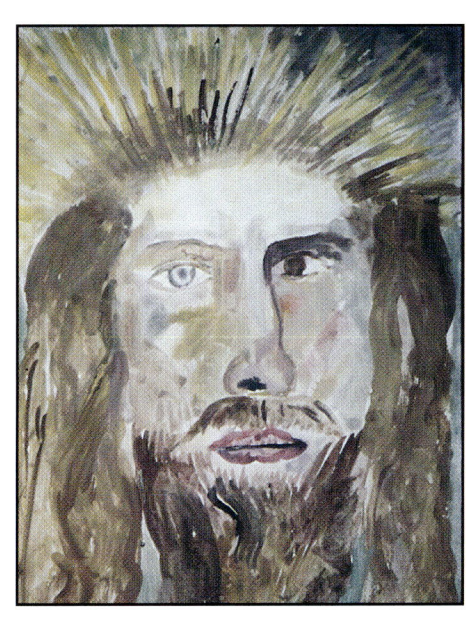

Case 16 - Fig. 146b
Tempera on cardboard. 42x30

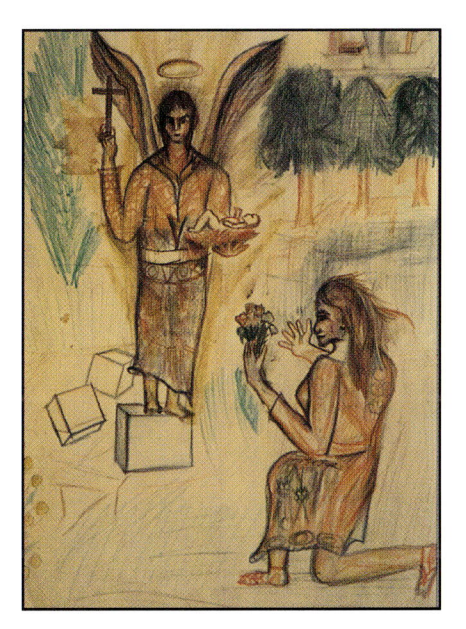

Case 16 - Fig. 146c
Colored crayon. 42x30

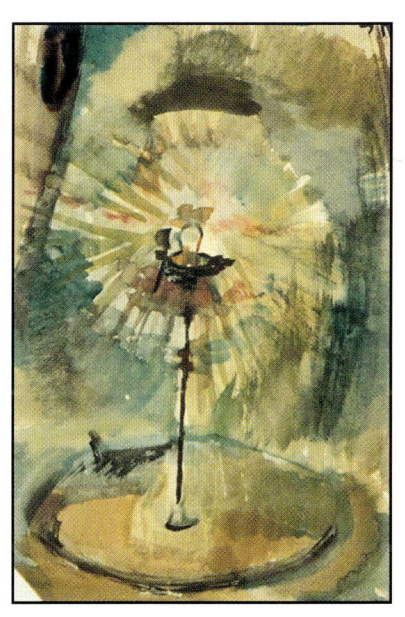

Case 16 - Fig. 146d
Tempera on cardboard. 42x30

139

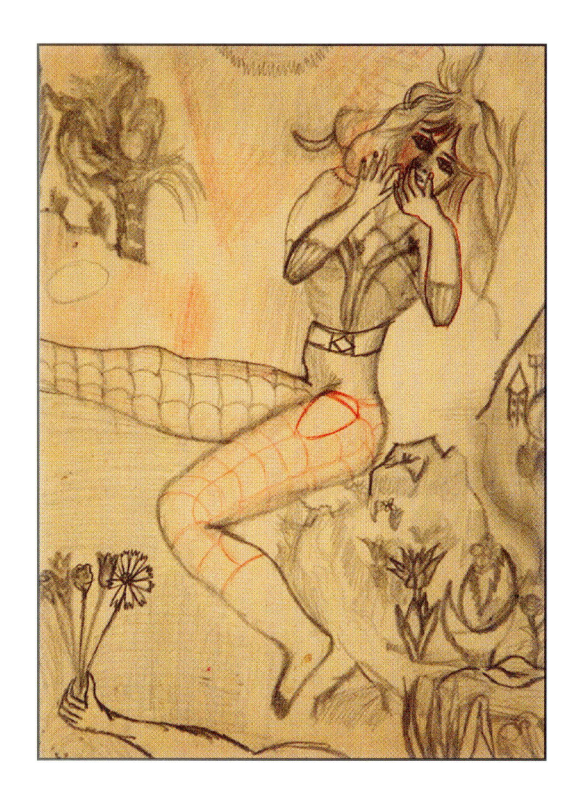

Case 16 - Fig. 147
Colored crayon. 42x30

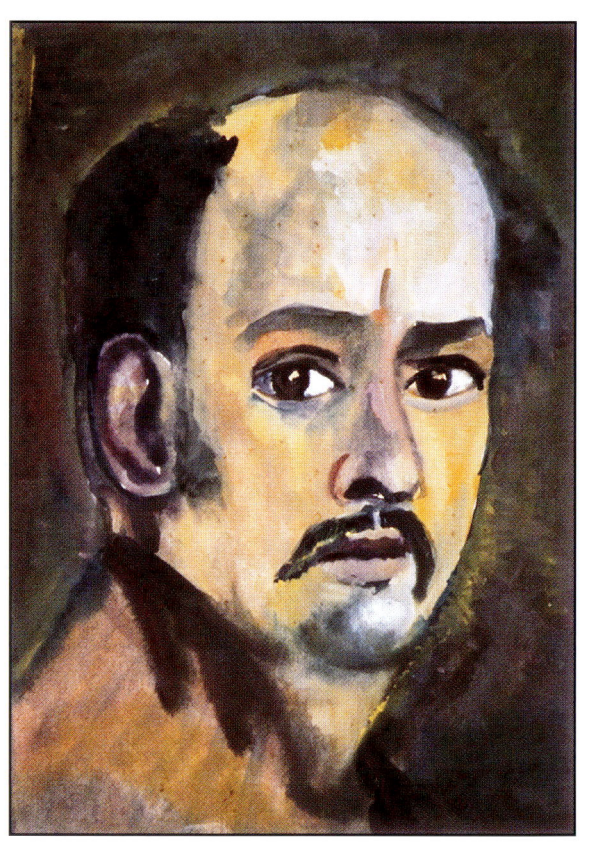

Case 16 - Fig. 148
Tempera on cardboard. 42x30

patory stress and anxiety about the success of the exhibit produced a relapse from which he recovered with a temporary increase in his medication.

In 1994 I visited the Psychiatric and Neurological University Hospital in Pécs where Zs. H. was my patient during his first hospitalization. Upon my return to Pécs, I inquired about some of my former patients; thus I found out about Zs. H.'s progress from his physicians at the hospital and at the outpatient clinic.

My visit to Pécs in 1994 coincided with the time of Zs. H.'s exhibit. The exhibit had just closed a few days before my arrival. When the doctor at the outpatient clinic told Zs. H. that I was in town and was interested in his artwork, he was ready to bring some of his paintings to the clinic. He remembered me very well (after 28 years!) and when he left his paintings in care of the clinic staff he left a message for me to select any of his paintings that I liked to take home to the United States with me. I did not have the opportunity to reach Zs. H. at that time, but enjoyed seeing his paintings and selected two of them offered to me as gifts by the painter, a self-portrait and a flower still life.

The self-portrait produced in 1994 is a very good likeness of the painter as I was told by his doctor at the clinic. Even I could recognize him by comparing his "adult face" to the self-portrait he painted at fourteen years of age. It is a well-composed painting. The picture is well balanced and the use of colors enhances the aesthetic appeal of the painting done with secure and strong tracing *(Fig. 148)*. Several consecutive self-portraits are performed with equal skill *(Figs 149a, 149b)*.

The flower still life I selected is one of several very well composed paintings. The geraniums (an often represented flower in Hungarian folk art) are arranged in a ceramic vase ornamented with stylized flowers, also a typical example of Hungarian folk art. The colors of this painting are harmonious and the centered motif of flowers in a vase is enhanced by a background done in soft colors. The painter was able to give the appearance of solid weight to the vase as compared to the light softness of the flowers. The use of light adds shape and dimension to this well balanced painting *(Fig. 150)*.

In 1995, I returned to Pécs as a visiting professor at the Psychiatric and Neurological University Hospital. During this stay I had the opportunity to visit Mr. Zs. H. at his home. He and his mother and one of his brothers graciously received me. Mr. Zs. H. called me Madame Doctor as he did at the time he was my patient. (I asked whether I should call him Mister H. or Zs. as I knew him as a youngster. He preferred to be called by his first name.) I was accompanied by his present physician who told the family that I was now a retired professor. From then on, I was addressed as Madame Professor—when occasionally during the conversation Mr. Zs. H. addressed me as Madame Doctor, he apologized and corrected himself, saying Madame Professor. He was visibly pleased to meet me after such a long time and, with excellent social graces, offered refreshments while he showed me his paintings. Some of his paintings are framed and decorate the walls of his home.

A large collection of several hundred drawings and paintings produced throughout the years is piled up on top of tables, and on the floor in his room where he works at a small table by the window. I was allowed to take a picture of the painter surrounded by his art work.

Furthermore, Mr. *Zs. H.* agreed to my photographing a large number of his drawings and paintings which I selected for their interest in revealing the phases of the changes in his style. While I was looking through his collection Mr. *Zs. H.* asked if he could draw a portrait of me. In a very short time he produced a pencil sketch of very good likeness and donated it to me.

Both he and his mother confirmed that he is rather a loner, although he occasionally goes to the meeting of the local artist painters.

His appetite is good (he is even concerned about being overweight). He sleeps well. His routine physical and laboratory checkups are within normal limits. He smokes one to two packs of cigarettes a day—sometimes more.

He likes to read art books and occasionally copies the pictures of ancient or classical medieval art works. These are excellent copies, some painted in oil, some done in crayon *(Figs 151a, 151b)*. These are copies made of pictures of different sizes, and are all enlarged by the artist as he copied them to fill the papers of 29.5 × 42 cm he uses for most of his drawings.

I visited Mr. *Zs. H.* again in 1996 and 1997 and I was received warmly by the patient and his family. Mr. *Zs. H.* showed me his drawings and paintings produced since my last visit. He also allowed me to take photographs of several of these artworks selected by me, based on the same criteria as previously, to illustrate the different styles he was attempting.

**The analysis of the drawings and paintings of *Zs. H.* is based on a 28-year follow-up of the clinical history and the pictorial material.**

*The artwork of Zs. H. can be assigned to several categories* differing both in their style and in the content of the representations.

*Group 1. Self-portraits* painted throughout the years. They are done in different media: tempera, acrylic or oil. Each is a good likeness in realistic style *(Figs 148, 149a, 149b)*.

Lately, he also made a series of twenty self-portraits in crayon on very small and thin paper squares. The facial expression in his self-portraits is somber, maybe somewhat depressed and occasionally giving the impression of aloofness, but in general they reflect the artist possessing self-esteem and holding eye contact with the viewer (the mirror).

*Group 2. Portraits of the painter's mother*

These are well balanced pictures in warm colors. Throughout the years they show the gradually aging face of the mother *(Figs 152a, 152b)*.

*Group 3. Paintings of a woman's head or torso*

There are more than one hundred paintings of this subject (an imaginary woman). A few are executed in naturalistic colors, but the majority of these are pictures with a rigid facial expression done in unusual even bizarre colors. It is always the same picture with a somewhat stylized face, producing a disquieting impression. According to the artist, he likes to "paint her" in different colors as he sees and as he likes it. This is an imaginary painting, not a hallucination *(Figs 153a–h)*.

*Group 4. Paintings of hermaphrodites*

These are huge naked human figures with explicit male genitalia and female breasts. The figures are outlined in color but in general they appear two-dimensional and rigid, almost statue-like instead of being realistic human shapes. The only comment of the artist on these

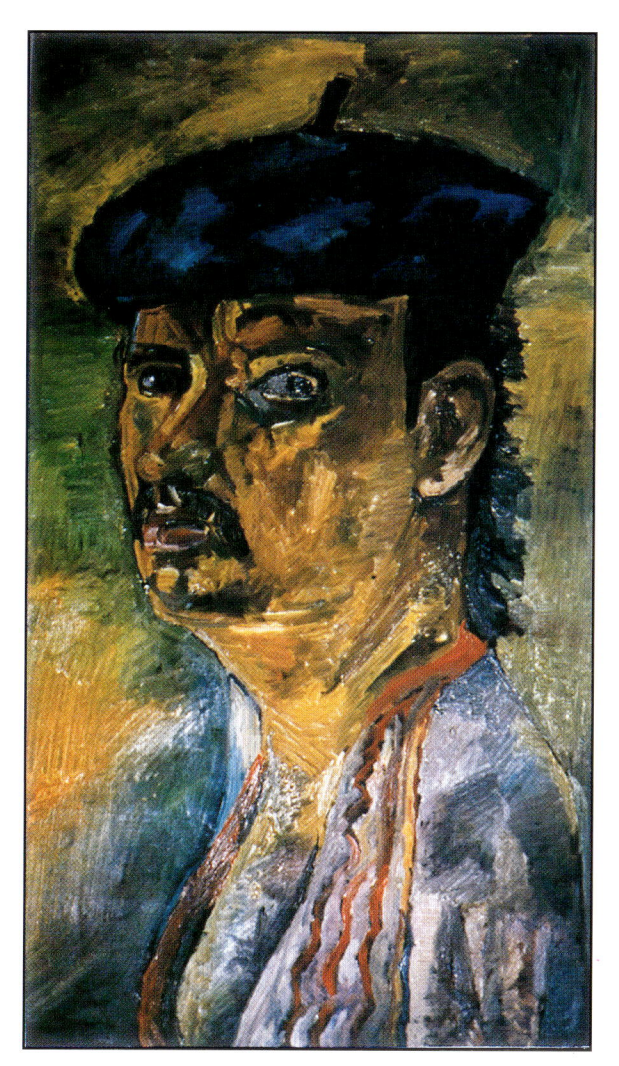

Case 16 - Fig. 149a
Tempera on cardboard. 42x30

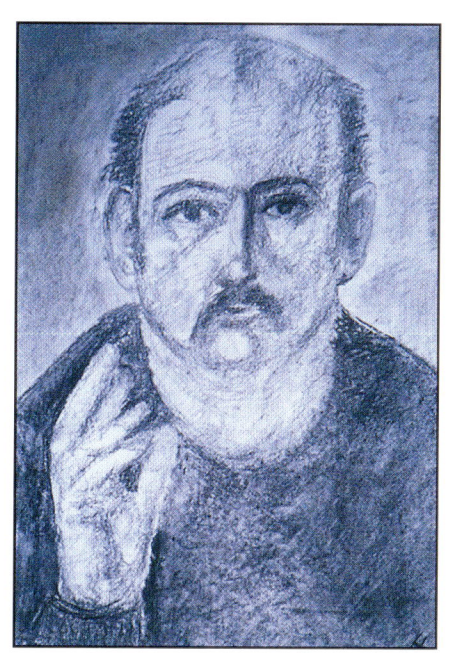

Case 16 - Fig. 149b
Pencil drawing. 42x30

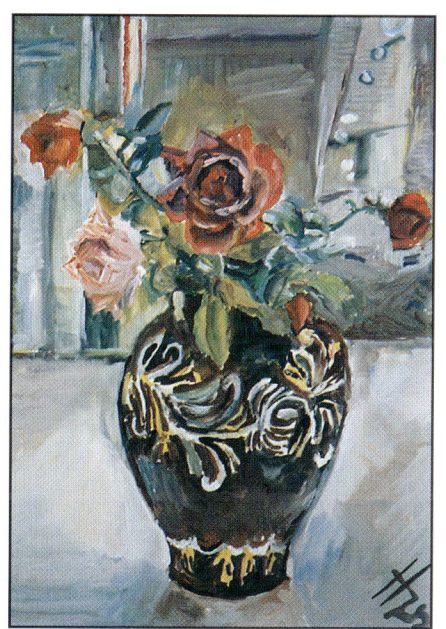

Case 16 - Fig. 150
Oil on canvas. 57x32

143

Case 16 - Fig. 151a
Pencil drawing. 29.5x42

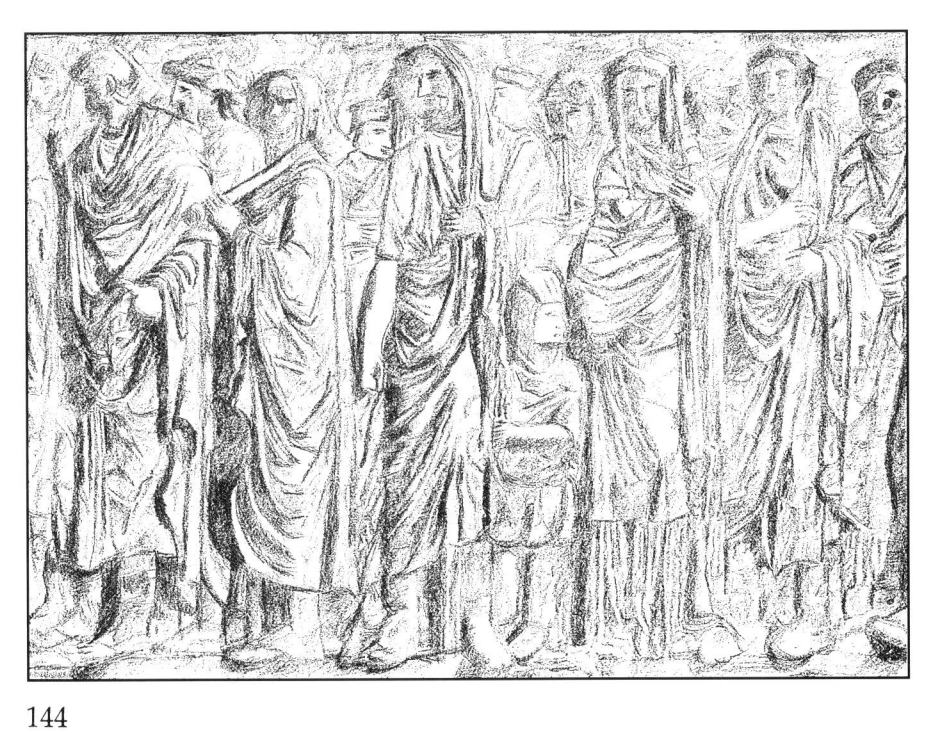

Case 16 - Fig. 151b
Pencil drawing. 29.5x42

Case 16 - Fig. 152a
Oil on canvas. 42x30

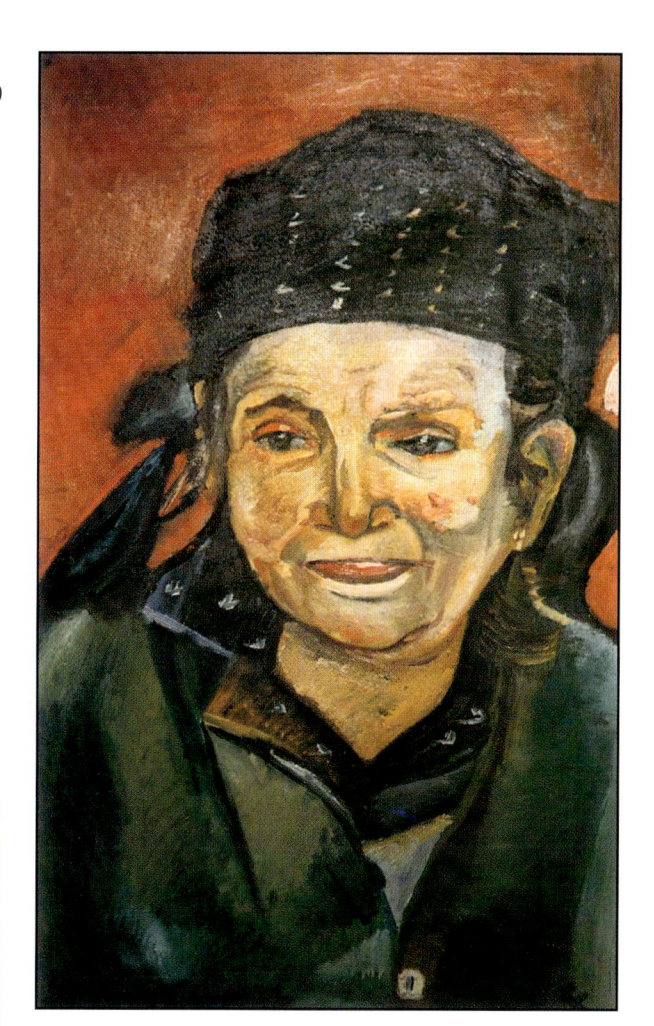

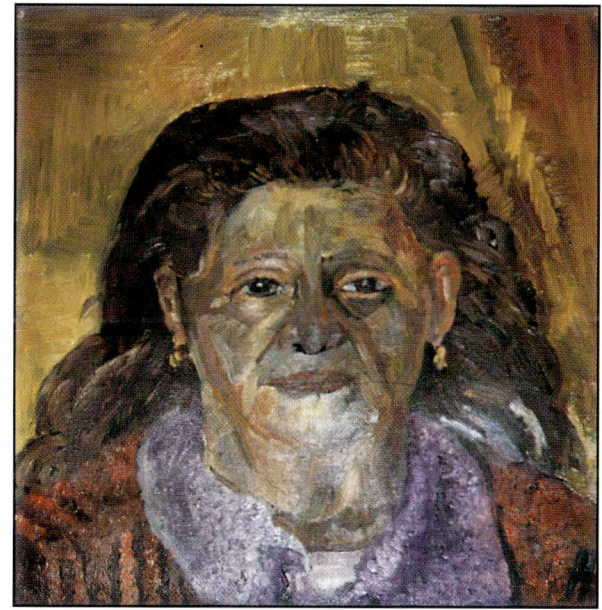

Case 16 - Fig. 152b
Oil on canvas. 42x30

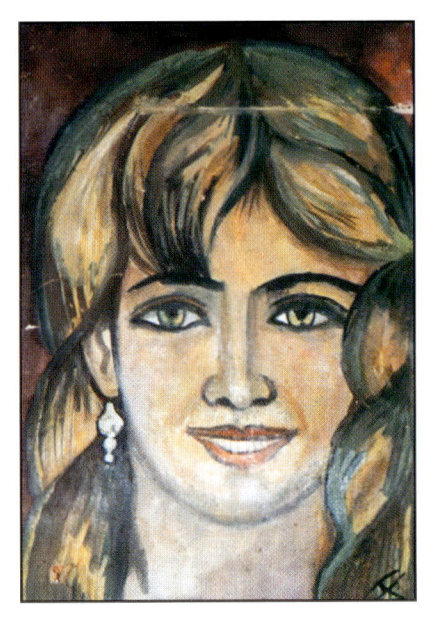

Case 16 - Fig. 153a
Tempera on cardboard. 42x30

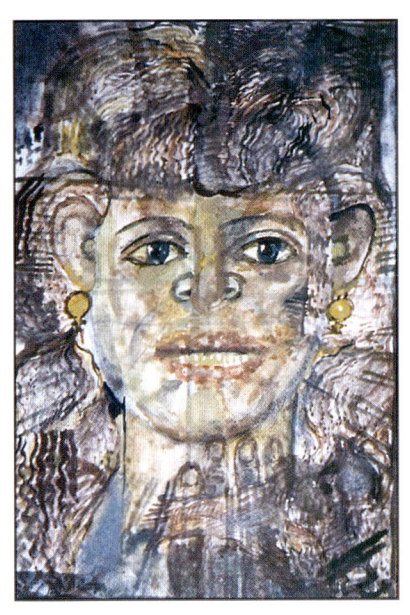

Case 16 - Fig. 153b
Tempera on cardboard. 42x30

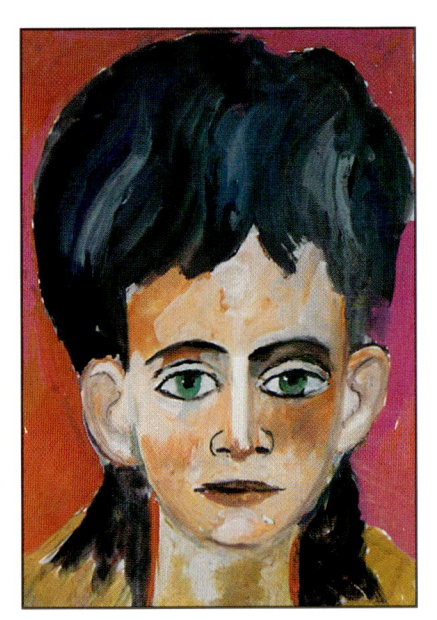

Case 16 - Fig. 153c
Tempera on cardboard. 42x30

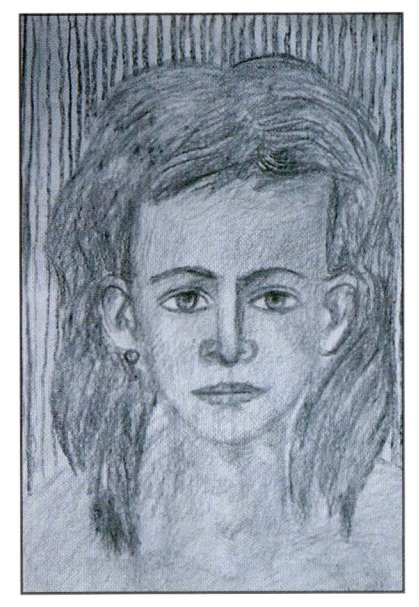

Case 16 - Fig. 153d
Pencil drawing. 42x30

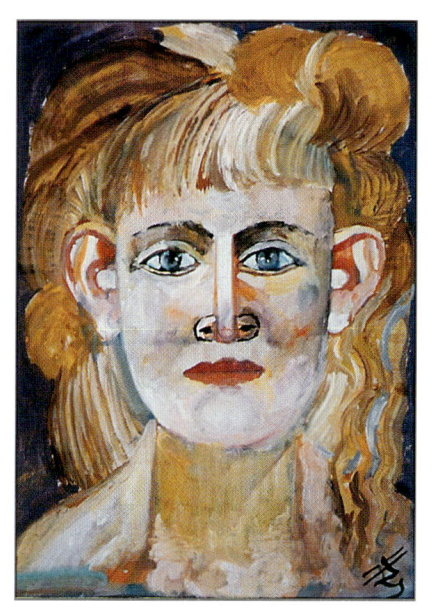

Case 16 - Fig. 153e
Tempera on cardboard. 42x30

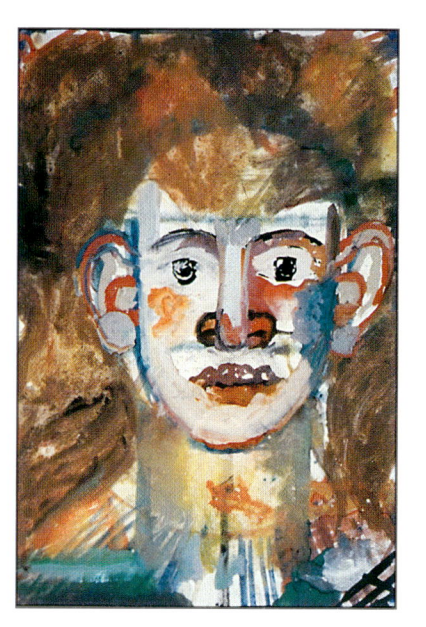

Case 16 - Fig. 153f
Tempera on cardboard. 42x30

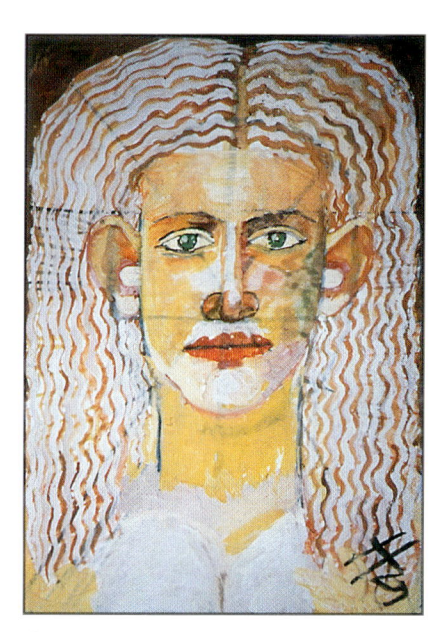

Case 16 - Fig. 153g
Tempera on cardboard. 42x30

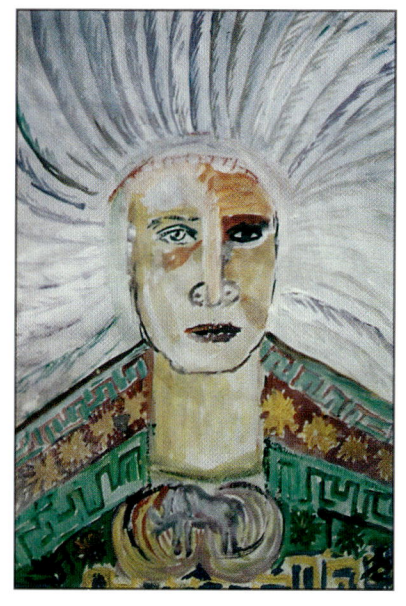

Case 16 - Fig. 153h
Tempera on cardboard. 42x30

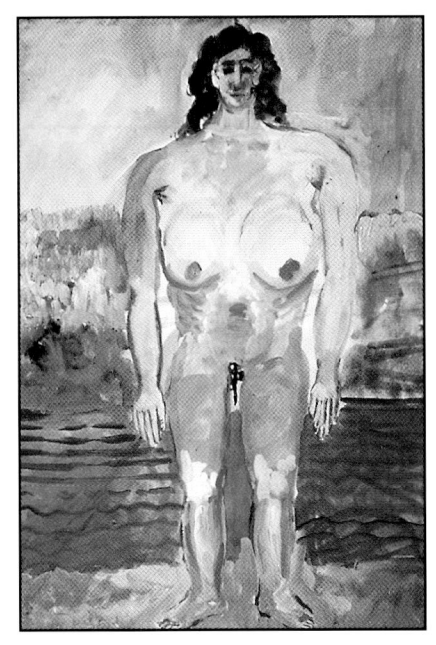

Case 16 - Fig. 154a
Tempera on cardboard. 42x30

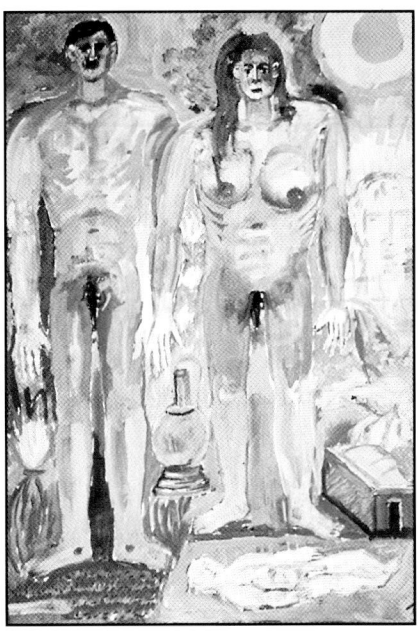

Case 16 - Fig. 154b
Tempera on cardboard. 42x30

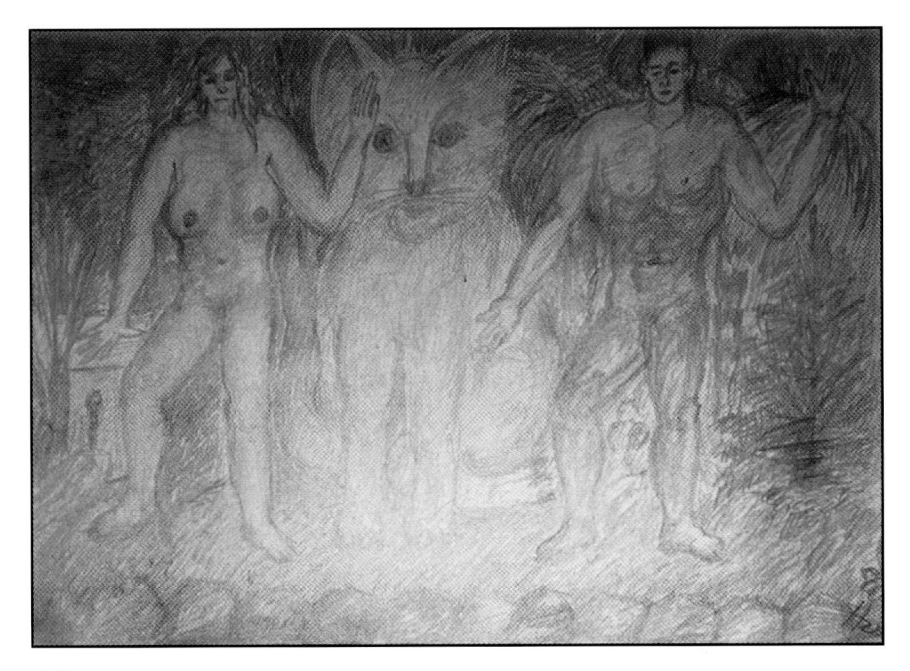

Case 16 - Fig. 154c
Pencil drawing. 30x42

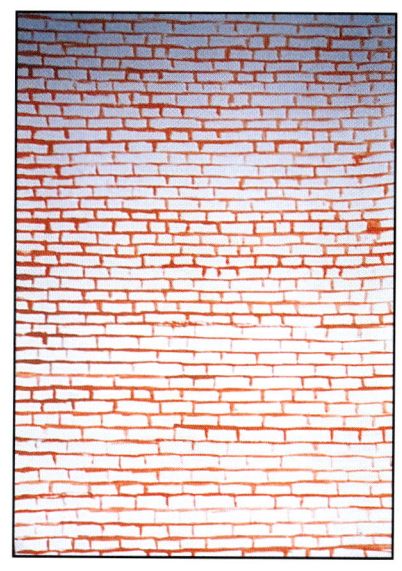

Case 16 - Fig. 155a
Tempera on cardboard. 42x30

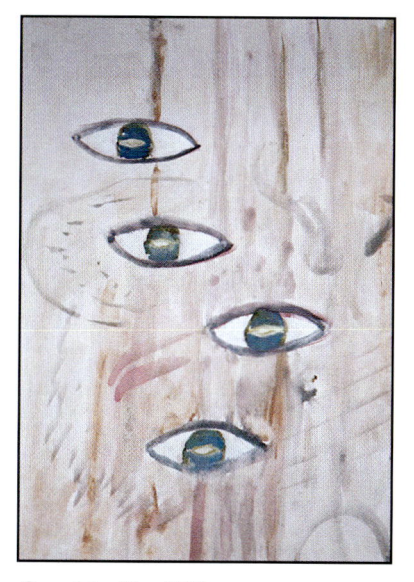

Case 16 - Fig. 155b
Tempera on cardboard. 42x30

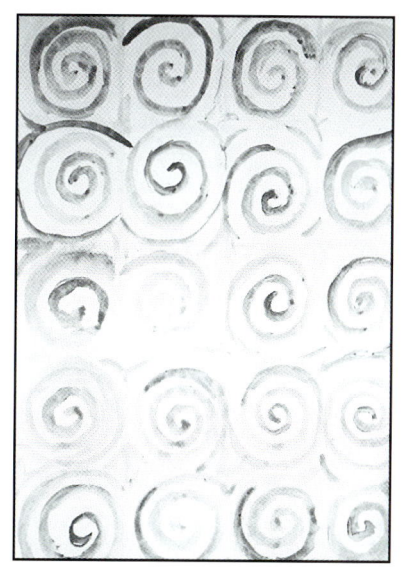

Case 16 - Fig. 155c
Tempera on cardboard. 42x30

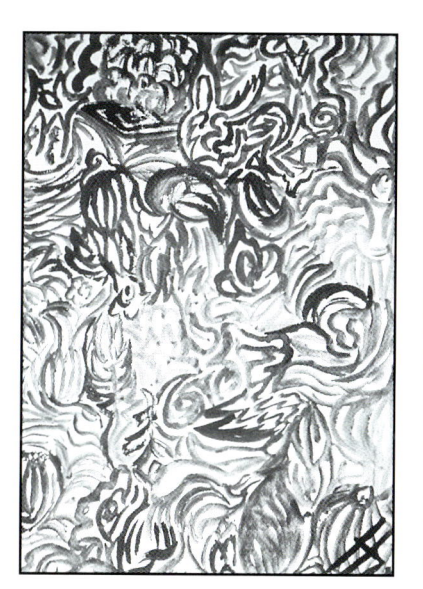

Case 16 - Fig. 155d
Tempera on cardboard. 42x30

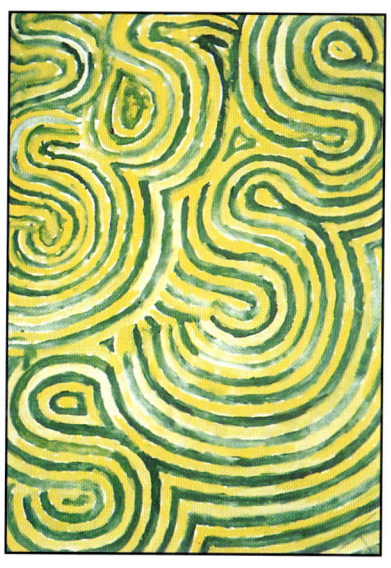

Case 16 - Fig. 155e
Tempera on cardboard. 42x30

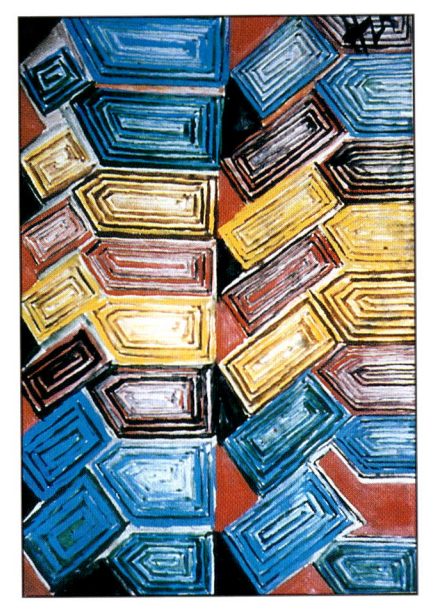

Case 16 - Fig. 156a
Tempera on cardboard. 30x42

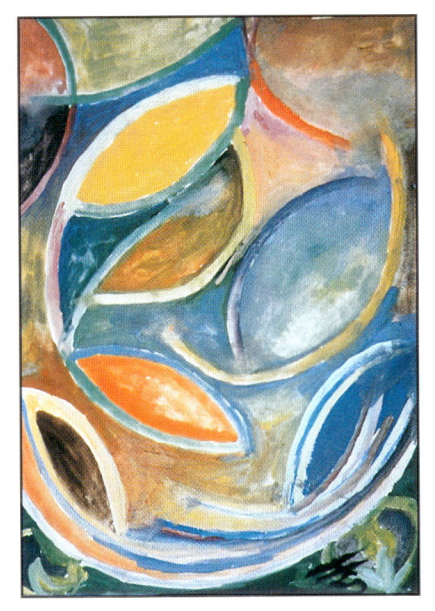

Case 16 - Fig. 156b
Tempera on cardboard. 42x30

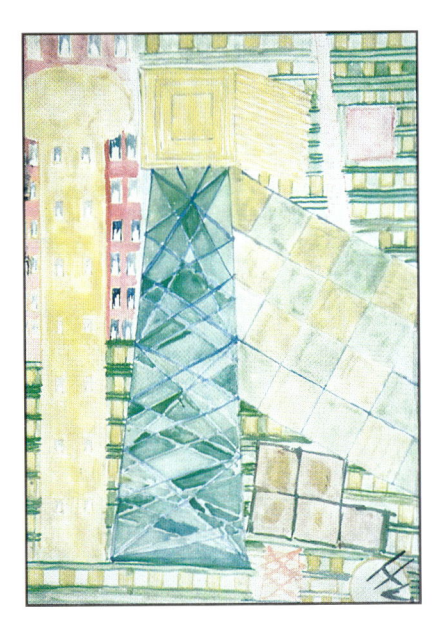

Case 16 - Fig. 156c
Tempera on cardboard. 42x30

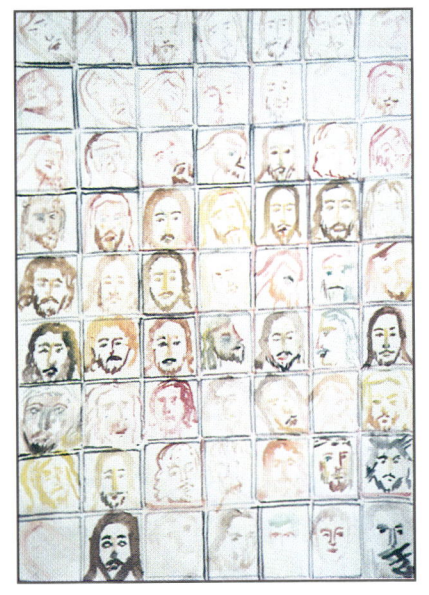

Case 16 - Fig. 156d
Tempera on cardboard. 75x55

Case 16 - Fig. 157a
Tempera on cardboard. 42x30

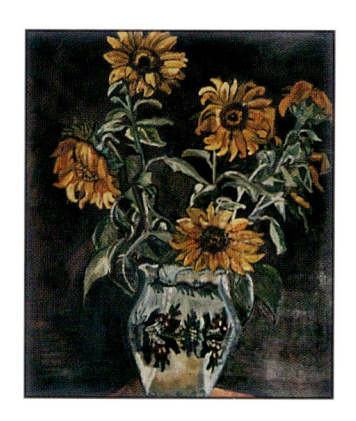

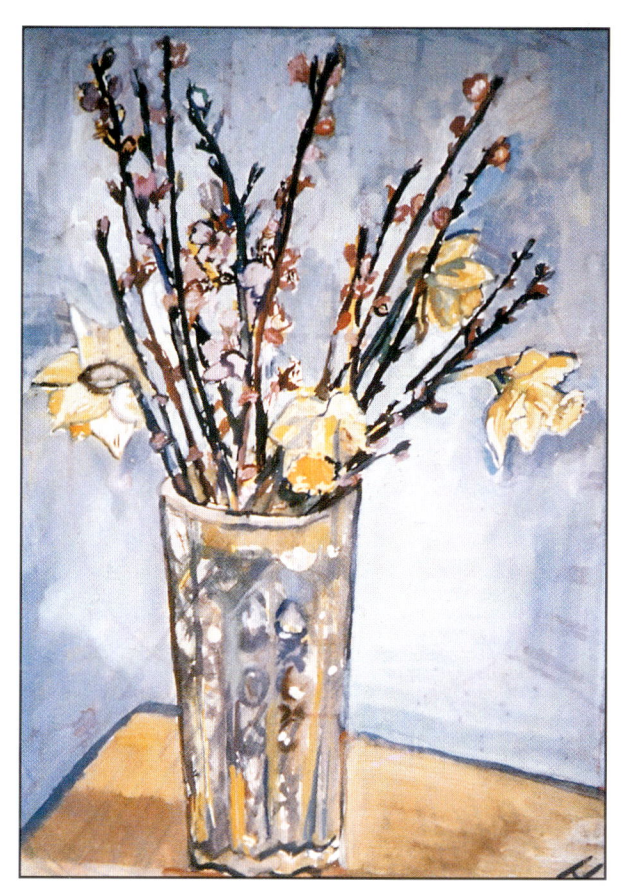

Case 16 - Fig. 157b
Tempera on cardboard. 42x30

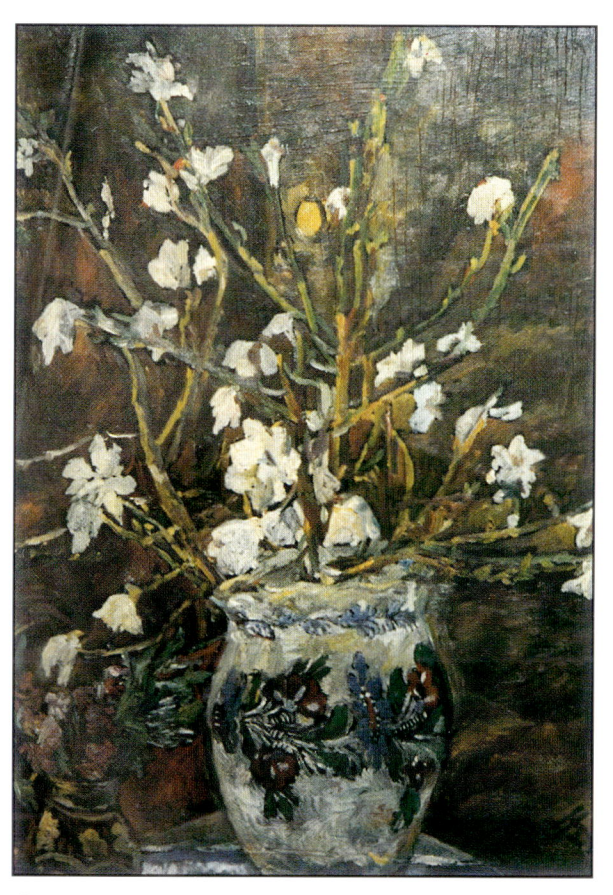

Case 16 - Fig. 157c
Tempera on cardboard. 42x30

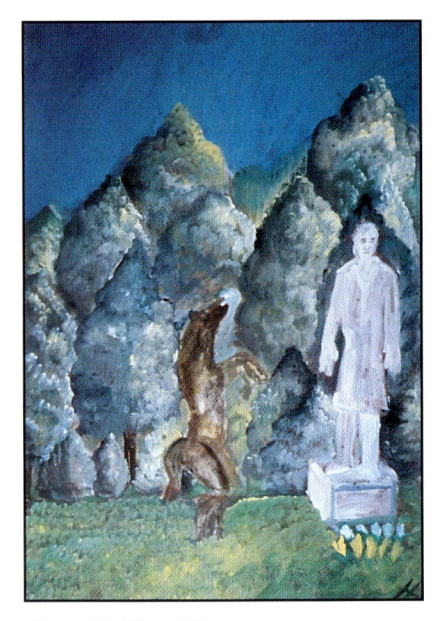

Case 16 - Fig. 158a
Tempera on cardboard. 42x30

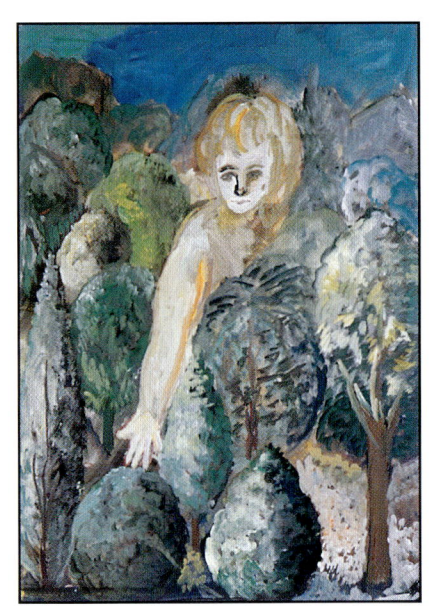

Case 16 - Fig. 158b
Tempera on cardboard. 42x30

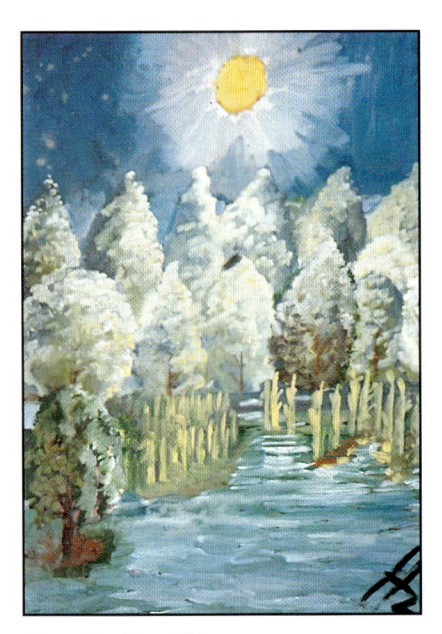

Case 16 - Fig. 158c
Tempera on cardboard. 42x30

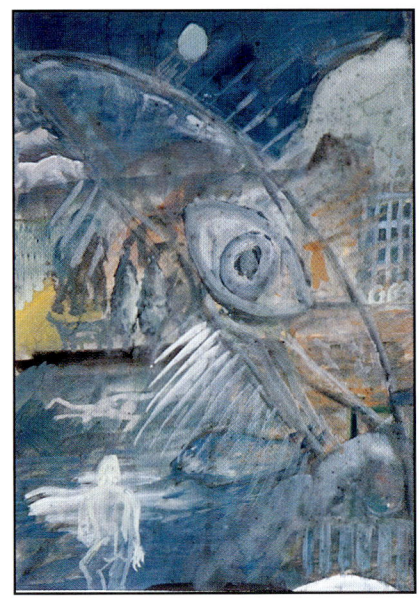

Case 16 - Fig. 158d
Tempera on cardboard. 42x30

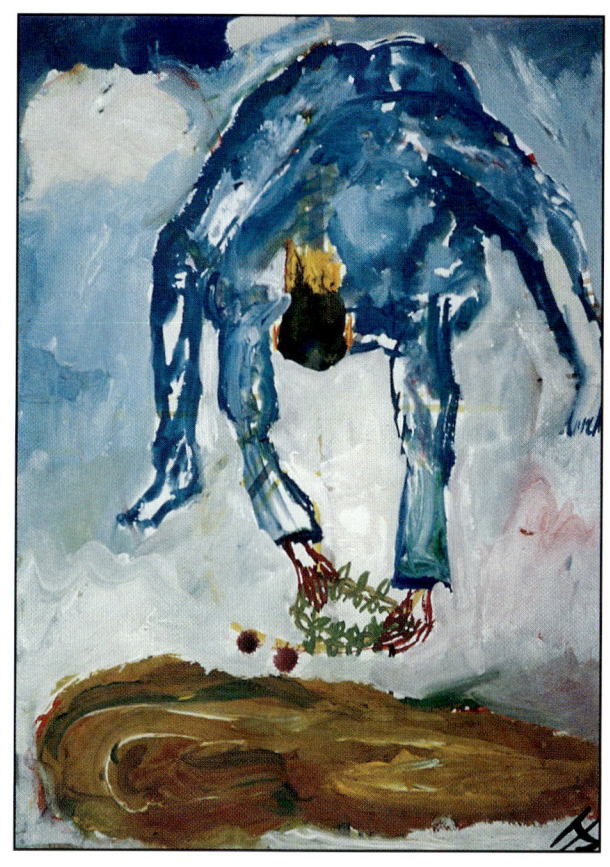

Case 16 - Fig. 159
Tempera on cardboard. 42x30

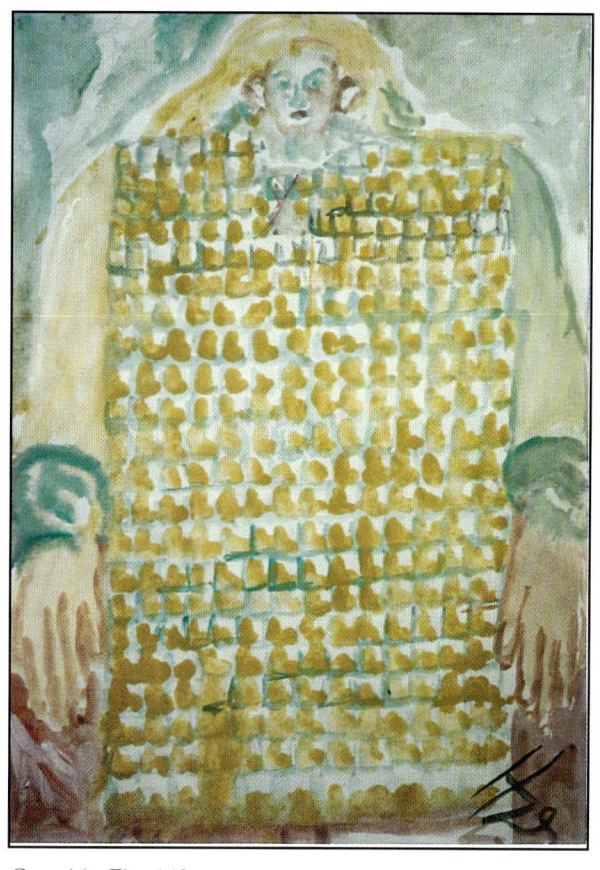

Case 16 - Fig. 160
Tempera on cardboard. 42x30

pictures was "sometimes I just feel like painting these" *(Figs 154a–c)*.

*Group 5. Stereotype nonfigurative paintings*
The whole surface is covered by repeated lines and geometrical shapes: among these works we find some which show a compulsive neatness of the repeated forms like the "brick wall" *(Fig. 155a)*, done in red tempera, or blue eyes with a purple background *(Fig. 155b)*. Sometimes the lines form spirals *(Fig. 155c)*, or masses of lines in different brown tones *(Fig. 155d)*. He produced a similar picture of interwoven yellow and green wavy lines *(Fig. 155e)*.

Others are pleasing colorful compositions of sometimes harmonizing colors *(Figs 156a, 156b)*. *Figure 156c* is a mosaic of colorful geometrical shapes and lines on which a high and narrow house with many windows and a "mushroom cap" are also represented. As a contrast to these

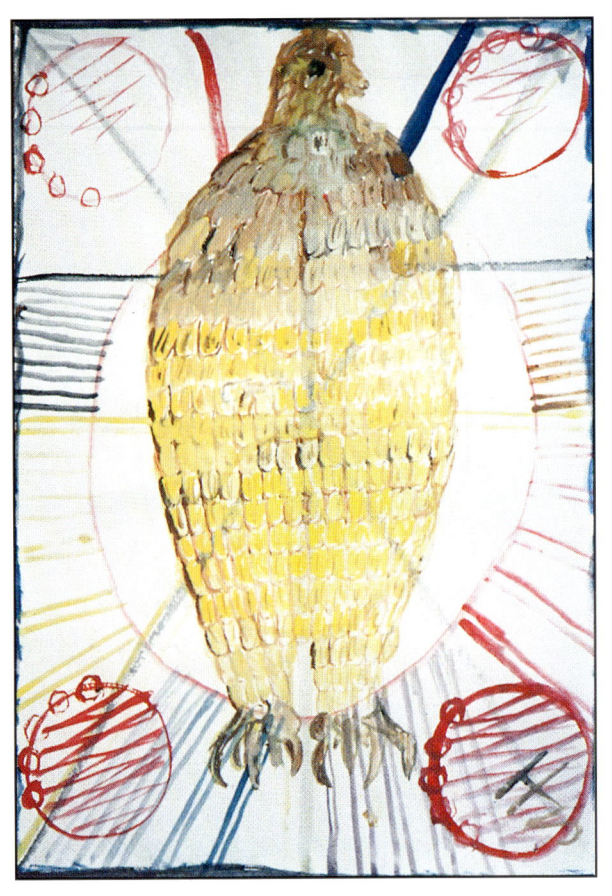

Case 16 - Fig. 161
Tempera on cardboard. 42x30

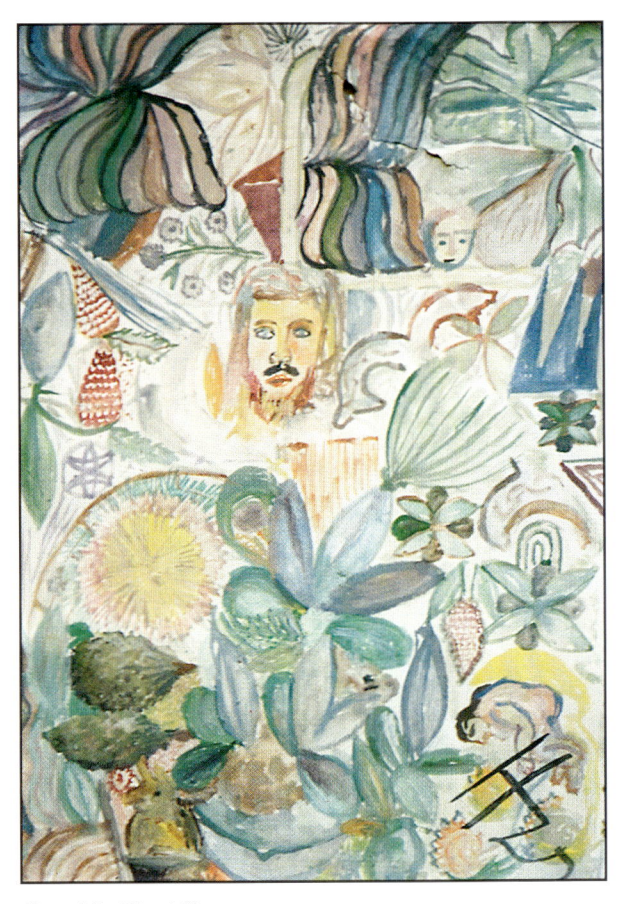

Case 16 - Fig. 162
Tempera on cardboard. 42x30

pictures, in *Fig. 156d* there are several portraits in a grid.

*Group 6. Naturalistic landscapes and flowers still lives*

Zs. H. painted several landscapes. Some are representations of different views of the city of Pécs and of its environs done in naturalistic style. He also has three sketchpads filled with paintings of the cabin on the small vineyard owned by his family where he spent time during several summers. Some of these paintings are naturalistic representations; others are quite gloomy, almost surrealistic and certainly give the impression of a depressed mood.

The naturalistic landscapes are less accomplished than his portraits—the composition is still balanced but the perspective may not al-

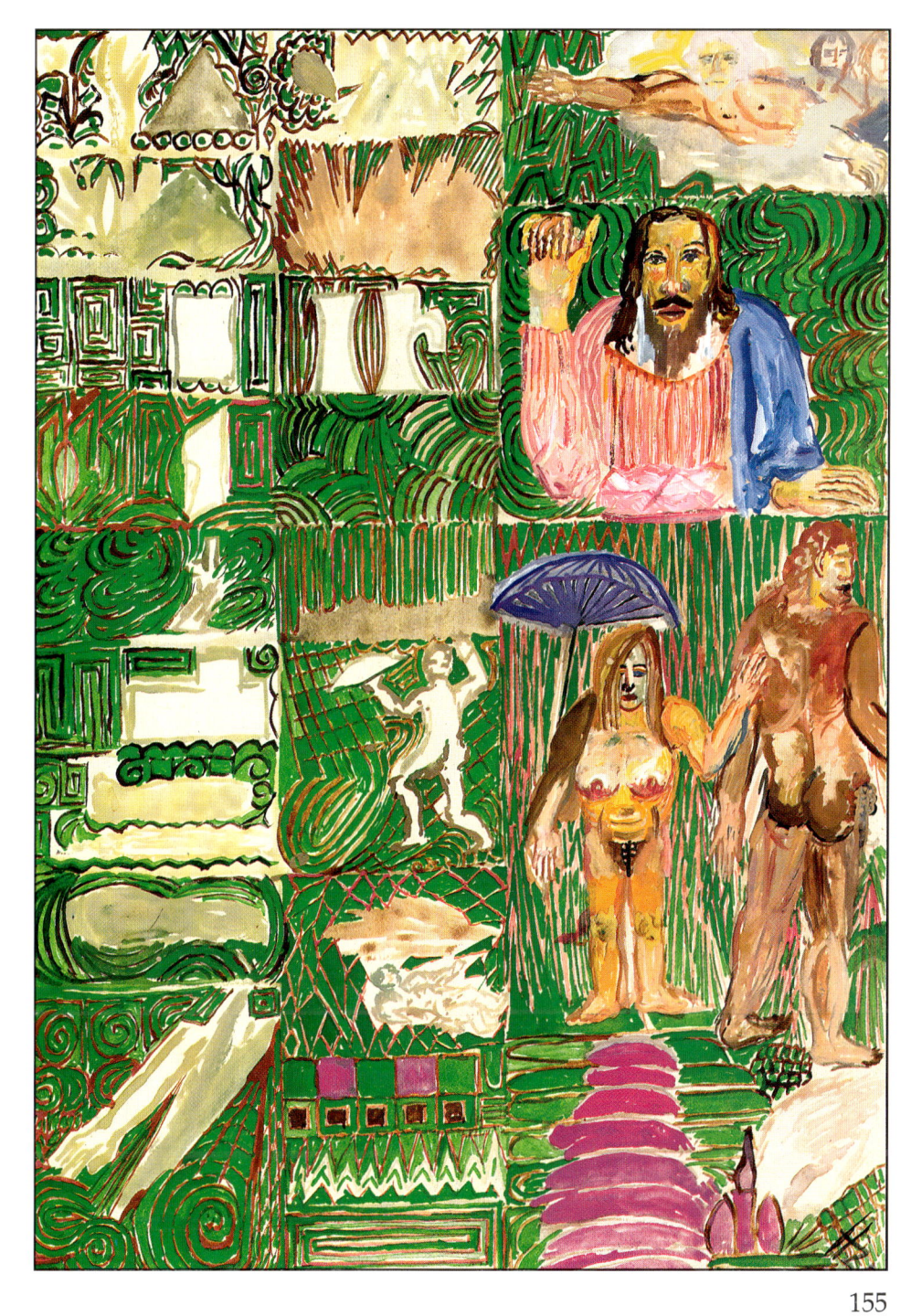

Case 16 - Fig. 163
Watercolor
on cardboard. 42x29.5

155

ways reflect the depth in the relationship of the different elements of the composition. The colors are naturalistic. The foreground and background may blend into a two-dimensional detail in some parts of the pictures.

The flower still lifes are very delicate naturalistic representations. The patient likes to collect the flowers himself (*Figs 157a–c* and the previously shown picture of geranium, *Fig. 149*).

*Group 7. Fantasy landscapes*

There are only a few such paintings among the hundreds of his artworks. Their style is the closest to surrealistic painting. These are some of his latest works. The shapes are well outlined but the relative size of objects is unnatural; for example, a horse standing on his hind legs is as tall as the trees of the forest surrounding the clearing on which this mythical animal is depicted. The composition is balanced. The colors are soft, mostly muted bluish green. The whole picture has a dreamlike quality (not a nightmare) with a pleasant and almost serene appearance *(Fig. 158a)*.

On *Fig. 158b* which is also a dreamlike landscape of a forest in very delicate green color, a woman's figure is emerging from among the trees. This certainly is to be considered a surrealistic painting. In *Fig. 158c* stereotypic rows of trees stand in water illuminated by a large sun centered above them. This is not a serene, but a disquieting picture.

*Figure 158d* is truly a surrealistic landscape with ghostlike figures swimming or standing in the water in the foreground, while a transparent shape of an "eye" (as explained by the patient) merges from the water. The background of this scene consists of a landscape with a building and trees. It is a night-scene illuminated by the moon. This may be the representation of a vision.

*Group 8. Symbolical paintings*

*Figure 159* represents a man (the artist) holding a laurel wreath "falling into an abyss from the height of the sky". It is a depressive scene of losing self-confidence, a vision.

*Figure 160* is unique in style among this patient's paintings. He gave no explanation as to what (or whom) it represents. The enormous body clothed in a dress of a stereotypic pattern (almost like a chain armor) supports a relatively very small head of a woman with long blond hair. The arms and hands are also massive shapes. The figure stands in a rigid posture. Is it some goddess, or just a very powerful woman?

*Figure 161* shows a huge bird covered by a stereotypical, regular plumage which is similar to the dress of the woman in the previous picture. Maybe this huge bird also represents some kind of an idol. The bird is surrounded by radial lines, while the four corners of the picture are decorated by red circles. The artist gave no explanation to this picture.

*Figure 162* is a surrealistic picture in which human faces and body and motives of plants are painted in harmonious colors. The space between the motives is filled with abstract forms.

*Figure 163* is also surrealistic in style. According to the painter it is the representation of a vision of the figure and the head of Christ as he has seen it and then filled the background in colorful abstract designs. This is one of his latest paintings made in 1997.

After reviewing these paintings and drawings made in different styles, it is important to point out that this artist does not have any periods of certain length of time in which he would work in any given style, as it is seen in the works of other painters who changed styles in different phases of their illness or recovery (FERDIÈRE 1951, MEYER 1954). *Zs. H.* changes the style of his artworks several times a day. He alternates between the representations of fantasies or visions stereotype geometrical products, naturalistic portraits or still lifes and miniature copies of pictures of classical art. Similar rapid changes in style were observed during several consecutive art therapy sessions by JAKAB (1968). That patient suffered from paranoid schizophrenia with depressive traits. While in a psychotic state, she draw pictures in three different styles within the hour of art therapy session, always in the same sequence: first, a confused scribbling, followed by a rigid geometrical design in a frame and finally a symbolical naturalistic representation of her feelings or of other paranoid ideas. The scribbling was id-material, the next geometrical design provided ego control and finally, she could face and represent her painful emotions in conveying these in a naturalistic style.

We may infer that the rapid changes in style of *Zs. H.* may have a similar psychological background, although we have not done an extensive interview about the actual sequences of the changes in his style. It is possible that after painting some intensive and occasionally disturbing visions, the painter takes refuge from the overwhelming emotions in producing stereotype, rigid, geometrical drawings, or copying pictures from books on classical art. When this later style achieved a calming effect (ego boundaries re-established), he was again able to produce realistic works, some of which may be symbolical compositions. The rapid changes in style may well be part of the self-healing produced by integrating the surfacing id material into a structured and conscious artistic expression.

As an explanation to his selection of different subjects and style *Zs. H.* says: "I just feel like painting one thing or another and I do it so that it would be right". Apparently the choice of subject and of style reflects his affective state at the time of producing the artwork. He does agree that his mood is fluctuating and that it influences his paintings.

In general he is satisfied with his paintings although when talking about them he is very modest about their artistic value.

Neither the quality of his artistic talent and his technical ability nor his drive to create have been influenced negatively by the use of medications. This case is certainly a success story about the recovery from psychosis and about long-term maintenance on psychotropic medication.

# THE CHARACTERISTICS OF DRAWINGS AND PAINTINGS OF PSYCHIATRIC PATIENTS FROM THE ARTISTIC POINT OF VIEW

The majority of works of mentally ill patients published up to 1956 do not attempt to assess the art of the mentally ill person from the artistic point of view, except in some individual cases. As mentioned by ANASTASI and FOLEY (1941), in the literature we find only rarely a systematic analysis of the art of the mentally ill from the artistic point of view.

An exception is the work published by VOLMAT in 1956. In general, the authors are preoccupied in an arbitrary way by one or another of the artistic qualities of the works. In the majority, they call attention only to the change in style in those cases where that is very evident (FERDIÈRE 1951, KAPLAN and SAKHEIM 1955, MEYER 1954). Others are content with indicating the originality of the use of colors. According to PRINZHORN (1922), in some cases the colors choke off the forms of the composition. Furthermore, the motives of forms, meant originally as representations, go beyond this original meaning, giving an ornamental character to the work. Other authors show the strange way of tracing the lines; ZIESE (1953) refers to the isolation of formal elements and the replacement of the logical subordinations by simple mechanical repetitions. According to ZIESE, in the works of schizophrenic patients there is no "movement" and there are no "nuances". The colors are only placed side by side, and instead of contributing to the harmony of transition they produce an effect of separation. REITMAN (1948) describes the following characteristics of the mentally ill patients' drawings: condensation, symbolism, pictorial agglutination, stereotypy and perseverance, while at other times the lack of integration, a chaotic organization and the choice of inadequate colors is characteristic. FERDIÈRE (1947a, 1951) analyzes the drawings of schizophrenic patients from the point of view of the form and the fashion of tracing the lines. According to him, the schizophrenics who draw for the first time in a state of psychosis create a new style with a morbid and original technique.

In our opinion, the patients express themselves by insufficient media; nonetheless they make remarkable efforts at expressing themselves while, at the same time, disregarding the rules and principles of the aesthetics of the arts. They express themselves at all costs, and the result, although without a specific style and even without a real artistic goal, is frequently a touching expression of their experiences.

The totality of these works provides the physician with a rich ground for research: one can discover the symptoms of the illness. Below we describe only certain characteristic traits based on our observations.

# THE CONTENT

Based on the study of the works of our patients we faced the following questions: Are there any subjects in the patients' art which have not yet been expressed in the fine arts? Our answer is negative. The psychological field of the works of the mentally ill is more restricted than that of normal works of art. Nonetheless, we may see an enriched content in the patients' art, when they represent their hallucinations, and the bizarre symbolism born of their illusions. The works of the mentally ill have most frequently a repressed (latent) content disguised by the manifest subject.

## *Manifest Content*

Our collection is lacking in ornamental designs.

The themes are stereotyped: landscapes without figures or with human figures and, if there are human figures they are in general not represented in action.

Some of our patients have drawn the city and the view of the garden of the clinic *(Figs 46a–c, 47, 90, 126)*.

Works on religious subjects are relatively rare in our material. F. B. (Case 14) represented Saint Anthony in the form of a monk in a kneeling position *(Fig. 125)*. Mrs. A. P. (Case 3) did some portraits of Saint Anthony *(Figs 32 and 33)* in the form of postage stamps which is an unusual manner of representation among religious paintings.

S. F. (Case 11) represented his religious vision through weak lines in crayon which are almost imperceptible on a dark blue background *(Fig. 107)*. This is probably based on the recollection of an antique painting—evoked in his delirious state. That same patient drew the holy family in a bizarre way on an Easter greeting card *(Fig. 102)*. The strange symbolism of Miss R. A. (Case 8) appears to us in the very presentation of the "Celestial Rose" *(Fig. 85)*. Zs. H. (Case 16) often represents his religious visions *(Figs 138, 146a–d, 163)*.

Among the works of our patient L. I. (Case 1) who had been a student at the engineering college, we find some mechanical structures *(Figs 11 and 13)*, which are as incomprehensible as the fantastic and primitive machines of A. J. (Case 5) who had no technical education *(Figs 54 and 55)*.

Action scenes are rare. The movement is missing in the pictures which, through the presence of several figures, should give the impression of scenes. They produce the effect of "living tableaux" instead of looking like a piece of an action.

The greatest variety and the most striking effects are produced by the representations of hallucinations. This is explained by the fact that their subject is most distant from any sensation experienced by normal persons. This is a world which approaches that of dreams and of children's fantasies.

The subject of the drawings only rarely correlates with the delusions of our patients. Nonetheless, they disclose their megalomania in their self-portraits where they represent themselves as kings, film stars, generals, etc. and express their identities in added writing [*Figs 16a* and

*17d* by L. I. (Case 1) and *Fig. 120* by L. V. (Case 13)]. Some of the works of N. N. (Case 15) were inspired by his hallucinations and by his delusions of jealousy connected to them.

## Symbolic Content

According to PRINZHORN (1922), the drawings of the mentally ill are autistic hieroglyphs, the key to which is only known by the patient. We agree also with the opinion of DELAY (1952) who declares that one cannot interpret the symbols of patients unless the patient himself gives information about them. UHLIN (1969b) points out the descriptive character of symbols in the art of a schizophrenic girl. With reference to the fine arts PRUYSER (1968) interprets the symbol of the Holy Ghost and its emblems.

We do not plan to enter into detailed psychoanalytical interpretations of the symbolism of the art works in our collection, although this is a tempting way of understanding their symbolism.

Among the works of our schizophrenic patients we find several symbolical expressions which are not comprehensible with the help of conventional symbols. Here are some examples.

Mrs. A. P. (Case 3) expressed her suffering in self portraits in *Figs 29* and *30*: Blood is dripping from the stone heart attached to her neck, while a little angel is chiseling it. Her self-portrait in *Fig. 31* acquires a strange significance through the discrepancy between the saintly halo and the blasé expression of the woman with a cigarette between her lips.

The pictures of L. I. (Case 1) resembling a torpedo are conceived as female figures with accentuated genital organs. Their abstract schematic forms have a double symbolical meaning if one considers the frame itself as a phallic symbol (*Figs 17a–d*).

From the medical records of A. J. (Case 5) we find out about his obsessional idea that "they have illegitimately retained my shoes". This is the reason for presenting his portrait barefoot. (*Figs 59* and *60*).

On *Fig. 109* by S. K. (Case 12) it is only through the explanations of the patient that the triple meaning can become evident—a single object which is at the same time "the ear of the profile, an electric shock machine, and a kitchen stove". This is unique in our collections. This drawing, without having the unity of an artistic composition, reminds us of the works of abstract painters.

The discordance between the manifest subject and the symbolism of *Fig. 110* by S. K. is so strong that, without the explanations of the patient, we would be totally unable to arrive at even an approximate explanation of the meaning of this composition. This drawing is similar to the representation of the "World of Planets" of the schizophrenic patient of CESAR (1951).

KRETSCHMER (1941) in his Fig. 14 gives an impressive example of the explanation of the symbols in the pictures of the mentally ill. He remarks that the synthesis of images occurs in the outer sphere of the conscious mind of the cultured man, while the symbolic images occupy the center of consciousness of the schizophrenic patient. In addition to their central place, the symbols acquire a significance different from the usual conventional meaning.

According to MÜLLER-SUUR (1954), in the symbols of schizophrenics the normal meanings are lost while abnormal meanings take the place of the normal ones. This is the case, for example, in *Figs 109* and *110* of our patient *S. K.* (Case 12).

The great symbolism of our Case 12, *S. K.* is similar to that of the patient A. Kotz of PRINZHORN (1922) and to a patient of FERENCZY (1935). All three patients attributed special meanings to the numbers, for example, "the number 2 is equal to richness because two is more than one". Our patient gave symbolical interpretation only after he had completed his painting in a psychotic state, saying that "each figure has a special meaning". He extends the symbolism itself to the colors: "my red means something completely different from that of other painters". He wants to express through his colors the mystical concepts of a world of dreams which he cannot explain in words. Once he states that he wants "to be able to paint the different musical tones of the flute". This shows his tendency to synesthesia, similar to that of the patient of FERENCZY (1935) who made an embroidery in the colors of the Hungarian flag and said: "I have embroidered the national hymn". The same patient said, later: "I hear the needle singing ... the beauty of a work is not essential. The essential is the song ... ." Another patient of FERENCZY gives a special meaning to colors, for example: the green represents the voice of an acquaintance. These cases reveal how the emotional background determines the use of the symbols.

BURSTIN (1946) considers the symbols to be "the concept of affective thinking". The symbols may serve as basis for the creations of artistic values. "They can be an original creation and, as such, achieve the highest psychological level. This is the case of the creation of poets which indicate each time a new and harmonious synthesis. The symbol is what one makes out of its contents." CHRISTOFFEL (1952) points to the importance of the role of a mythical world in dreams and in the arts, while this way of thinking also plays an essential role in the world of mentally ill patients. According to CARUSO (1953), the symbols represent different elements of the personality and, thus, become deranged in psychiatric illnesses. This observation is sustained also by the opinion of STÖRRING (1955) who believes that illusions and hallucinations are possibly based on the constitution of patients who have eidetic properties. Furthermore, according to STÖRRING, psychoneuroses of eidetic patients are more severe, because of pre-existing problems of adaptation to reality which are further aggravated by the psychosis. ANGYAL (1941) states that the premorbid personality traits of patients have a determining role in the symptom-building in schizophrenia, mostly at the beginning of the psychosis.

# THE COMPOSITION

The problem of the composition and of the "contrapposto" must be raised regarding any art work. Even in the works of untrained painters, the problem of visual relationship is apparent. The contrapposto is a goal-directed function of the mind which consists in the creation of equilibrium which includes the component parts in the artistic dynamism.

In the works of our patients created during the active stage of the exacerbation of their illness we do not find any proof of this conscientious construction. The lack of balance is related to the disintegration of the personality. Although the contrapposto means the balance of visual relationships, it cannot be achieved, for example, in the drawings consisting of a system of horizontal and vertical lines, forming a kind of mesh, which give the sense of equilibrium as in *Figs 6* and *8*) by *L. I.* (Case 1), and in the drawings of Mrs. *J. U.* (Case 7).

The drawings of schizophrenic patients are characterized by the fact that they cover the whole surface at their disposition. This is very evident in the case of MORGENTHALER (1942) who called it horror vacui. It has been called by FERDIÈRE (1947) "plenitude". MINKOWSKA (1947) has suggested for the same concept, the term "filling out" (the surface) ("remplissage"). Our patient *Zs. H.* (Case 16) fills the whole surface even in cases where he completes figure-drawing with geometrical motives.

According to FAY (1912), serious qualities are mixed with gross defects in the works of schizophrenics, due to a lack of criticism and because the patients represent what they want to see rather than what they see in reality.

The lack of intellectual control leads to the surfacing of elements in the artworks of patients which do not exist in the fine arts. The lack of technique gives to some of their artworks a liveliness of colors and a special freshness in appearance.

# THE STYLE

From the point of view of the style, one can classify the works of mentally ill patients in several categories, by the similarity of the drawings of patients who suffer from the same illness.

Based on these common traits, several authors have attempted to categorize the paintings of the mentally ill into different groups. We do not have the intention of establishing a new system. We consider that, for our purposes, the division of the works into four groups following the classification of CESAR (1951) is useful:

1. Symbolical linear drawings similar to archaic works and to those of children;
2. Geometrical linear drawings with characteristics similar to the traits of abstract works;

3. Works with Freudian symbols, similar to the artworks of the Middle Ages and the Byzantine period;

4. Light-dark drawings of academic character.

Regarding our collection, we want to emphasize that the art of the mentally ill has no relationship to the known styles of the fine arts in spite of certain apparent similarities.

In our works, the objects and human figures, in their majority, are represented in their greatest surface *(en face)* or in profile. For example, see the drawings by *J. U.* (Case 7), *Figs 76, 77, 79*, and by *A. J.* (Case 5) as well as the drawings of *L. V.* (Case 13). Nonetheless, this maximal view is not exclusively used by the mentally ill. It occurs also throughout the history of art.

Even when patients' pictures represent objects from their milieu, for example, the hairstyle and clothing, or automobiles in the style of the times, those have only accessory relevance for the style. The representation of the imaginary, such as that of monsters, goes back to the earliest epochs of art history.

In accordance with the data in the literature (BERGERON and VOLMAT 1952, CAMERON 1938, KAPLAN and SAKHEIM 1955, MEYER 1954, TOMPKINS 1952), we can establish the lack of naturalistic presentations in the drawings made in a psychotic state. Our collection is composed in part of symbolical works, and in part by works which represent reality only partially through their strange style.

We must consider art as a live function which, during its evolution, always presents itself in new forms. In looking at an object in the fine arts, we recognize the characteristic style of the era and the geographic area of its origin. This is not the case in the artistic works of the mentally ill.

We can establish that the works of patients who suffer from the same type of psychosis are similar, irrespective of the time and place of their origin. There is a certain similarity between the works of our patients and of the patients with a similar diagnosis published in other collections.

We can establish from the series of *S. K.* (Case 12) that this painter worked before his illness in a naturalistic style, while during his psychosis he produced symbolical works (*Figs 109 and 110*). During the treatment, his style changed again. He gradually approached the naturalistic style he used before his illness. It is of special interest to note that his style during the time of post-convulsive amnesia, after electric shock, became similar to children's drawings—a sign of regression of the mental functions in this state *(Fig. 118)*. Was it the same mechanism (of amnesia) which made him "forget his delusions?" Two weeks after his temporary amnesia, his style changed again; he abandoned completely the primitive technique, and again painted in his naturalistic style as he had before his illness. At that time, he declared that he could not remember having painted anything during his period of amnesic confusion and that those paintings were so primitive that they were as if not done by him. Following the electric shock treatments, he did not produce symbolical compositions any more, although we asked him to do so. We will return to this case during the discussion of the prognosis.

SCHOTTKY (1936) reports a change of style in the works of a teacher of practical arts. The patient suffered from a schizophrenic form of illness. Her style changed twice. The works produced at the onset of her illness show a definitive regression as compared to her artwork of before the illness. The pictures after the onset of her illness are primitive—"schematic and constructive"—, their content and form are similar and attest to lack of goal-orientedness. The large surfaces of colors flow into each other. The colored areas are not contained within the contours; several places remain free of color. A few months later the patient became more tranquil and produced a variety of artworks carefully done with delicate broad tracing, corresponding to the actually represented object. Finally, at the end of the psychotic state she returned to her "usual technique": the works produced at this stage are like conventional illustrations.

Meyer (1954) states that the realistic style and technical media of his schizophrenic patient changed during the process of illness into a symbolical style and, at the same time, the technical aspects also changed similarly. The method of using colors and forms corresponded to the symbolical representation. The enriching effect of the psychosis on his works was only transitory.

## THE WAYS OF EXPRESSION (TECHNIQUE)

### The Line

The line is a medium of artistic expression. Artists always change their lines under the influence of affective and logical motives. On the other hand, in the majority of our material we can establish an unchanging way in the using and drawing of the lines. The tracing of it is characterized (considering the line as a fixed movement) by uniformity, totally devoid of accent and rhythm, especially in the art of schizophrenic patients. The uniform lines of schizophrenic art cannot be found in the drawings of children or in the folkloric art although the creations of the mentally ill have some resemblance to these.

We have already mentioned the resemblance among hypnagogic states, dreams, and some psychotic states. According to Pawlow (1926), in the hypnagogic state, the balance between stimulus (excitation) and reaction is lost. As a result of equalization, the stimuli (excitation) of different intensities provoke similar reactions. Maybe the uniform lines and the washed out colors are caused by such phases. In the paradoxical phase, a stimulus (excitation) of minimal intensity may gain great importance—a fact which shows in bizarre effects in the drawings.

The works of our patients are frequently characterized by interrupted lines. The mesh of lines produces a striking originality in these works. The characteristic traits listed above are relevant mostly for the works of schizophrenic patients.

The lines made by manic patients have a different character. This type of line gives the impression of a hasty gesture. It is the patients' attempt to realize everything in the shortest time possible. While they are tracing one line, their attention is already on the next action *(Figs 123, 125, 126)*. For example, the double contour of the hairstyle in *Fig. 121* produced by a continuous single line is full of elan and vitality.

We must ask ourselves if the patients touch the surface with their tools in the same way as the sane person does. The condition of harmony is that the motion through which the line is produced must do justice to both the intellectual and the affective functions. If this balance is disturbed in favor of one of these factors, then a surprising effect can be produced. From this point of view the following observations can be made about our collection:

The patients reach and touch the surface in a way different from the way the sane person does, and they also apply the colors in a strange manner. This is due to their different psychomotor activities. In the patients' works, the affective factor predominates. The intensity of the affect is extended to an enormously large scale, from the strongest impulse *(Fig. 34)* to the weakest signs caused by inhibition in which the motions of the body and of the arm are minimal *(Fig. 43)*.

We concur with the opinion of PRINZHORN (1922) when we establish that in the case of mentally ill patients this fashion of working is not caused only by lack of practice or of artistic training. They frequently have no aesthetical concepts. Unlike the lines appropriate for the intended goal of the artist, the movement initiated by morbid affectivity—which almost tears the paper or only barely touches it—characterizes the expression of the graphic material of the mentally ill.

Regarding the characters of the lines, we see an important similarity between our observations and the conclusions of BREIL (1953) based on the graphological analysis of the handwriting of schizophrenics. BREIL states that for schizophrenics there are two groups of movements in their way of tracing the lines. One can be seen as typical of schizophrenic handwriting: abnormally large size of the tracing or abnormally small traces and arrhythmic movement of tracing. The psychological tension and the inability to observe as well as the affective coolness show in these irregular traces. A second group of the method of tracing (such as ataxic and misguided connection and derailed lines) can be found mostly in the handwritings of other mentally ill patients. Basically, we find that compared to the writings of schizophrenic patients analyzed by BREIL the same disturbances occur in the drawings and paintings of schizophrenic patients. The characteristics of the second group noted by BREIL are found in the technique of manic depressive patients.

## *The Creation of Form*

The psychotic patients are not preoccupied with the aesthetical or the technical completion of forms. Neither are they concerned with the method of achieving the contact between different surfaces. The forms are frequently conventional; nonetheless they may have an individual usage. The "torpedo women" of *L. I.* (Case 1) show a good example of this *(Fig. 17a–d)*. Otherwise, the tendency to represent schematically and the use of geometrical forms are also characteristic. Almost everywhere we see examples of hills and trees drawn by our patients in a stereotyped fashion. The same is valid for some ornamental designs.

We also see examples in which the lines of the contour of one image are part of another image *(Fig. 72* of Case 5).

In the representation of human figures, the lack of naturalistic presentation is most striking. Regarding this characteristic, the same tendencies can be observed in patients from different cultures and different geographical locations. We can see such examples in the human figures presentation of *A. J.* (Case 5), and also by *L. I.* (Case 1), whose works are similar to those presented in the book by PRINZHORN (1922) and in other publications.

## Colors–Effects of the Light

Psychology attributes specific significance to individual colors. These characteristics of the colors will change in the hands of the mentally ill through their unusual and original usage. Thus, their artworks may have an unexpected and surprising effect *(Figs 64, 92 and 99)*. In our patients' cases, the colors do not have an important role in giving form to the objects.

In our collection, the role of the effect of light cannot be considered to be identical to that known in the artworks of normal persons where the light is a most important medium of modeling. *Zs. H.* (Case 16) uses light correctly for modeling only in his precise copies of ancient and medieval artworks *(Figs 151a, 151b)*.

In the hands of our patients, the modeling is uncertain and the repartition of the light and dark surfaces as well as the choice of colors is very individual. The arbitrary use of light and shade and half-shade between identically traced lines in the drawings of *F. Cs.* (Case 6) *(Figs 73, 74)* are examples of this. In *Fig. 36* of the picture made by Mrs. *A. P.* (Case 3) we see sharp contours of light surfaces on surrounding dark areas. Such works produce a striking effect through their coloring *(Figs 92 and 94)*. The colors of *Fig. 98* have an unsettling effect. On the other hand, the colors of *L. T.* (Case 4), through their delicate and gentle nuances, project a calm serenity *(Figs 47 and 48)*.

## The Space

We intend to discuss here the depth which is expressed through the method of the perspective in the artworks.

According to ROY (1958), schizophrenic patients intend to preserve in their artworks the image of a stable world and of the filling of the space.

In the majority of our collections the artworks have a two-dimensional character without the effect of depth. This is not surprising since the use of perspective is unknown to the patients who have not received professional instruction. The disappearance of perspective in the case of artists who became mentally ill is therefore even more characteristic of the illness. The drawing of *S. K.* (Case 12), made during his period of amnesia *(Fig. 118)*, which we have already discussed, is characterized by the loss of the effect of depth, in spite of his previous art training. During his recovery the works of *Zs. H.* (Case 16) have changed from two-dimensional to three-dimensional representations with correct perspective *(Figs 157a–c)*.

The inadequate representation of depth in schizophrenic patients' drawings may be based on problems in their depth perception. LAMPONI (1949) has demonstrated in a stereoscopic experiment that the perception of depth (the view in perspective) is present only in 50% of hebephrenics, 53.3% of paranoids, and in 16.6% of catatonics. The problems of representing depth occur also in organic brain damage, for example, in patients who suffer from constructive apraxia (JANOTA 1938, LHERMITTE and MOUZON 1942). These observations are significant with regard to the attempt of certain authors to characterize different forms of schizophrenia according to the experience gained from the cortical localizations of neurological deficits.

The absence of correlation between surface and depth characterizes the art of the mentally ill, in contrast to the fine arts characterized by the balanced interplay of surface and depth.

## Body Proportions and Movement

In the art of mentally ill patients the proportions do not correspond to the requirements of anatomical representation. This is true both for stationary figures and figures in movement. The artistic anatomy is unknown to these patients.

However, these defects are no reason for denying the works of the mentally ill the quality of "work of art". We find similar deficiencies also in folk art.

The ability to represent movement in action is missing in the art of the mentally ill. MORGENTHALER (1942) has found, in his detailed studies of the works of schizophrenics, that "actions are relatively rarely represented". Later studies have given this observation a more general meaning. Also, in our material we find representations both of human and of animal figures in a motionless position. These figures do not evoke the impression of movement in its evolution. They represent a movement stopped at the moment of registering it. There are exceptions such as the lively battle scenes full of movement by *L. T.* (Case 4) *(Figs 48–51)*.

The rigid representation of actions finds its explanation in the mannerism of the schizophrenic patients. It is, however, striking that manics full of vigor and movement represent their figures in the same frozen attitudes, producing a static impression instead of a dynamic representation of action.

In our collection, the representation of monsters is characterized by enormous heads on a disproportionately small body and by weak extremities *(Figs 19–23, 57, 102, 124)*. The monsters produce their effect mostly through the expression of exaggerated proportions of the head instead of the gestures or movements of the body *(Figs 14, 127–135)*. In the representations of hermaphrodites of *Zs. H.* (Case 16) the head is too small in relation to the body *(Figs 154a–c)*.

# SPONTANEITY AND PERIODICITY OF THE ARTISTIC ACTIVITY, THEIR RELATIONSHIP TO PSYCHOSIS

Several authors deal with the question whether during mental illness a certain latent talent reveals itself, or whether it is the case of the birth of a new talent during the process of the illness. According to KRETSCHMER (1941), based on SCHILDER's concept (1918), the intuitive artistic inspiration could feed itself off the "sphere of the consciousness" (periphery). He points out that the "creative, genial persons, especially artists and poets ... make the analogy between their productive achievements and the dreams ... thus we can consider this relationship as an acknowledged fact". The image of a word could produce an agglutination with the help of this sphere of the consciousness. A similar synthesis of images is at the center of the consciousness of schizophrenics. The distorted affect of these patients and their irrational and strange judgment may have an enhancing effect on their religious, artistic, and poetic productions in the view of KRETSCHMER (1941).

The "light or borderline" stages of manic depressive illness increase the productivity since the hypomanic states facilitate the associations and produce an abundance of ideas. ZSAKÓ and JÓ (1931) state that mental illness has a certain influence on the productivity as far as it increases the inclination toward activity and decreases the inhibitions. JUDA (1953) denies that mental illness enhances the development of a creative talent.

In our opinion, mental illness does not produce artistic talent. We have seen that the works of mentally ill patients do not reach the level of true works of art based on criteria of the fine arts. Nonetheless, we accept the opinion of EY (1948) who says: "The aesthetical pathological production that originates directly from mental illness is a special structure." It is not "an artwork", but "a natural object of art".

We may assume that patients in a state of psychosis prefer drawing as a medium of expression to other more conventional media such as speech or writing. One of the causes of this tendency may be that the graphic expression offers the easiest and best way to express symbols.

Nonetheless, several of our patients draw and write at the same time. In these cases, the discordance between the expressive power of these two different media is evident. The patients' graphic expression is more instinctive and more primitive, but this makes it more understandable than their writings which frequently remain incoherent and incomprehensible. The patients attempt to express through their drawings the content of their mind, which they are unable to express otherwise. The drawings of *L. L.* (Case 2) express simpler subjects through more comprehensible methods than his simultaneous text which is almost unintelligible.

In regard to the desire of the mentally ill to express themselves in drawings, DELAY (1952) states: "The fact itself that the mentally ill person uses a method of expression, although it may be quite strange, is a sign that he is not totally alienated and that he has preserved a conscious part of his psyche that allows him specifically to express the mental illness itself." The drawing has achieved the value of a new "language" in a patient of UEBERSCHLAG (1947). SZÉCSI (1935) is of the opinion that mentally ill patients do not make premeditated artistic compositions, rather they are driven by a strong emotional necessity to express the content of their psyche.

According to EMERY (1929), the "non-objective" paintings of patients allow the repressed content to enter the surface of consciousness. This conscious content then becomes available for verbal expression. BIEBER and HERKIMER (1947/48) state that the drawing as a new expressive medium facilitates the contact with the outside world. KEMPF (1920) considers the artistic productions as a symbolical language available to psychoanalytic interpretations.

We may approach the problem of artistic inspiration from the point of view of its periodicity and spontaneity as we review the history of some of our cases. In Case 6 *(F. Cs.)*, it becomes evident that the patient's interest in drawing was not continuous. He was treated at our hospital for thirteen years and, during this long period of time, he only drew for two months. During this period, according to his medical record, he spontaneously requested paper and pencil to draw. He produced a large number of impressive works. In some of these works he may have represented his hallucinations *(Fig. 75)*. His psychological state remained unchanged during the whole period following his admission; nonetheless his interest in drawing became extinct from one day to the other without any notable outside influence. Later, he had no interest at all in drawing, even if he was asked to draw. He was never able to explain the cause of his impulse to draw. He found an original expression to define his productivity and his talent: "I am taken over by such a spell of dizziness that a drawing drops out of my head".

Our patient *A. J.* (Case 5) was hospitalized from 1910 and he only spontaneously requested drawing instruments in 1922, "to paint what I feel". At other times, he stated that his drawings were "fantasies born from my brain".

For *Zs. H.* (Case 16) painting and drawing have become a daily and continuous activity in an otherwise withdrawn life-style.

The impulse to draw was preserved by Mrs. *A. P.* (Case 3) even during the periods of her greatest agitation. During these periods of aggressivity and agitation, when it was impossible to establish contact with her, at a certain moment she withdrew into a corner to produce one of her art works with delicate traits.

The lobotomy did not decrease her ability to draw. We may not be mistaken when we imply that after the lobotomy her artistic ability even improved.

In the case of *L. T.* (Case 4), the continuous drive to draw did not become extinct even during the last phase of his illness. Even while in a bad mood, and in an affective stupor, he continued without interruption his incomprehensible smearings. His strength of artistic expression had weakened and finally it ceased during his illness. The knowledge of the history of his illness allows us to conclude that the decline of his artistic expression and the quality of his works were consistent with the severity of his illness.

As a problem somewhat removed from our subject, the question of a cerebral localization of artistic qualities will only be referred to briefly. Even the destruction of the angular gyrus of the dominant hemisphere does not completely extinguish artistic abilities. This observation is sustained by the case of BONVICINI (1926): the painter D. Urrabieta (Vierge) at age thirty-one, suffered a stroke which caused right-sided hemiplegia, motor aphasia, alexia, agraphia, and ataxia without sensory aphasia and without apraxia. In spite of this illness, he was able to resume drawing with his left hand. The works produced during this period (six months after the stroke and with the motor aphasia unchanged) had the same artistic quality as the works done before his illness. Thus the circumscribed lesion of the brain had not destroyed his special artistic talent.

# DIAGNOSTIC VALUE OF THE PICTORIAL PRODUCTS

The clinical diagnosis is based on the observation of symptoms which are regularly found in the same illness.

One should not neglect in the diagnosis of the mentally ill patients the analysis of the drawings and paintings, because they show similarities in the same category of illness. These works help us in the interpretation of the special structure of a morbid personality. If we are successful in discovering the characteristic traits which are recurrent in the artworks of patients suffering from the same illness, we have then discovered the diagnostic value of these artworks.

Naturally, one should not draw conclusions about the presence of mental illness in an artist solely on the basis of the artistic expression of his works. This fact is underlined by the example in the work of WEYGANDT (1926) about the hundreds of marble and limestone statues found in the palace of the prince of Palagonia and which represent fairytale-like monsters. According to WEYGANDT, these bizarre statues were not sculpted by one, nor by several mentally ill artists suffering from the same mental illness. These are sculptures which were executed according to the requirements of their patron, the prince, who was paranoid schizophrenic.

Some authors questioned whether it is right, based on the artistic qualities of pictorial works, to draw conclusions about the mental illness of their creators. We are skeptical about such a simplistic explanation considering the great variety of individual characteristics of the artworks in different categories of illnesses. Our reservation of judgment is further substantiated when we realize that the psychological mechanisms, which gain an overwhelming significance in mental illness, are not strange in normal psychological conditions.

According to PRINZHORN (1922), there are no sure signs to distinguish the works of sick artist painters. STAVENITZ (1939) finds that one must know the social and individual history of an artwork in order to judge whether its author is mentally ill or not. Similarly, according to ZELDENRUST (1951), it is impossible to establish the illness of an artist based on his work without knowing the artist himself.

DELAY (1952), in his presentation of the artwork of the mentally ill at the World Congress of Psychiatry in 1950, established that only a few artworks have not shown regression in comparison with the previous qualities of the work of these artists, while, in another group of patients the artistic level of the work increased following the psychosis. According to DELAY, the relationship of the illness and the quality of the works, is very inconsistent.

In psychoanalysis, PANETH (1929) finds most useful the abstract works which are formally not tied in to the representation of nature. The psychoanalytic value of drawings, he says, is the greatest in patients whose verbal associations are inhibited and thus it is difficult to establish contact with them, "because, in this expression, one cannot lie".

BACH (1952), based on the fact that spontaneous artworks represent the whole personality, recognizes the diagnostic and prognostic value of the pictures of the mentally ill.

According to BIEBER and HERKIMER (1947/48), the recognition of the structure of the personality is facilitated by the artistic productions.

The actual question in psychiatric research is whether there are recognizable aspects in the graphic expression which are characteristic in certain mental illnesses. KÜRBITZ (1912) has expressed his opinion on this issue: "It is possible to find differences in the pictorial presentation which is more or less typical for a certain illness, thus providing a differential diagnostic value". (More on this subject with an update of the literature is presented in the historical overview of the Introduction.)

In the drawings of the mentally ill, published by GILYAROVSKI (1954), we find the symbolical and bizarre representations by schizophrenics, brisk tracings and vivid colors of manic patients and even the representation of a nightmare by a patient in alcoholic delirium.

BERGERON and VOLMAT (1952) have published three drawings by a patient suffering from manic depressive psychosis. The portrait produced in the manic phase is scribbled over by lines drawn in different directions. The portrait produced in the depressive phase is characterized by deep shadows. The artwork drawn during the normal period represents a pleasant and somewhat exotic face. It is known from the case history of a schizophrenic patient (No. 12 of the same authors) that at the beginning of his illness the schizophrenic patient drew motifs of flowers. After lobotomy, he attempted to paint landscapes of different kinds—actually without success—and finally he contented himself by copying pictures representing landscapes. During a recurrence of this illness his drawings became chaotic and symbolical. It is interesting that this change in style preceded the clinical symptoms of relapse.

RÉGIS (1882/1883) recognizes the prognostic value of the drawings of manic-depressive patients. WADESON and BUNNEY (1969) present the characteristics and psychodynamic interpretations of manic depressive art.

The question of the diagnostic value of drawings has been raised not only in relationship to the art of the adult mentally ill patients but also in child psychiatry (SEHRINGER 1992). The majority of authors who were interested in this topic have discovered a parallelism between the qualities of the drawings and the psychological state of the child. An excellent book on disturbed children's drawings by AUBIN (1970) supports his theories with relevant case histories and 80 pictures. STERN (1923), TRAUBE (1937) and LEMBERGER (1951) have documented that the whole personality is manifested in, and can be studied with the help of, children's drawings. KLÄGER (1990) describes the pictorial thinking in his richly illustrated book on children's drawings.

From the point of view of the psychological development DALLA VOLTA (1951) found that the representation of the world correlates with the intellectual development of the child.

DIAZ ARNAL (1950) established a parallelism

between the qualities of the drawings and the level of mental development of retarded children. NIKITIN (1930), based on a large sample, found that the artistic talent is less developed in psychopathic children with characterological difficulties than in normal children. GERBER (1968) gives case examples of the compulsive use of drawings by very young children.

The spontaneous drawings made the early diagnosis possible in the case of childhood schizophrenia published by AHNSJÖ (1952). The understanding of the signs specific for schizophrenia in this case have a special interest because of the similarity of normal children's drawings to those of the drawings of schizophrenic adults. Anthropomorphism, a characteristic trait of some adult psychiatric patients' artworks, is also found frequently in children's drawings (JARREAU 1991).

By analyzing the artworks of the mentally ill, we may conclude that they represent—within the limits of their technical ability—the world corresponding to the concepts and sensations they have, like all other artists who produce only what they have experienced.

Naturally, the feelings of the mentally ill do not always correspond to the real sensory stimuli of the environment. Thus, some of their representations cannot be naturalistic. They frequently use strange symbolical representations, difficult or impossible to comprehend. One can understand these works only with the explanation given by the patients themselves, or not even then.

In the study of our material we found that the composition and the methods of technical expression, the type of the trace, the use of the touch by pencil or brush, are similar in all our patients who belong to the same diagnostic category of the psychosis.

Three of our patients took courses at the Academy of Fine Arts before their hospitalization. The others received no special professional education. The quality of the artworks of our patients who had studied art regressed during their illness.

## DIAGNOSTIC QUALITIES OF THE ARTWORKS OF SCHIZOPHRENICS

BÜRGER-PRINZ (1932) has attempted to determine the "artistic behavior" of schizophrenic patients based on BLEULER's (1911) fundamental symptoms of schizophrenia.

As expected, the majority of the works in our collection are produced by schizophrenic patients. In the artworks we find the characteristic signs of the illness. The cooling of the affective life is manifested by unaccentuated lines. The bizarre thinking shows in the symbolical compositions constructed frequently with geometrical forms, characterized by discordance between the expressed subjects and the latent meaning. Inasmuch as schizophrenic patients are characterized by stereotypy and mannerism, their traces are affected, unskilled and rigid. The same motifs are repeated with the same gestures *(Figs 6–8, 40, 45)*.

DELAY (1952) also recognizes, with certain reservations, that the drawings of schizophrenics reflect autism, ambivalence, and a tendency to abstraction.

Based on the study of the embroideries of mentally ill women, VIÉ and SUTTEL (1944) have distinguished two types of morbid technique: either a variant of the normal technique, or a new technical form where the novelty consists in the choice of materials or in the technique. FERENCZY (1935) also finds that anomalies in the needlework are similar to the characteristics of other works of schizophrenics. The individual details are isolated instead of being constructive elements of the composition. FERENCZY describes the characteristic traits as follows: negativism, ambivalence, troubles of rhythm and aggregation. The dissolution of the original motifs and the disregard for their compatibility culminate in the selection of colors. The harmony and the logical use of colors is missing in the works of patients who are guided by their momentary impulses. "Thus, the different colors divide the unified elements of the motifs into fragments."

From among the characteristics of the schizophrenics' drawings, FERDIÈRE (1947) analyzes the stereotypy which is revealed in the repetition of the same drawing for several days or weeks, with little variation, or with the addition of insignificant details. FERDIÈRE described this trait by using GIRAUD's expression (1936), "invariable fixation".

In his monograph about the creative activity of his schizophrenic patient, MORGENTHALER (1942) emphasized that this patient repeated the same theme for years, practically unchanged.

The stereotypical repetition of the same figure for weeks characterizes the works of our patient *L. I.* (Case 1) *(Figs 15a, 17d)*. Also *L. T.* (Case 4) repeats the same subjects several times during his illness *(Figs 46a–50)*.

BERGERON and VOLMAT (1952) established, based on the data of YAHN (1950), that the patient's tendency of repetition increases with the chronicity of the illness.

The exactness of the dividing lines, without structural function, the minutious and patient method of working on the creation of ornamental frames, indicate a morbid pedantry in the drawings of Mrs. *J. U.* (Case 7).

The content of the representation of hallucinations is pathognostic for the artistic products of schizophrenic patients. See the detailed observations on this subject in the next Chapter.

# DIAGNOSTIC CHARACTERISTICS OF THE WORKS OF MANIC PATIENTS

The drawings of manic depressive patients differ from those of the schizophrenics. The spectator is astounded at first by the precipitous movements and the brusqueness of the tracing.

As the manic psychosis is characterized by the acceleration of associations, sometimes to the level of incoherence, the lines of the manic patients are brutal and totally independent from one another, without supporting each other mutually in the totality of the work *(Fig. 124)*. In the case of KAPLAN and SAKHEIM (1955), the drawings of a thirteen-year-old patient suffering from a manic depressive psychosis were disorganized, confused, and traced roughly during his psychosis. This was also evident in the drawings of our patient *F. B.* (Case 14).

The palette of the manic patients is totally different from that of the schizophrenics. The latter often show a gentle harmony of colors while in the works of manic patients the contrast of colors is exaggerated. If they remind us of the colors of the *trecento*, this is only an apparent resemblance, and they are in no relationship with the well-balanced color contrast of that era.

The primitive joy of colors of the manic patients has an infantile character. NAGY (1905) sees the expression of playful childish fantasies in their tendency to change colors. He mentions that children often use several colors on the same drawing. They even represent the same object in different colors.

The majority of the works of schizophrenic patients are black and white pencil drawings. While giving up the colors they attempt to model the forms in a precise fashion. In contrast, manic patients produce pictures in lively colors. It is interesting to compare these observations with those of LANGNER (1936) according to whom the adjectives and the adverbs used by schizoid poets frequently indicate a form while, to the contrary, those of cyclothymic refer to colors. This characteristic can be viewed as a constitutional characteristic of the personality. Similarly, in the RORSCHACH (1946) projective tests the cyclothymic personalities have a greater affinity to the colors while the schizothymes have a greater affinity to forms.

KIBLER (1925) has demonstrated in tachistoscopic experiences, with syllables in color, that schizophrenic individuals have a greater aptitude for abstraction than cyclothymes, the latter group being influenced more by the difference of colors during the experiment.

KARPOV (1926) established a parallelism between the manic state and the artistic inspiration.

Our patients *L. V.* (Case 13) and *F. B.* (Case 14) as well as *Zs. H.* (Case 16) in the early psychotic stage of his illness produced figurative drawings in eccentric colors. Their artworks are characterized by unskilled spatial representation, lack of composition, wrong proportions, wrong accentuation, brutal traces and the way of applying the colors in a linear graphic form. The heads are too big in relation to the extremities and sometimes even in relation to the trunk. If we disregard these negative characteristics, we cannot deny the suggestive force of the pictures. These works disregard the laws of reality and the objective observation of nature. The graphic qualities dominate the pictorial qualities. The tracing, as a result of movement, is related to the superficiality and quick changes of the emotions. They explain the brusque traces, which are inappropriate for modeling.

## THE WORKS OF A PATIENT SUFFERING FROM ALCOHOLIC HALLUCINOSIS: RELATIONSHIP TO THE PSYCHOSIS

The representations of hallucinations will be discussed in more detail in the next chapter. Here we intend to mention only that the characteristic trait of the alcoholic delirium is actually the vision of terrifying animals which our patient *N. N.* (Case 15) succeeded in representing. The psychosis of the delirium was combined with paranoid traits corresponding to the paranoid ideas of the patient about "the devils" and other supernatural creatures which are represented by him. The great number of visions and the repetition of some nightmares are characteristic of the psychosis itself, as well as of the drawings of this patient. From the drawing of *Fig. 130*, one can assume that this is not a representation of a real hallucination, but rather that of an illusion, also a characteristic symptom of patients in delirium. The order in which a clock is transformed, at first into a bizarre monster, next into a tent, is similar to the fleeting visions in mescaline intoxication.

# CHARACTERISTICS OF THE REPRESENTATION OF HALLUCINOSIS

In the literature, we find only a small number of graphic representations of true hallucinations. The likely cause of this is, as Prinzhorn (1922) has also said, that the patients cannot define their visions in the same fashion as the real and palpable objects, either by words or by another method of expression, such as, for example, drawing. Prinzhorn published some drawings of hallucinations with the remark that we cannot state about a picture that it is the representation of a vision unless the patient himself gives us this information.

To approach the problem of hallucinations and their psychopathological mechanism, we may use some examples from the literature on experimental intoxications which provoke hallucinations.

One can find phenomena similar to the hallucinations of the mentally ill in dreams, in hypnagogue states, and in the symptoms of intoxication by mescaline (Baruk and Joubert 1953, Beringer 1927, Heuyer and Lebovici 1950, Pennes 1954, Staehelin 1941).

As a hypnagogue appearance, Smythies (1953) found in mescaline intoxication, for example, a certain colored blotch to be floating in the air, which can be transformed into objects just to fade away and disappear ultimately in the darkness. The visions may appear on one side of the visual field and then disappear on the other side.

Delay and Gérard (1948) have established that during mescaline intoxication, ecstatic states occur. The experimental subjects see sparkles, the objects change place, and everything is in motion. Even the day after the intoxication they are overwhelmed by colored objects and in their dreams they see fabrics of wonderful colors. Delay and Volmat (1963) provide a general overview on painting and chemotherapy.

Porot et al. (1942) also emphasize the symptom of hyperexcitability in relationship to colors, a symptom that also appears in intoxication by *Cannabis sativa* (hashish). The intoxicated person sees also grotesque changes in the size of objects, for example, greatly elongated extremities.

Alliez (1953), in an experimental intoxication with Ortedrine (r-phenylisopropylamine), has observed a slowing of the thought processes, a tendency to perseveration, distrust of the environment, disturbances of the body scheme, illusions, and hallucinations.

According to Ey and Rancoule (1938), in mescaline intoxication and in chronic encephalitis, one cannot distinguish between hallucinations and illusions. "This is a confusion between the subjective and the objective. It is an excess of the subjective in the perception which is the basic nature of an illusion and of all the phenomena described as illusions, hallucinations, or pseudo hallucinations."

Häfner (1954) is of the opinion that perceptions, thoughts and feelings could become hallucinations by losing their 'ego quality' ("Ich-Qualität"). In schizophrenic patients the hallucinatory experiences move into the unmitigated sphere of perceptions or they may even be experienced as such. Morel (1939/41) considers that different elementary excitatiory processes—as inadequate excitations—may cause perceptions without objects, that is hallucinations.

According to Maurel and Wilhelm (1955), mescaline exaggerates the manifestation of the morbid symptoms of the mentally ill, without making permanent the hallucinations thus provoked.

During intoxications and in the mentally ill patients' hallucinations, the consciousness is frequently clouded or at least limited. In the organic lesions of the brain, optical hallucinations and sometimes multi-sensorial hallucinations can occur in a lucid state of consciousness (Gloning and Weingarten 1954). Wadeson and Epstein (1975) describe the intraphysic effects of amphetamine in hyperkinesis.

Derwort (1953) has shown in his experiments that during vestibular stimulation, the subjects report directional distortions in space, tilting and unsystematic dysmorphic visions. Partial changes of forms occur; for instance, a knife appears to bend and a hatchet presents a deformed appearance, similar to the beak of a bird.

We observe in the representations of hallucinations of our patients their misunderstandings of the body proportions. The most striking examples are the deformed little people of *L. L.* (Case 2) who appear as if seen in a bent mirror *(Figs 19, 20, 22)*.

We dwelled on the phenomena of intoxications in order to explain the difficulty of recording in drawing the impressions of fleeting hallucinations which are vague and of variable intensity. The patient frequently forgets them just as we forget our dreams. After the disappearance of a vision, the patient frequently does not remember it anymore. *Zs. H.* (Case 16) stated about his vision depicted in *Fig. 163*: "I had to draw it *immediately* as I saw it."

Another possible cause of the rarity of representations of hallucinations is the fact that, in the state of delirium, the vision captivates the whole attention of the patient, to the point where he is incapable of distancing himself from it at that moment in order to draw. During the state of hallucinating, the patients cannot distance themselves from it to engage in drawing.

This is similar to the experience by which we try to analyze our emotions through introspection, from a psychological point of view. At the moment of the conscious analysis, the affective tone weakens and we can judge its intensity only by remembering the accompanying phenomena. A very strong emotion fills the consciousness completely and excludes a simultaneous intellectual analysis of the quality of that emotion. It is known that hallucinations overcome the consciousness completely with such an intensity that at those moments nobody can establish contact with these patients. Naturally, in that state, the patient does not even get the idea of drawing his visions.

After the delirium some patients are capable of evoking their visions to talk about them or, rarely, to represent them through drawing (Bertschinger 1911). However, in these drawings a certain tendency to confabulate may be manifested.

We find a possible psychological explanation of the representation of hallucinations in the case histories published by NAGLER (1952). His patient suffering from a paranoid psychosis found true relief after he drew an animal which he thought to be persecuting him.

According to MARCHAND (quoted by VIÉ and SUTTEL 1944) some of the works of the mentally ill are inspired by their paranoid ideas. Other patients represent in their drawings, or in their embroideries, their visual hallucinations. For example, one of his epileptic patients painted the visual hallucinations seen during the "aura". ZSAKÓ (1908) published some pictures in which the patients illustrated their paranoid ideas. Excellent illustrations substantiate the representations of hallucinations of a schizophrenic patient of MARINOW (1971).

KRIS (1933) has analyzed busts with tightly closed lips and deformed lips produced by the sculptor F. Xaver Messerschmidt during a period of schizophrenic psychosis. One of these faces has lips in the form of a beak. It was based probably on the sculptor's recurrent vision which suggested to him that a bad spirit attacked his mouth. Apparently these are not representations of actual hallucinations in themselves. Rather, they are self-portraits reflecting the reaction of the patient suffering the tortures of his hallucinations.

The drawings of our patient *N. N.* (Case 15) suffering from alcoholic hallucinosis show that the patient linked some of his visions to his paranoid ideas of jealousy, with the intention of threatening his wife by means of the monsters he drew and by convincing her of their existence *(Figs 131a, 131b, 131d)*. To protect his children, he drew at the same time a monster with benign demonic properties *(Fig. 131c)*. Through these qualities, the drawings acquire a meaning equivalent to the idols of primitive people.

It is unique that throughout his hospitalization this patient never drew any other subject but his hallucinations; from a psychiatric point of view this is of great importance.

Among the drawings of our other patients we can only sporadically discover some hint of hallucinations, for example, in *Figs 109* and *110* of *S. K.* (Case 12). Among the drawings of *L. I.* (Case 1) we find only at the margin of a page some bizarre animals which may be interpreted as images of a vision *(Fig. 14)*. About *Fig. 44* of *L. T.* (Case 4) and *Fig. 37* of Mrs. *A. P.* (Case 3), we can only assume that they were done under the influence of a vision, similar to *Figs 23* and *25* of *L. L.* (Case 2). It becomes evident from the text produced by the patient *S. F.* (Case 11) about *Fig. 107* that it is a representation of a "dream-face". Some paintings of *Zs. H.* (Case 16) are identified by him as visions *(Figs 138, 146a–d, 163)*.

Mrs. *A. P.* describes some of her works done after the lobotomy as "brain-ghosts". However, we have difficulties in distinguishing her planned "fairy-tale world" from those representing hallucinations. The patient herself states that the drawings in blue-green shades "are brain-ghosts done in the colors of craziness". In their technical execution these are nonetheless very similar to her other pictures produced in naturalistic colors.

# PROGNOSTIC SIGNIFICANCE OF THE STYLE AND OF THE TECHNICAL QUALITIES

It is to be proven whether a comparison of the changes in the pictorial work with the process of the illness could be used as a basis for prognosis.

There is an early report in the literature by Régis (1882/83) that the drawings of manic depressive patients lead to some conclusions regarding the development of their illness, especially its transitional phases. For this reason, Régis believes that the drawings have a prognostic value.

The drawings of a paranoid schizophrenic patient of Tompkins (1952) have been symbolical at the beginning of his illness while during recovery they became conventional. In the case of a patient with paranoid psychosis of Cameron (1938) the pictures which were done during his psychosis were original while those done after the course of the illness and recovery have shown conventional expressions. During the psychosis curved lines were most evident and the recurrence of these allowed the physician to recognize the recurrence of the illness. In another case by Cameron, in the most severe phase of the psychosis, the drawings were only concrete objects; the perspective was missing; the background was stereotypical and only black color was used. The clinical improvement led to a realistic representation of the environment. A similar change in style occurred during the psychosis of the schizophrenic patients of Meyer (1954). Anastasi and Foley (1941) found the changes in the collection of Nijinsky's drawings to be characteristic of the development of his illness.

Our collection has a special value from this point of view. The patients were hospitalized for a long time or followed for decades after discharge (Case 16). With the help of their case histories we have the opportunity to follow the changes in their personality, and the fluctuations during the different stages in the severity of their illness.

The quality of the drawing in relationship to the changes in the illness would permit prognostic conclusions. From this point of view, our patient L. T. (Case 4) merits some attention. He had studied at the Academy of Fine Arts. Looking at his works, we can recognize some traits which indicate his artistic education, in spite of the scarcity of subjects and the stereotyped repetition of the same forms (*Figs 40* and *41*). His drawings became more and more stereotyped with faint tracing and poverty of form as his illness progressed. His emotions become rigid and cool, as he becomes increasingly uninterested and indifferent to the impressions of the world. In his last drawings one cannot see anything but colored patches or vague silhouettes which show through the mesh of lines drawn in pencil. The series of works in which the same subject was used from the beginning to the end of his illness is demonstrative. For example, one sees the contrast between the battle scenes, executed earlier, full of dynamism *(Figs 48 and 49)* and the fading drawings of the same subjects produced a few years later *(Fig. 51)*. One can find a similar, or an even more striking, contrast between the colored pictures representing the view of the city of Pécs *(Fig. 47)* and the drawings, poor in form, of the same scene produced a few years later during a more advanced stage of his illness *(Figs 46a–c)*.

The case of our patient Mrs. *A. P.* (Case 3) is of similar prognostic interest. Before her illness she worked as a sculptress. During her illness her drawings show an incontestable regression. Like other patients, she expressed herself through a reduced number of subjects drawn with monotonous traces. With the exception of some bizarre subjects, her drawings resemble, in general, the postcards in fashion at the beginning of the century.

Sometimes an affective explosion is reflected in her works *(Fig. 34)*. Her drawings lack the plastic modeling and the effects of light and shade that one expects of a sculptor *(Fig. 36)*. Her works became increasingly stereotyped during the course of her illness.

Six months after her discharge from the hospital where she underwent a bilateral prefrontal lobotomy, we received a letter from her husband informing us that his wife had again started her work as a sculptor, and that the quality of her works had attained the prepsychotic level.

We established that seven years after the lobotomy, the schizophrenic traits were clearly recognizable in her behavior and in her artworks. Nonetheless, her works became more systematic and she produces unified scenes. In these she integrates otherwise diverse elements as seen in the illustrations of children's fairy-tale books. Her initiative to draw has increased following the lobotomy. It is of interest that early after the lobotomy her drawings became more naturalistic—so much so that the representations of her home and the portraits of the members of her family are well recognizable and of almost photographic exactitude.

The chronological order of the works of *S. K.* (Case 12) reflects the longitudinal aspect of his illness. *Fig. 108* dates from the time before the manifestation of the psychosis. Its unfinished and strange atmosphere is the sign of the painter's impatience. *Figures 109* and *110*, produced during the most severe phase of the psychosis, are unique among his works from the point of view of the technique and style because of their symbolical abstract representation. This strange style disappeared after electric shock treatment, when he returned to the naturalistic style *(Figs 111–116)*.

The transitory effect of the shock treatment, which manifested itself clinically in amnesia, was reflected in works similar to children's drawings *(Figs 117* and *118)*. The drawing of *Fig. 114*, produced two weeks after the completion of the electric shock, marks the transition in the style of his works. The restless effect of this painting, the use of exaggerated colors, and the vividness of the whole picture, are exceptional among his products.

The stereotyped repetition of geographical maps and of female figures for months and years is characteristic of the chronicity of the illness of *L. I.* (Case 1).

# SOME RELATIONSHIPS TO CHILDREN'S DRAWINGS

The comparison of the drawings of the mentally ill and those of children returns frequently in the literature. We do not intend to treat this problem in detail here. The similarity of the works of psychotic patients to the drawings of children lies in the projection of perceptions and feelings which differ from the experiences of non-psychotic adults.

The drawings of children vary according to their age. It is well documented by BENDER (1952) that the drawings are similar in children of the same age, regardless of the culture or the land and time of their origin. This is observed also in the case of the works of the mentally ill. Those who suffer from the same psychosis produce works that are similar in style and in technique.

Children intend to represent the real world. Nonetheless, they only reflect their insufficiently developed concepts about things, instead of a true representation of nature. Children emphasize the details that appear important to them.

KÜRBITZ (1912) sees the similarity of children's drawings and those of the mentally ill in the fact that they do not work from sensory observations. "Their representations are influenced by innumerable ideas and scattered associations. Therefore, instead of representing the object as actually seen, they represent a combination of their experience, their ideas, and knowledge of the object. The ideas dominate not only the person doing the drawing but they also dominate the drawing itself."

Through the distorted, unreal view of the world, the works of psychotic patients are far from being naturalistic representations. They attest to the patient's inability to understand and judge the surrounding world, since their concept of the world is changed by the psychosis so that objects may have a strange appearance.

We should note also that realistic painters use a gradation of values. They accentuate some details, depending on their importance, while they only sketch other details. The artist never reproduces with the impartial exactitude of a photograph. Nonetheless, his judgment would never allow him to enter the bizarre world of the mentally ill. FLEISCHMANN quotes Goya's words about the artistic creation: "Painting, just like poetry, selects from the universe what it finds most appropriate for its goals. The paintings unify and concentrate in a single fantastic figure, situations and characters which are disseminated by nature in different individuals. Through this wise and creative combination the artist deserves the title of inventor and ceases to be a subordinated copyist."

The child's development leads to an evolution of the drawing from the technical point of view (GOODENOUGH 1926). In the case of the mentally ill, the drawings of adults show a regression, which makes the works similar to those of children. In hysterical states, similar characteristics have been described in drawings which do not show real intellectual regression. For example, according to DELAY (1952), the hysterical patient, whose behavior has regressed to that of an eight-year-old child, during this period of regression drew in a manner characteristic of that age. ANGYAL (1941) demonstrated that an individual regressed to a certain younger age through hypnosis draws according to the criteria of that age.

According to the research of GYÁRFÁS (1939), the drawings of schizophrenic patients, following insulin coma, frequently show a regression to the level of children's drawings.

# CERTAIN RELATIONSHIPS WITH ARCHAIC DRAWINGS AND WITH THE DRAWINGS OF PRIMITIVE PEOPLE

Several authors have established a certain archaic character in the art of the mentally ill. Some traits of these drawings can also be found in the drawings of primitive people in our age and in prehistoric art. Already LOMBROSO (1887) and KIERNAN (1892b) have seen the analogy between the drawings of the mentally ill and primitive art in the symbolism, the lack of perspective, and the affinity to colors.

According to KRETSCHMER (1929), the differentiation between the external world and the self is missing among primitive people. They cannot distinguish with certainty what happens outside of them and what is projected by themselves. This is how magical thinking evolved.

The catathymic mechanism erases the limits between the external world and the self, and thus it leads to magical thinking, where the facts are combined in a certain mesh of special correlations. These thought processes and their primitive representations lead towards the agglutination of images. According to KRETSCHMER (1936), this is different from the symbols of civilized people who can also project abstract ideas into a certain form. Nonetheless, the latter are always conscious of the symbolical character of this form, which is never assumed to be identical with the object itself. Regarding the symbols, LHERMITTE (1938) arrives at a similar conclusion about the development of primitive language when he says, "The primitive mime forms his gestural activity to express abstract concepts. Thus his gestural language arrives through analogy to the symbol."

According to HAMILTON (1918), the symbolical art of children, of primitive people, and of the mentally ill, indicate concepts organized at a lower level, or concepts resulting from a morbid process.

PFEIFER (1923) believes that in pathological cases, the patients approach a primitive genius. This is different from the mentality of children who represent in drawings the objects of the world in a fashion resembling the drawings of primitive people. Nonetheless, according to DESPERT (1948), the three-year-old child can already distinguish between fantasy and reality.

KÜRBITZ (1912) finds an analogy between the works of the mentally ill, of the children, and of primitive people. We may designate all these similar traits as intellectual realism.

SCHILDER (1918) states: "We must realize that the world of the primitive people and of psychotics may show a broadening of the meaning, and of the importance of the meaning, of the world. Nonetheless, the structural interdependence of the details on which the complicated structure of reality is built is missing. The reality adaptation of the thinking is absent."

One cannot state, based on the artwork, that the thought processes of the mentally ill have regressed to the level of prehistoric man, even if some drawings remind us of archaic and primitive drawings *(Fig. 66)*. Magical and symbolical expressions characterize the schizophrenic patients' drawings, but in spite of this it is evident that their thought processes have not suffered a uniform regression to a primitive level. Patients who are not in delirium may show bizarre behavior, although even in their negativistic state they are conscious of social conventions against which they rebel.

The artworks of primitive people are clearly object-related and understandable, their goal being to express real objects.

In the art of the mentally ill, we find most of all a certain unresolvable tension, which emanates primarily from the need for a symbolical solution. However, the patients use original expressions (the meaning of which is only known to themselves) instead of conventional symbols. This is exactly what determines the individual character of their drawings. Through this trait, the creations of the mentally ill are different from prehistoric works which were comprehensible in their time, just as they are today because their essential characteristic is the representation of reality. According to PRINZHORN (1922), the characteristic ambivalence of schizophrenia is missing in the artworks of children and of primitive people. VERWORN (1917) established that prehistoric art is based on sensory perception and thus, as a consequence, it is "physioplastic" and appears realistic, while the method of representation which characterizes children's drawings is ideoplastic, that is, the consequence of a certain abstraction. SCHENK (1939) finds a similarity between the children's drawings, the drawings of the mentally ill, and the drawings of some patients suffering from aphasia, in their ideoplastic representation. Among the characteristic traits of the drawings of the mentally ill, MORSELLI (1885, 1894) mentions the use of ideographism.

Regarding the artwork in our collections, the position of the figures on the sheet like "totem poles" *(Figs 19, 20, 22 of L. L.)* (Case 2) and the idols of Case 15 *(Figs 133–135)* remind us of the artworks of primitive people.

# SUMMARY

Artistic productions are the reflections of the thought processes and the impressions of their creators. However, the impressions of the mentally ill frequently do not correspond to reality. Therefore, their representations cannot be naturalistic. The majority of their works based on special abstractions use a personal symbolism. They are based on strange concepts that the sane person cannot understand, sometimes even with the explanation given by the patients themselves.

The expression through abstract and symbolical forms allows a comparison of the schizophrenic patient's drawings with those of the surrealist. Nonetheless, the lack of artistic composition distinguishes the art of the mentally ill from modern art. This lack of artistic composition and of the contrapposto is related to the incoherence of the associations and to the perseveration and stereotypy of schizophrenic patients. Manic patients are incapable of realizing a balanced composition because their attention span is decreased and their associations become superficial and accelerated.

In the patients' artwork, the morbid mechanism of their associations is reflected, as are also the strange content of their consciousness and certain traits which characterize their psychomotor activity. In one word, the artwork represents the total personality of its creator, a fact which gives the works of the mentally ill a certain diagnostic and prognostic value.

We find in the drawings of schizophrenic patients the characteristic signs of the illness. The coolness of the affective life is manifested by unaccented tracings. The split personality is reflected in bizarre and symbolical compositions, constructed frequently of geometrical figures and characterized by lack of harmony between the expressed subject and its hidden meaning. Just as the behavior of schizophrenic patients is characterized by stereotypy and mannerisms, their lines are manneristic, unskilled, and rigid. The primitive archaic thinking of schizophrenic patients provides a link between their art and that of primitive people and archaic drawings.

The drawings of manic depressive patients are different from those of the schizophrenics. At first appearance, the quickness of the movement and its brusqueness are striking. In mania the acceleration of associations and of the thought processes, sometimes to the level of incoherence, causes the tracing to be presented brutally, the lines twisting around by themselves, as it were, without sustaining a sense of unity such as would be found in the fine arts. The palette of the manics is totally different from that of schizophrenics. In the work of manics the contrast of colors is always shocking. One never finds the gentle harmony of colors which characterizes a good number of the drawings of schizophrenics.

In the artworks of the psychotic ill, especially in schizophrenia, one can discover also the expression of paranoid ideas and hallucinations. One of our patients, suffering from alcoholic hallucinosis, never drew anything throughout his hospitalization except his hallucinations which he linked to his paranoid ideas of jealousy. Through his drawings he intended, on the one hand, to menace his wife through the monsters he drew and to try to convince her of their existence and, on the other hand, he intended to protect his children by means of monsters of good will. He attributes demonic properties to the 'monsters' drawn, thus they become equivalent to the idols of primitive people.

The works of the psychotic ill are characterized by the absence of a balanced composition and the lack of representation in accurate perspective. They are unskilled also in the expression of movement. Nonetheless, these traits are not only due to the lack of skill. One can find these defects in the case of painters who had studied art and who, during the time they were mentally ill, lost their ability to create a unified composition, achieved through adequate technical methods. Even if the continuous exercise conserves the technical ability developed in their training, the range of the content becomes narrowed during the mental illness.

Considering the relationship between the gravity of the illness and the quality of the artwork executed at different times by the same patient during his psychosis, we can arrive at prognostic conclusions. The drawings set in a chronological order reflect the longitudinal course of the illness. The figures produced by a schizophrenic patient in the most severe phase of the psychosis are isolated among the artworks of the patient by their symbolical abstract representations as well as by the technique and the style *(Figs 10, 11)*. This strange style disappeared following electric shock treatment and was replaced by works done in the naturalistic style. The transitory effect of the electric shock is manifested from the clinical point of view by amnesia. As a consequence, his artwork showed a regression to the level of children's drawings. Throughout the years the patient's drawings became more and more stereotyped with faded traces and poor forms, parallel with the progression of the illness (Case 12).

The follow-up of our lobotomized patient (Case 3) is quite interesting. The schizophrenic characteristics of her artwork are just as evident after the surgery as they were before. However, the content is more normal; her figures are now organized, in relation to each other, forming scenes. Some drawings have acquired an important dynamic aspect. She produced a series of drawings as illustrations to fairy tales. In these we can recognize without a doubt the conscious and adequate composition. *The lobotomy apparently has strengthened her creative ability.*

The spontaneity and periodicity of the artistic activity in the mentally ill are not caused by the appearance of a new talent or the revelation of a latent talent in the patient. Patients often draw to avoid boredom and through a certain need for activity and, finally, sometimes they prefer, as a method of expression, the drawings as compared to other conventional methods such as talking and writing.

On looking at an artwork in the fine arts, the

style of the work indicates the time and geographical place of its origin. This is not valid in the case of the art of the mentally ill. There is a certain rapport between the artworks of our patients and those of patients with a similar diagnosis, regardless of the time and of the land of origin of the paintings.

A comparison of the art of the mentally ill with children's drawings, archaic artworks, and those of primitive people, can establish a similarity mostly in the ideographic manner of their representation rather than in their subjects.

From our observations based on the above described sixteen cases, it is evident that the drawings and paintings of mentally ill patients can be analyzed according to the same criteria as the works in the fine arts.

Detailed clinical observations and long-term follow-up of both the clinical course and the art products lead to empirical data which are characteristic traits of different psychiatric disorders.

The patients' art products may serve as a diagnostic tool, as an aid in designing the treatment program and in defining the prognosis.

The patients described in these collections have not been provided with the newest methods of art therapy; at the time of their hospitalization art therapy as such did not exist as a specialty. Patient art was nonetheless used during individual psychotherapy and in psychoanalysis as an excellent tool of communication.

In the last decade the works of some painters and sculptors who have been mentally ill at some point in their lives became recognized as "outsider art", "visionary art" or "art brut", recognized entities in the fine arts.

Certainly some of our patients' works would qualify for being recognized on their own merit as a pictorial expression of emotions.

# BIBLIOGRAPHY

AHNSJÖ, S. (1952): Spontaneous paintings. *Compt. rend. I. Congr. mond. Psychiatr.* 7, 115

ALLIEZ, J. (1953): Délire amphétaminique. *L'Encéphale* 42, 21

*American Journal of Art Therapy.* Published by Vermont College of Norwich University, Montpelier: Vermont.

ANASTASI, A., FOLEY, J. P. (1941): A survey of the literature on artistic behavior in the abnormal, II: Approaches and interrelationships. *Ann. New York Acad. of Sciences* 42, 1

ANDREOLI, V. (1996): *Carlo a mad painter*. Venice: Massilio

ANGYAL, L. (1937): Über die verschiedenen Insulinschocktypen und ihre neuropsychopathologische Bedeutung. *Arch. f. Psychiatr.* 106, 662

ANGYAL, L. (1941): A rajzolás változása, korsuggestiós kísérletekben (Le changement des dessins dans les experiences à suggestion d'âge.) *Magyar Pszichológiai Szemle* 14, 113

ARNHEIM, R. (1986): The artistry of psychotics. *American Scientist* 74 (Jan/Feb)

ASSAEL, M. (1990): The eye. In I. JAKAB (ed.), *Art Media as a Vehicle of Communication*. Proc. 1990 Int. Congr. Psychopathol. Expr., Montreal 1990. Brookline, Mass.: American Society of Psychopathology of Expression, pp. 189–196

ASSAEL, M., GABBAY, F., ROSEMAN, J. (1975): Spontaneous painting in group, in I. JAKAB (ed.), *Psychiatry and Art*, Vol. 4, Transcultural Aspects of Psychiatric Art. Basel: S. Karger, pp. 1–5

AUBIN, H. (1952): *L'homme et la magie*. Paris: Desclee de Brouwer

AUBIN, H. (1970): *Le dessin de l'enfant inadapté*. Toulouse: Privat, pp. 193–194

BACH, S. R. (1952): Peintures et modelages spontanés dans les établissements pour malades. *Rev. Suisse de Psychol.* 11, No. 3

BADER, A. (1966): Le cas du peintre Suisse: Louis Soutter. *Vie méd.* 47, 37

BADER, A. (1968): *Louis Soutter—eine pathographische Studie*. Stuttgart: Eckhardt

BADER, A. (1971): Découverte psychopathologique de Charles Filiger, peintre symboliste. *Confinia Psychiatrica* 14, 18–35

BADER, A. (1972): *Geisteskranker oder Künstler?* Bern: Verlag Hans Huber

BADER, A., NAVRATIL, L. (1976): *Zwischen Wahn und Wirklichkeit—Kunst–Psychose–Kreativität*. Luzern: Bucher

BARANYAI, M. (1978): Bosch és az emberi szem (Bosch and the human eye). *Művészet* 19, 6. 36–41

BARUK, H., JOUBERT, P. (1953): Actions thérapeutiques et dangers des amphétamines ou amines psychotoniques. *Ann. Med. Psychol.* 111, I. 305.

BAUDOUIN, CH. (1929): *Psychoanalyse de l'art*. Paris: Alcan

BEHRENDS, K. (1976): *Karl Junker. In Imaginary Dwellings* (film). Basel: Sandoz

BENDER, L. (1952): *Child Psychiatric Techniques*. Springfield, Ill.: Thomas

BERGERON, M., VOLMAT, R. (1952): De la thérapeutique collective par l'art dans les maladies mentales. *L'Encéphale* 41, 143

BERINGER, K. (1927): *Der Meskalinrausch*. Berlin: Springer

BERTSCHINGER, H. (1911): Illustrierte Halluzinationen. *Jb. f. Psychoanal. u. Psychopathol. Forsch.* 3, 69

BIEBER, I., HERKIMER, J. K. (1947/48): Art in psychotherapy. *Am. J. Psychiatry* 104, 627

BILLIG, O. (1968): Spatial structure in schizophrenic art. In I. JAKAB (ed.), *Psychiatry and Art*. Proc. IVth Int. Coll. Psychopathol. Expr., Washington, D.C., 1966. Basel–New York: S. Karger, pp. 1–16

BILLIG, O., BURTON-BRADLEY, B. G. (1975): Cross-cultural studies of psychotic graphics from New Guinea. In I.

JAKAB (ed.), *Psychiatry and Art.* Vol. 4, Transcultural Aspects of Psychiatric Art. Basel: S. Karger, pp. 18–47

BILLIG, O., BURTON-BRADLEY, B. G. (1978): *The Painted Message.* New York: Halsted Press

BLEULER, P. E. (1911): *Dementia praecox oder Gruppe der Schizophrenien.* Aschaffenburg, Handb. d. Psychiatrie, 4. Abt. 1. Hälfte. Leipzig–Vienna: Deuticke

BONVICINI, G. (1926): Die Aphasie des Malers Vierge. *Wien. Med. Wochenschr. 76,* 88

BRAUNER, A., BRAUNER, F. (1994): *L'accueil des enfants survivants.* Paris: Groupement de Recherches Pratiques pour l'Enfance

BREIL, M. A. (1953): Graphologische Untersuchungen über die Psychomotorik und Handschriften Schizophrener. *Monatschr. f. Psychiatrie 125,* 193

BRÜCKMANN, I. (1932): Antoni Gaudi. Ein pathographischer Versuch. Zugleich ein Beitrag zur Genese des Genieruhms. *Z. Neurol. 139,* 133

BULTMANN, B. (1960): *Oskar Kokoschka.* Salzburg: Verlag Galerie Welz, p. 42

BÜRGER-PRINZ, H. (1932): *Über die künstlerischen Arbeiten Schizophrener.* Bumke, Handb. d. Geisteskrankheiten 9. Berlin: Springer, 668

BURSTIN, J. (1946): Le symbole en psychiatrie. *Ann. Med. Psychol. 104, II.* 1

CAMERON, N. (1938): Individual and social factors in the development of graphic symbolization. *J. Psychol. 4,* 165—Cited by ANASTASI and FOLEY

CARUSO, I. A. (1953): Le symbole dans la psychologie profonde. *Studium generale 6,* 296

CERLETTI, U., BINI, L. (1938): L'Elettroschock. *Arch. Gen. Neurol. Psychiat. Psicoanal. 19,* 266

CESAR, O. (1951): Contribution à l'étude de l'art chez les aliénés. *Arqu. Assistencia Psicopatas S. Paulo 16,* 51—Ref.: *Zbl. Neurol. 124,* 154 (1953) and *Ann. Med. Psychol. 112, I.* 403 (1954)

CHRISTOFFEL, H. (1952): Psychiatrie und Kultur. *Monatschr. f. Psychiatrie 123,* 178

CONRAD, K. (1953): Der zweite Sündenfall. Psychiatrische Betrachtungen zur modernen Kunst. *Ann. Univ. Saraviensis 1,* 3

CORRONS, P., GIDEON, K. (1968): Directed artistic creativity as an accelerating technic in dynamic group therapy. 4th Int. Coll. Psychopathol. Expr., Washington, D.C., 1966. Abstract in I. JAKAB (ed.), *Psychiatry and Art.* Basel–New York: S. Karger, p. 208.

DALLA VOLTA, A. (1951): La représentation de l'univers infantile. *Arch. di psicol. neur. e psichiatr. 12,* 163

DAX, E. C. (1953): *Experimental Studies in Psychiatric Art.* London: Faber and Faber, pp. 1–100

DAX, E. C. (1991): Schizophrenic images. In I. JAKAB (ed.), *Art Media as a Vehicle of Communication.* Brookline, Mass.: American Society of Psychopathology of Expression.

DELAY, J. (1952): Art psychopathologique et médecine. *Semaine méd. Suppl. 32,* 10

DELAY, J., GÉRARD, H. P. (1948): L'intoxication mescalinique expérimentale. *L'Encéphale 37,* 196

DELAY, J. VOLMAT, R. (1963): *Psychopathologie und bildnerischer Ausdruck; I. Serie: Malerei und Chemotherapie.* Basel: Sandoz

DELAY, J., VOLMAT, R., PICHOT, P. (1959): *Le cas d'un peintre amateur atteint d'une névrose narcissique profonde.* I Symp. sull'Arte Psicopathologica. Verona: Société Internationale de Psychopathologie de l'Expression

DELONG, W. B., ROBBINS, E. (1961): The communication of suicidal intent prior to psychiatric hospitalization: a study of 87 patients. *Am. J. Psychiatry 117,* 695

DERWORT, A. (1953): Über vestibulär induzierte Dysmorphopsien. *Dtsch. Z. Nervenheilk. 170,* 294

DESPERT, J. LOUISE (1948): Delusional and hallucinatory experiences in children. *Am. J. Psychiatry 104,* 528

DIAZ ARNAL, I. (1950): Le psychisme du déficient à travers le dessin. *Revista de Psicol. Madrid. 6,* 735

DIGIOVANNI, J. (1990): Georgia O'Keefe: The artist as self-healer. The Phoenix Effect. In I. JAKAB (ed.), *Stress Management Through Art.* Brookline, Mass.: American Society of Psychopathology of Expression, p. 135

DIGIOVANNI, J., MCINTIRE-MANGO, H. (1991): Bonnard's mirrored view of women. In I. JAKAB (ed.), *Art Media as a Vehicle of Communication.* Brookline, Mass.: American Society of Psychopathology of Expression, pp. 53–89

DRACOULIDES, N. N. (1952): *Psychanalyse de l'artiste et de son oeuvre.* Collection Action et Pensée. Aux editions du Mont-Blanc

DRACOULIDES, N. N. (1953): Répercussions de sevrage précoce sur les tableaux d'un peintre moderne. *Acta Psychother. Basel 1,* 23

DREIFUSS, G. (1978): Artists in the creative process of Jungian analysis. *Confinia Psychiatrica 21,* 45–50

DROBEC, E., STROTZKA, H. (1951): Narkodiagnostische Untersuchungen bei Surrealisten. *Z. Psychother. 1,* 64

Dupré, E. Devaux (1910): La mélancolie du peintre Hugo van der Goes. *Nouv. Iconogr. Salpêtrière 23*, 605

Ehrenzweig, A. (1948): Unconscious form-creation in art. *Br. J. Med. Psychol. 21*, 185

Ehrenzweig, A. (1953): *The Psychoanalysis of Artistic Vision and Hearing.* New York: Brazillier

Elgar, F., Maillard, R. (1956): *Picasso.* Zürich: Ex Libris

Emery, M. (1929): Color in occupation therapy. *Occup. Ther. Rehab. 8*, 421—Cited by Bergeron and Volmat

Evlachow, A. (1937): Léonard de Vinci n'était-il un épileptoïde? *Arch. gen. di Neurol. 18*, 343—Ref.: *Zbl. Neurol. 89*, 217 (1938)

Ewald, G. (1950): Abstrakte Malerei. *Psychol. Rdsch. 1*, 133—Ref.: *Zbl. Neurol. 120*, 416 (1952)

Ey, H. (1948): La psychiatrie devant le surréalisme. *L'Evolution Psychiatr.* Paris *4*, 3

Ey, H., Rancoule, M. (1938): Hallucinations mescaliniques et troubles psychosensoriels de l'encéphalite épidémique chronique. *L'Encéphale 33*, II. 1

Fay, H. M. (1912): Réflexions sur l'art et les eliénés. *Aesculape 2*, 200—Cited by Anastasi and Foley

Ferdière, G. (1947a): Les dessins schizophréniques (première communication): leurs stéréotypies (vraies ou fausses). *Ann. Med. Psychol. 105*, I. 95

Ferdière, G. (1947b): Introduction à la recherche d'un style dans le dessin des schizophrènes. La forme opposée au contenu et les limites de l'analyse. Intérêt de l'étude du style. Considérations méthodologiques. Le musée-laboratoire de l'avenir. *Ann. Med. Psychol. 105*, II. 35

Ferdière, G. (1951): Le dessinateur schizophrène (Présentation d'un créateur). *L'Evolution Psychiatr.* Paris 215.

Ferdière, G. (1976): Pique Assiette. *In Imaginary Dwellings* (film). Basel: Sandoz

Ferenczy, J. (1935): Parallele zwischen den Handarbeiten weiblicher Geisteskranken und der Volkskunst. *Jackson Memorial Vol.* Debrecen

Fernandes, G. (1933): Surrealismo e esquizofrenia. *Arch. Assist. Psicopat.* Pernambuco 3, 140—Cited by Anastasi and Foley

Fischer, R. (1969): On creative, psychotic and ecstatic states. In I. Jakab (ed.), *Psychiatry and Art.* Vol. 2, Art Interpretation and Art Therapy. Basel–New York: S. Karger, pp. 33–65

Fischer, R. (1975): The art of madness and madness of art. In I. Jakab (ed.), *Psychiatry and Art.* Vol. 4, Transcultural Aspects of Psychiatric Art. Basel: S. Karger, pp. 61–63

Fleischmann, B. (n.d.): *Francesco Goya.* Wien: Otto Lorenz

Foy, J. L. (1968): On self portraiture. In I. Jakab (ed.), *Psychiatry and Art.* Vol. 1, Basel: S. Karger, p. 209

Foy, J. L. (1971): The deafness and madness of Goya. In I. Jakab (ed.), *Psychiatry and Art.* Vol. 3. Basel: S. Karger, pp. 2–15

Foy, J. L. (1990): Paul Klee. Creativity with the left and right hand. In: I. Jakab (ed.), *Stress Management through Art.* Proc. Int. Congr. Psychopathol. Expr., Boston 1988. Brookline, Mass.: American Society of Psychopathology of Expression, p. 134

Foy, J. L. (1991): The enigma of Giorgio de Chirico. In I. Jakab (ed.), *Art Media as a Vehicle of Communication.* Brookline, Mass.: American Society of Psychopathology of Expression, pp. 23–36

Freeman, J. (1964): Introduction. In Jung, von Franz, Henderson, Jacobi, Jaffe (eds), *Man and His Symbols.* Garden City: Doubleday, pp. 9–15.

Freud, S. (1910): Leonardo da Vinci and a memory of his childhood. In *Standard Edition*, Vol. 11, 59–137. London: Hogart Press

Freud, S. (1958): The dynamics of transference. In *Standard Edition*, Vol. 12, London: Hogarth Press

Friedman, L. (1969): The therapeutic alliance. *Int. J. Psychoanal. 50*, 139–153

Gedo, J. (1980): *Picasso: Art as Autobiography.* Chicago: University of Chicago Press

Gerber, M. (1968): The compulsive use of nonverbal expressions by three very disturbed young children. In I. Jakab (ed.), *Psychiatry and Art.* Proc. IVth Int. Coll. Psychopathol. Expr., Washington, D.C., 1966. Basel: S. Karger, pp. 61–67

Gilyarovski, V. A. (1954): *Psichiatriya.* Moskva: Medgiz

Giraud, P. (1936): Analyse du symptôme stéréotype. *L'Encéphale 30*, I. 229—Cited by Ferdière, *Ann. Med. Psychol. 105*, I

Gloning, I. K., Weingarten, K. (1954): Über optische Halluzinationen. *Wien. Z. Nervenheilkd. 10*, 58

Gomirato, G., Gamna, G. (1954): Sul significato psicopatologico dei disegni degli schizofrenici. *Giorn. Psichiatr. 82*, 261

Goodenough, F. L. (1926): *Measurement of Intelligence by Drawings.* New York: World Book Co.

Gyárfás, K. (1939): Disturbances of drawing in hypoglycemia. *Confin. Neurol. 2*, 148

Häfner, H. (1954): Zur Psychopathologie der halluzinatorischen Schizophrenie. *Arch. f. Psychiatr. u. Neurol. 192*, 241

HALBREICH, U. (1978): A nonverbal dialogue as a treatment of schizophrenic patients. In I. JAKAB, L. MILLER (eds), *Creativity and Psychotherapy*, Proc. 8th Int. Congr. Psychopathol. Expr., Jerusalem, 1976. *Confinia Psychiatrica* 21, pp. 58–67

HALLIDAY, D. (1981): Doodles or scribes. In: I. JAKAB (ed.). *The Personality of the Therapist*. Pittsburgh, Penn.: American Society of Psychopathology of Expression, p. 112

HAMILTON, A. M. (1918): Insane art. *Scribner's Mag.* 63, 484—Cited by ANASTASI and FOLEY

HAMMAN, R. (1935): *Geschichte der Kunst*. Berlin: Knaur, p. 459

HANSER, S. B. (1997): A decade of music therapy research in anxiety and pain reduction. In R. PRATT, Y. TOKUDA (eds), *Arts Medicine*. Michigan: International Arts Medicine Association, pp. 60–62

HÁRDI, I. (1968): Phänomenologie des Alkoholismus im Lichte der dynamischen Zeichnungsuntersuchungen. In I. JAKAB (ed.), *Psychiatry and Art*. Proc. IVth Int. Coll. Psychopathol. Expr., Washington, D. C., 1966. Basel–New York: S. Karger, pp. 75–85

HÁRDI, I. (1990): Dynamic examination of animal-drawing. In I. JAKAB (ed.), *Art Media as a Vehicle of Communication*. Proc. 1990 Int. Congr. Psychopathol. Expr., Montreal 1990. Brookline, Mass.: American Society of Psychopathology of Expression, pp. 197–206

HÁRDI, I. (1992): Forty years of dynamic examination of drawings. In I. JAKAB, I. HÁRDI (eds), *Psychopathology of Expression and Art Therapy in the World*. Budapest: Animula, pp. 81–92

HÁRDI, Lilla (1992): Pictures of a psychoanalytic treatment. In I. JAKAB, I. HÁRDI (eds), *Psychopathology of Expression and Art Therapy in the World*. Budapest: Animula, pp. 145–148

HARDING, P., JONES, D. (1975): Bernard Stone, "Sequential Graphic Gestalt". In I. JAKAB (ed.), *Psychiatry and Art*. Vol. 4, Transcultural Aspects of Psychiatric Art. Basel: S. Karger, pp. 216–229

HARROWER, M. (1972): *The Therapy of Poetry*. Springfield, Ill.: Ch.C. Thomas Publ.

HEUYER, G., LEBOVICI, S. (1950): Une nouvelle toxicomanie: le maxiton. A propos de deux observations. *Ann. Med. Psychol.* 108, II. 353

HOFFMAN, R. E. (1987): Computer simulations of neural information processing and the schizophrenia–mania dichotomy. *Arch. Gen. Psychiatry* 44, 178–187

HOFFMAN, R. E. (1992): Attractor neural networks and psychotic disorders. *Psychiatr. Ann.* 22, 3. 119–124

IJUIN, S. (1992): Therapeutic meanings of compositive drawing methods for schizophrenics: From a viewpoint of their sky-earth expressions and psychic fields. In I. JAKAB, I. HÁRDI (eds), *Psychopathology of Expression and Art Therapy in the World*. Budapest: Animula, pp. 149–166

IMORI, M. (1997): Poetry therapy in Japan: Haiku-therapy for schizophrenics. In R. PRATT, Y. TOKUDA (eds), *Arts Medicine*. Michigan: International Arts Medicine Association, pp. 124–131

IN DER BEECK, M. (1966): *Wahnsinn, Ironie und tiefere Bedeutung*. Leverkusen: Bayer

IN DER BEECK, M. (1975): Vincent van Gogh and James Ensor. Epileptoid-ictaffin and defect-schizophrenic structures. In I. JAKAB (ed.), *Psychiatry and Art*. Vol. 4, Transcultural Aspects of Psychiatric Art. Basel: S. Karger, pp. 8–9

IRWIN, E. (1981): A study of effects of abuse over time. In I. JAKAB (ed.), *The Personality of the Therapist*. Brookline, Mass.: American Society of Psychopathology of Expression, pp. 154–169

IRWIN, E. C., SHAPIRO, M. I. (1975): Puppetry as a diagnostic and therapeutic technique. In I. JAKAB (ed.), *Psychiatry and Art*. Vol. 4, Transcultural Aspects of Psychiatry Art. Basel: S. Karger, pp. 86–95

JACOBI, J. (1964): In JUNG, VON FRANZ, HENDERSON, JACOBI, JAFFE (eds), *Man and His Symbols*. Garden City: Doubleday, pp. 272–303

JACOBI, J. (1969): *Vom Bilderreich der Seele*. Olten, Germany: Walter-Verlag AG

JACOBI, J. (1971): Compulsive symptoms in pictures from the unconscious. In I. JAKAB (ed.), *Psychiatry and Art*. Vol. 3, Conscious and Unconscious Expressive Art. Basel: S. Karger, pp. 103–104

JAKAB, I. (1956a): *Dessins et peintures des aliénés*. Budapest: Akadémiai Kiadó, 145 pp.

JAKAB, I. (1956b): *Zeichnungen und Gemälde der Geisteskranken*. Budapest: Akadémiai Kiadó, 168 pp.

JAKAB, I. (1960): Die Wirkung des Elektroschocks und der Leucotomie auf die bildnerischen Darstellungen Schizophrener. *Das Medizinische Bild* 3, Heft 5, 129–142

JAKAB, I. (1967): Graphic expression of the emotional troubles of retarded children. *Confinia Psychiatrica* 10, 16–27

JAKAB, I. (1968): Coordination of verbal psychotheraphy

and art therapy. In I. JAKAB (ed.), *Psychiatry and Art*. Basel: S. Karger, pp. 92–101

JAKAB, I. (1969a): Art and psychiatry. Their influence on each other. In I. JAKAB (ed.), *Psychiatry and Art*. Vol. 2, Art Interpretation and Art Therapy. Basel–New York: S. Karger, pp. 90–123

JAKAB, I. (1969b): Az aesthetikai választás tényezői (Aesthetical choices made by school children). *Ideggyógyászati Szemle 22*, 519–525

JAKAB, I. (1970): Graphischer Ausdruck und Prognose: Wissenschaft oder Intuition. *Confinia Psychiatrica 13*, 81–98

JAKAB, I. (1976): The Watts towers. In *Imaginary Dwellings* (film). Basel: Sandoz

JAKAB, I. (1978): Imaginary dwellings. In I. JAKAB, L. MILLER (eds), *Creativity and Psychotheraphy*. Proc. 8th. Int. Congr. Psychopathol. Expr., Jerusalem, 1976. *Confinia Psychiatrica 21*, 73–91

JAKAB, I. (1979): Creativity and mental illness. *Bull. Menninger Clin. 43*, 4, 365–378

JAKAB, I. (1986): Graphic expression of feelings by a heart transplant patient and his family. In I. JAKAB (ed.), *The Role of the Imagination in the Healing Process*. Proc. 1984 Int. Congr. Psychopathol. Expr., Boston, 1984, Pittsburgh, Penn.: American Society of Psychopathology of Expression, pp. 51–72

JAKAB, I. (1990a): Stress management through art, an overview. In I. JAKAB (ed.), *Stress Management through Art*. Proc. Int. Congr. Psychopathol. Expr., Boston, 1988. Brookline, Mass.: American Society of Psychopathology of Expression, pp. 5–22

JAKAB, I. (1990b): Therapeutic aspects of family video art therapy. In C. STEFANIS, C. SOLDATOS, A. RABAVILAS (eds), *Psychiatry: A World Perspective*. Vol. 4. Proc. VIIIth World Congr. Psychiatry, Athens, 12–19 October 1989. Amsterdam–New York: Elsevier Science Publishers B. V., pp. 178

JAKAB, I. (1990c): Medical practice and medical research. In M. WHITE, J. GOLDSMITH (eds), *Standards and Review Manual for Certification in Knowledge Engineering. Handbook of Theory and Practice*. Rockville, Md.: The Systemware Corporation, pp. 399–411

JAKAB, I. (1992): The role of art expression in psychiatry. The past, the present, and the future. In I. JAKAB, I. HÁRDI (eds), *Psychopathology of Expression and Art Therapy in the World*. Budapest: Animula, pp. 11–32

JAKAB, I. (1994a): Childhood Schizophrenia Persisting into Adult Age. In *Proc. '94 Int. Symp. Psychopathol. Expression and Workshop for Art Therapy*. Seoul, Korea: The Korean Assoc. for Clinical Art

JAKAB, I. (1994b): The influence of environmental and personal events on psychiatric patient's artwork. In *Proc. '94 Int. Symp. Psychopathol. Expression and Workshop for Art Therapy*. Seoul, Korea: The Korean Association for Clinical Art, pp. 33–40

JAKAB, I. (1996): Environmental influences on patient's art. In I. JAKAB (ed.), *The Influence of Recent Socio-Political Events on Fine Arts and on Patient's Art*. Brookline, Mass.: The American Society of Psychopathology of Expression

JAKAB, I., HOWARD, M. C. (1971): The artistic talent of an adolescent with borderline psychoneurotic life adjustment. In I. JAKAB (ed.), *Psychiatry and Art*. Vol. 3, Conscious and Unconscious Expressive Art. Basel: S. Karger, pp. 32–51

JANOTA, O. (1938): Sur l'apraxie constructive et sur les troubles apparentés de l'aperception et de l'expression des rapports spatiaux. *L'Encéphale 33, II*. 173

*Japanese Bulletin of Arts Therapy*. Published by The Japanese Society of Psychopathology of Expression & Arts Therapy, Tokyo, Japan

JARREAU, G. (1991): L'anthropomorphisme dans les dessins d'enfants. In I. JAKAB (ed.), *Art Media as a Vehicle of Communication*. Brookline, Mass.: American Society of Psychopathology of Expression, pp. 255–268

JASPERS, K. (1922): *Strindberg und Van Gogh*. Leipzig: Ernst Bircher—Ref.: *Zbl. Neur. 29*, 250, 1922.

JILEK, W. G. (1995): Emil Kraepelin and comparative sociocultural psychiatry. *Eur. Arch. Clin. Neurosci. 245*, 231–238

JÓ, J. (1933): Intézeti múzeumunk fejlődése (The development of the museum of the institute). In *Angyalföldi Emlékkönyv*. Budapest, p. 61

JUDA, A. (1953): *Höchstbegabung*. München–Berlin: Urban und Schwarzenberg

JUNG, C. G. (1953): *Collected Works*. Vol. 12: *Psychology and Alchemy*. New York: Pantheon, pp. 1–563

JUNG, C. G. (1964): Approaching the unconscious. In JUNG, VON FRANZ, HENDERSON, JACOBI, JAFFÉ (eds), *Man and His Symbols*. Garden City: Doubleday, pp. 18–103

KAITO, A. (1994): The landscape montage technique. In *Proc. '94 Int. Symp. Psychopathol. Expression and Workshop for Art Therapy*. Seoul, Korea: The Korean Association for Clinical Art, pp. 65–74

KAPLAN, A., SAKHEIM, G. (1955): Manic-depressive psychosis in a 13-year-old boy: psychologic test findings. *J. Nerv. Ment. Dis. 121,* 140

KARPOV, P. I. (1926): *The Creative Activity of the Insane and its Influence on the Development of Science the Art and Technics.* Ed. Monog. Moscow: First Exemplary Typography, Sovereign Pub.—Cited by ANASTASI and FOLEY

KEMPF, E. J. (1920): *Psychopathology.* Mosby, St. Louis, 1, 762—Cited by ANASTASI and FOLEY

KERNBERG, O. (1965): Notes on countertransference. *J. Am. Psychoanal. Assoc. 13,* 38–56

KIBLER, M. (1925): Experimentalpsychologischer Beitrag zur Typenforschung. *Z. Neurol. 98,* 524

KIERNAN, J. G. (1886): Genius not a neurosis. *Neurol. Rev. 1,* 212—Cited by ANASTASI and FOLEY

KIERNAN, J. G. (1887): Genius not a neurosis. *Alienist and Neurol. 8,* 341—Cited by ANASTASI and FOLEY

KIERNAN, J. G. (1892a): Is genius a neurosis? *Alienist and Neurol. 13,* 119—Cited by ANASTASI and FOLEY

KIERNAN, J. G. (1892b): Art in the insane. *Alienist and Neurol. 13,* 244, 684—Cited by ANASTASI and FOLEY

KLÄGER, M. (1990): *Phänomen Kinderzeichnung.* (2. Aufl.) Baltmansweiler: Pedag. Verlag Burgbucherei Schneider

KLÄGER, M. (1992): *Krampus: Die Bilderwelt des Willibald Lassenberger.* Baltmansweiler: Schneider Verlag Hohengehren

KLÄGER, M. (1993): *Die Vielfalt der Bilder.* Stuttgart: Konrad Wittwer

KRAMER, E. (1974): The unity of process and product. *Am. J. Art Ther. 14,* 15–16

KRETSCHMER, E. (1929): *Geniale Menschen.* Berlin: Springer

KRETSCHMER, E. (1936): *Körperbau und Charakter.* (11–12. Aufl.) Springer, Berlin: Springer

KRETSCHMER, E. (1941): *Medizinische Psychologie.* (6. Aufl.) Leipzig: Thieme

KRIS, E. (1933): *Ein geisteskranker Bildhauer (Die Charakterköpfe des Franz Xaver Messerschmidt). Imago,* 19, 384

KRIS, E. (1952): *Psychoanalytic Explorations in Art.* New York: International University Press

KÜRBITZ, W. (1912): Die Zeichnungen geisteskranker Personen. *Z. Neurol. 13,* 153

KWIATKOWSKA, H. Y. (1971): Family art therapy and family art evaluation. In I. JAKAB (ed.), *Psychiatry and Art.* Vol. 3, Conscious and Unconscious Expressive Art. Basel: S. Karger, pp. 138–151

LAING, J. H. (1975): Recurring fantasies in the paintings and writings by sadomasochists. In I. JAKAB (ed.), *Psychiatry and Art.* Vol. 4, Transcultural Aspects of Psychiatric Art. Basel: S. Karger, pp. 105–115

LALO, CH. (1940/41): Eugène Delacroix. *J. Psychol. Norm. Pathol.* Nos 4–6—Ref.: *Ann. Med. Psychol. 101,* II. 131 (1943)

LAMPONI, ST. (1949): La visione stereoscopia negli schizofrenici. *Acta Neurol. (Napoli) 4,* 523

LANGNER, E. (1936): Form- und Farbbeachtung und psychophysische Konstitution bei zeitgenössischen Dichtern. *Z. Menschl. Vererbgs. u. Konstitutionslehre 20,* 93

LEHEL, F. (1926): *Notre art dément.* Paris: H. Jonquieres et Cie

LEHTINEN, L. (1969): *Have You Ever Known a Perceptually Handicapped Child?* Los Angeles: Los Angeles chapter California Assoc. Neurologically Handicapped Children (Quoted by UHLIN 1969)

LEMBERGER, L. M. (1951): *L'étude de la personnalité infantile au moyen du dessin.* (Psiquis, organo oficial de la Liga mexicana de Salud mental, août 1951, p. 29)— Ref.: *Ann. Med. Psychol. 112,* I. 272 (1954)

LEWIS, C., MCLAUGHLIN, T. (1991): Leonardo da Vinci's use of prevision and early memory. In I. JAKAB (ed.), *Art Media as a Vehicle of Communication.* Brookline, Mass.: American Society of Psychopathology of Expression, pp. 37–40

LHERMITTE, J. (1938): Langage et mouvement. *L'Encéphale* 33, 1

LHERMITTE, J. MOUZON (1942): L'agnosie géométrique et la dyspraxie constructive dans les lésions de la sphère visuelle. *Ann. Med. Psychol. 100,* I. 54

LOMBROSO, C. (1887): *Genie und Irrsinn.* Leipzig: Reclam

LUCAS, X. (1991): Dynamics in art group psychotherapy. In I. JAKAB (ed.), *Art Media as a Vehicle of Communication.* Proc. Int. Congr. Psychopathol. Expr. Montreal 1990. Brookline, Mass.: American Society of Psychopathology of Expression, pp. 113–133

MACGREGOR, J. (1989): *The Discovery of the Art of the Insane.* Princeton, N.J.: Princeton University Press

MANDOLINI, H. (1925): Psychopathologie der Kunstschöpfung. *Rev. de criminol. psiquiatr. y med. leg. 12,* 146

MARCHAND, M.: Remarque de discussion à la démonstration de Vié et Suttel.

MARINOW, A. (1971): The schizophrenic patient draws his delusions. In I. JAKAB (ed.), *Psychiatry and Art.* Vol. 3, Conscious and Unconscious Expressive Art. Basel: S. Karger, pp. 69–77

MATERAZZI, M. (1990): Psicocine-psicoterapia grupal

programada. In C. STEFANIS, C. SOLDATOS, A. RABAVILAS (eds), *Psychiatry: A World Perspective.* Vol. 4. Proc. VIIIth World Congr. Psychiatry, Athens, 12–19 October 1989. Elsevier Sicence Publisher B. V.

MAUREL, M. H., WILHELM, M. (dr. Rouffach) (1955): Intérêt clinique de l'épreuve mescalinique au cours de certains syndromes psychiatriques. *Ann. Med. Psychol. 113, I.* 295

MELTZOFF, J., KORNREICH, M. (1970): *Research in Psychotherapy.* New York: Atherton Press

MENNINGER, K. A. (1938): *Man against Himself.* New York: Harcourt, Brace

MEYER, J. E. (1954): Stilwandel bildnerischer Produktion unter dem Einfluss einer Psychose. *Nervenarzt 25,* 237

MEYERSON, A. T., EPSTEIN, G. (1976): The psychoanalytic treatment centers as a transference object. *Psychoanal. Q. 45,* 274–287

MINKOWSKA, F. (1947): Van Gogh: les relations entre sa vie, sa maladie et son oeuvre. *L'Evol. Psychiatr. Paris 3,* fasc. I—Ref.: FERDIÈRE, G., *Ann. Med. Psychol. 105, II.* 35

MÖBIUS, P. J. (1901): *Ueber Kunst und Künstler.* Leipzig: Barth

MOREL, F. (1939/41): L'hallucination est-elle accesible à notre connaissance? *L'Encéphale 34, II.* 351

MORGENTHALER, W. (1921): *Ein Geisteskranker als Künstler.* Bern–Leipzig: Bircher

MORGENTHALER, W. (1942): Contribution à la psychologie du dessin. *Rev. Suisse de Psychol.* Fasc. 1–2

MORSELLI, E. (1885, 1894): *Manuale di semejotica delle malattie mentali. Guida alla diagnosi della pazzia per i medici i medici-legisti e gli studenti. Vollardi,* Milano, *1,* 1 (1885), *2,* 1 (1894)—Cited by ANASTASI and FOLEY

MOTTO, J. A., GREEN, C. (1958): Suicide and the medical community. *A. M. A. Arch. Neurol. Psychiat.* 80, 776–781

MOUSSONG-KOVÁCS, E. (1992): Temporo-spatial orientation's role in pictorial expression of emotions. In I. JAKAB, I. HÁRDI (eds), *Psychopathology of Expression and Art Therapy in the World.* Budapest: Animula, pp. 108–124

MÜLLER-SUUR, H. (1954): Die Wirksamkeit allgemeiner Sinnhorizonte im schizophrenen Wahnerleben. *Fortschr. Neurol.* 22, 38

MÜLLER-THALHEIM, W. K. (1975): Self-healing tendencies in creativity. In I. JAKAB (ed.), *Psychiatry and Art.* Vol. 4, Transcultural Aspects of Psychiatric Art Basel: S. Karger, pp. 161–170

NAGLER, I. (1952): Cited by BERGERON and VOLMAT

NAGLER, I. (1956): Cited by VOLMAT

NAGY, L. (1905): *Fejezetek a gyermekrajzok lélektanából* (Chapters on the psychology of children's drawings). Budapest: Singer & Wolfner

NAUMBURG, M. (1950): *Schizophrenic Art: Its Meaning in Psychotherapy.* New York: Grune and Stratton

NAUMBURG, M. (1953): *Psychoneurotic Art. Its Function in Psychotherapy.* New York: Grune and Stratton

NAUMBURG, M. (1966): *Dynamically Oriented Art Therapy: Its Principles and Practice.* New York: Grune and Stratton

NAVRATIL, L. (1958): Der Figur-Zeichen-Test beim chronischen Alkoholismus. *Z. Psychosom. Med.* 2, 95–103

NAVRATIL, L. (1965): *Schizophrenie und Kunst.* München: Deutscher Taschenbuch-Verlag

NAVRATIL, L. (1978): *Gespräche mit Schizophrenen.* München: Deutscher Taschenbuch-Verlag

NEIMAREVIĆ, D. (1969): Schizophrenie im bildnerischen Ausdruck der Malerin Marija Novaković (Mit Farbtafel IV). In I. JAKAB (ed.), *Psychiatry and Art.* Vol. 2, Art Interpretation and Art Therapy. Basel–New York: S. Karger, pp. 154–162

NEUMANN, E. (1959): *Art and the Creative Unconscious.* New York: Pantheon

NICHOLI, A. M., JR. (1978): The therapist–patient relationship. In NICHOLI (ed.), *The Harvard Guide to Modern Psychiatry.* Cambridge: Harvard University Press, pp. 3–22

NIKITIN, E. (1930): Intellektuelle und künstlerische (Musik, Dramatisation, Zeichen) Begabung schwererziehbarer Psychopathen. *Trudy defektol. Otdela psico-nerv. Akad. Samml.* 2, 148—Ref.: *Zbl. Neurol.* 59, 499 (1931)

NUCHO, A. (1986): A merging of verbal and creative therapies: Ikebana sculpturing. In I. JAKAB (ed.), *The Role of the Imagination in the Healing Process.* Pittsburgh, PA: American Society of Psychopathology of Expression (presently in Brookline, Mass.)

NUCHO, A. (1996): Art in Latvia after the collapse of the Soviet Union. In I. JAKAB (ed.), *The Influence of Recent Socio-Political Events on Fine Arts and on Patient's Art.* Brookline, Mass.: American Society of Psychopathology of Expression

OREMLAND, J. D. (1997): *The Origins and Psychodynamics of Creativity. A Psychoanalytic Perspective.* Madison, Conn.: International Universities Press Inc.

PANETH, L. (1929): Form und Farbe in der Psychoanalyse. Ein neuer Weg zum Unbewussten. *Nervenzarzt* 2, 326

PASTO, T. (1971): Phaëthon, Helios and the mental patient. In I. JAKAB (ed.), *Psychiatry and Art*. Vol. 3. Basel: S. Karger, pp. 78–85

PAVLOV, I. P. (1951): *Complete Works*. Moscow–Leningrad (in Russian)

PAWLOW, J. P. (1926): *Die höchste Nerventätigkeit (das Verhalten) von Tieren*. Übersetzt von G. Volborth. München: Bergmann

PENNES, H. H. (1954): Clinical reactions of schizophrenics to sodium amytal, pervitin hydrochloride, mescaline sulfate, and D-lysergic acid diethylamine ($LSD_{25}$). *J. Nerv. Ment. Dis.* 119, 95

PÉREZ, V. (1917): Valor semeiológico de las manifestaciones gráficas en la locura. *Siglo Medico* 74, 546—Cited by ANASTASI and FOLEY

PETŐ, Z. (1997): *Status praesens*. A selection from the poems of psychiatric patients. (In Hungarian.) Szeged: SOTE Nyomda

PFEIFER, R. A. (1923): *Der Geisteskranke und sein Werk*. Leipzig: Kröner

PICKFORD, R. W. (1967): *Studies in Psychiatric Art*. Springfield, Ill.: Ch. C. Thomas

PINEL, P. (1989): Traité médico-philosophique sur l'aliénation mentale ou la manie. In J. MACGREGOR (ed.), *The Discovery of the Art of the Insane*. Princeton, N.J.: Princeton University Press

PLOKKER, J. H. (1962): *Artistic Self Expression in Mental Disease*. London–The Hague: Skilton–Mouton

POKORNY, A. D. (1960): Characteristics of forty-four patients who subsequently committed suicide. *Arch. Gen. Psychiatry* 2, 314–323

POROT, A., BARDENAT, Ch., LEONARDON, P. (1942): L'encéphalite aigne mélitococcique. *Ann. Med. Psychol.* 100, I. 25

PRINZHORN, H. (1919): Das bildnerische Schaffen der Geisteskranken. *Z. Neurol.* 52, 307

PRINZHORN, H. (1922): *Bildnerei der Geisteskranken*. Berlin: Springer (2nd ed. 1968)

PRUYSER, P. W. (1968): Life and death of a symbol: A history of the Holy Ghost concept and its emblems. (Abstr.) In I. JAKAB (ed.), *Psychiatry and Art*. Basel: S. Karger, p. 211

RAPAPORT, I. F. (1968): The art of the retarded and nonverbal intelligence. In I. JAKAB (ed.), *Psychiatry and Art*. Proc. IVth Int. Coll. Psychopathol. Expr., Washington, D.C., 1966. Basel–New York: S. Karger, pp. 172–179

REDER, P., TYSON, R. L. (1980): Patient dropout from individual psychotherapy. *Bull. Menninger Clin.* 44, 3

RÉGIS, E. (1882/83): Les aliénés peints par eux-mêmes. *L'Encéphale* 2, 184, 373, 547 (1882); 3, 642 (1883)—Cited by ANASTASI and FOLEY

REINHARDT, S. (1971): The drawings of animals. Their use as an aid in distinguishing severe psychopathology. In I. JAKAB (ed.), *Psychiatry and Art*. Vol. 3, Conscious and Unconscious Expressive Art. Basel: S. Karger, pp. 112–116

REITMAN, F. (1948): Dynamics of creative activity. *J. Ment. Science* 94, 314

RÉJA, M. (1901): L'art malade: dessins de fous. *Revue universelle* 1, 913–915, 940–944

RENNERT, H. (1966): *Die Merkmale schizophrener Bildnerei*. Jena: Fischer

RHI, B. Y. (1994): Nostalgia expressed in the paintings of Lee Choong Sup—in concern with creativity in crisis. In *Proc. Int. Symp. Psychopathol. Expression and Workshop for Art Therapy*. Seoul, Korea: The Korean Association for Clinical Art, pp. 61–63

RIESE, W. (1926): *Vincent van Gogh in der Krankheit, ein Beitrag zum Problem der Beziehung zwischen Kunstwerk und Krankheit*. München: Bergmann—Ref.: *Zbl. Neurol.* 46, 651 (1927)

RIESE, W. (1959): Das Altern in farbpsychologischer Sicht. *Z. Altersforschung* 13

ROBBINS, E. et al. (1959): The communication of suicidal intent: a study of 134 consecutive cases of successful suicide. *Am. J. Psychiatry* 115, 724

RORSCHACH, H. (1946): *Psychodiagnostik*. Bern: Huber

ROUX, G. (1990): Images renversées. In I. JAKAB (ed.), *Art Media as a Vehicle of Communication*. Proc. 1990 Int. Congr. Psychopathol. Expr., Montreal 1990. Brookline, Mass.: American Society of Psychopathology of Expression, pp. 333–342

ROUX, G. (1991): Devils and wonders ... expression and psychosis. In I. JAKAB (ed.), *Art Media as a Vehicle of Communication*. Proceedings ASPE Congress, Montreal, 1990. Brookline, Mass.: American Society of Psychopathology of Expression, pp. 279–299

ROUX, G., LAHARIE, M. (1997): *Art et Folie au Moyen Age. Aventures et Enigmes d'Opicinus de Canistris (1296–vers 1351)*. Paris: Editions le Leopard d'Or

ROY, G. (1953): Analisi fenomenologica dell'assurdo

schizofrenico nei rapporti col surreale dell arte. *Arch. Psicol. Neurol. 14,* 605

ROY, G. (1958): *Arts fantastiques.* Paris: Delpire, p. 98

RUBIN, J. A., IRWIN, E. C. (1975): Art and drama: Parts of a puzzle. In I. JAKAB (ed.), *Psychiatry and Art.* Vol. 4, Transcultural Aspects of Psychiatric Art. Basel: S. Karger, pp. 193–200

RUBIN, J. A., MAGNUSSEN, M. G., BAR, A. (1975): Stuttering: symptom–system–symbol. In I. JAKAB (ed.), *Psychiatry and Art.* Vol. 4. Transcultural Aspects of Psychiatric Art. Basel: S Karger, pp. 201–215

RUSH, B. (1812): *Medical Inquiries and Observations upon the Diseases of the Mind.* Philadelphia. (New York: Reprinted by the Library of the New York Academy of Medicine, 1962)

SAARMA, YOU. M. (1953): Sur quelques formes des phénomènes de la hypnotèques chez les schizophrènes. *J. Nevropathol. et Psychiatr. Korsakov. 53,* 197

SAKAUE, M. (1997): Musical expressions of schizophrenics: Their meaning and the therapeutic consequences. In R. PRATT, Y. TOKUDA (eds), *Arts Medicine.* Michigan: International Arts Medicine Association, pp. 91–96

SANDLER, J. et al. (1975): Discussions on transference: the treatment situation and technique in child psychoanalysis. *Psychoanal. Study Child 30,* 409–441

SCHENK, V. W. D. (1939): Drawings of untrained and untalented adults. *Psychiatr. Neurol. Bull. Amst. 43,* 591—Cited by ANASTASI and FOLEY

SCHILDER, P. (1918): *Wahn und Erkenntnis.* Berlin: Springer

SCHMIDT-HEINRICH, E. (1953): Zur Psychologie des Surrealismus. *Arch. Psychol. 3,* 1

SCHNEDITZ, W. (1956): *Alfred Kubin.* Wien: Rosenbaum

SCHNEER, H. I. et al. (1961): Events and conscious ideation leading to suicidal behavior in adolescence. *Psychiatr. Q. 35,* 507–515

SCHNIER, J. (1950): The blazing sun. A psychoanalytic approach to Van Gogh. *Am. Imago 7,* 143

SCHOTTKY, I. (1936): Über einen künstlerischen Stilwandel in der Psychose. *Nervenarzt 5,* 68

SEHRINGER, W. (1992): Principles for the psychodiagnostic analysis of children's drawings. In I. JAKAB, I. HÁRDI (eds), *Psychopathology of Expression and Art Therapy in the World.* Budapest: Animula, pp. 46–80

SHAPIRO, M. (1958): *Van Gogh.* Zürich: Ex Libris, p. 12

SIMON, P. M. (1876): L'imagination dans la folie. Étude sur les dessins, plans, descriptions et costumes des aliénés. *Ann. Med. Psychol. 16,* 358–390

SIMON, P. M. (1888): Les écrits et les dessins des aliénés. *Archivio di antropologia criminelle, psichiatria e medicina legale 3,* 318–355

SMYTHIES, J. R. (1953): The "Base line" of schizophrenia. Part 1. The visual phenomena. *Am. J. Psych. 110,* 200

STAEHELIN, J. E. (1941): Pervitin-Psychose. *Z. Neurol. 173,* 598

STANNARD, K. (1991): Toulouse-Lautrec: Hephaestos as healer. In I. JAKAB (ed.), *Art Media as a Vehicle of Communication.* Brookline, Mass.: American Society of Psychopathology of Expression, pp. 41–52

STAVENITZ, A. R. (1939): Art and psychopathology. *Psychol. League J. 3,* 36—Cited by ANASTASI and FOLEY

STERN, W. (1923): *Psychologie der frühen Kindheit.* (3. Aufl.) Leipzig: Quelle & Meyer

STEWART, R. L. (1968): Tactile aesthetic perception among the blind: A comparison of blind and sighted subjects. In I. JAKAB (ed.), *Psychiatry and Art.* Proc. IVth Int. Coll. Psychopathol. Expr., Washington, D.C., 1966. Basel: S. Karger, 180–187

STEWART, R. L., BAXTER, J. (1969): Color preferences of three ethnic groups of elementary school children. In I. JAKAB (ed.), *Psychiatry and Art.* Vol. 2, Art Interpretation and Art Therapy, Vth. Int. Coll. Psychopathol. Expr. Basel–New York: S. Karger, pp. 186–190

STONE, B. (1969): Art therapy with nonverbal patients. In I. JAKAB (ed.), *Psychiatry and Art.* Vol. 2, Art Interpretation and Art Therapy. Basel–New York: S. Karger, pp. 191–204

STONE, B. (1975): Sequential graphic gestalt. In I. JAKAB (ed.), *Psychiatry and Art.* Vol. 4, Trans-cultural Aspects of Psychiatric Art. Basel: S. Karger, pp. 216–229

STÖRRING, G. E. (1955): Halluzinatorische und wahnähnliche Erlebnisse bei eidetischer Veranlagung. *Monatschr. Psych. Neurol. 129,* 261

SULLY, J. (1909): *Untersuchungen über die Kindheit.* Leipzig: Wunderlich

SZÉCSI, L. (1935): *On Works of Art of the Insane.* Widtown Galleries, New York, Catalogue of the exhibition of the Szécsi Collection. March 17–April 1, 1935—Cited by ANASTASI and FOLEY

SZILÁGYI, K. (1992): Drawings of the Goldsmith, A. W. In I. JAKAB, I. HÁRDI (eds), *Psychopathology of Expression and Art Therapy in the World.* Budapest: Animula, pp. 181–190

TAMURA, Y., ASANO, K. (1997): Renku as psychotherapy: Japanese traditional poetic forms adapted to poetry therapy. In R. Pratt, Y. Tokuda (eds), *Arts Medicine*. Michigan: International Arts Medicine Association, pp. 132–140

Tayal, S. (1968): Poems, paintings, porcelain and psychotherapy. In I. Jakab (ed.), *Psychiatry and Art*. Proc. IVth Int. Coll. Psychopathol. Expr., Washington, D.C., 1966. Basel–New York: S. Karger, pp. 188–193

Tayal, S. (1969): The communication of suicidal ideation in art therapy. In I. Jakab (ed.), *Psychiatry and Art*. Vol. 2. Art Interpretation and Art Therapy, Vth Int. Coll. Psychopathol. Expr. Basel–New York: S. Karger, pp. 205–209

Tényi, T., Trixler, M. (1992): Approaches to schizophrenic poetry. In I. Jakab, I. Hárdi (eds), *Psychopathology of Expression and Art Therapy in the World*. Budapest: Animula, pp. 208–210

Tényi, T., Trixler, M. (1996): The expression of magical influence in the art and delusions of schizophrenic Hungarian Gypsies. In I. Jakab (ed.), *The Influence of Recent Socio-Political Events on Fine Arts and on Patient's Art*. Brookline, Mass.: American Society of Psychopathology of Expression, pp. 247–258

Tokuda, Y. (1986): Recent trends in the development of image-including techniques in Japan and their significance in the therapeutic process. In I. Jakab (ed.), *The Role of the Imagination in the Healing Process*. Proc. Int. Congr. Psychopathol. Expr. Pittsburgh, Penn.: American Society of Psychopathology of Expression, pp. 30–33

Tokuda, Y. (1997): Therapeutic topos and their background dynamics: Applications of the techniques of arts therapy. In R. Pratt, Y. Tokuda (eds), *Arts Medicine*. Michigan: International Arts Medicine Association, pp. 43–52

Tompkins, H. J. (1952): Cited by Bergeron and Volmat

Traube, T. (1937): La valeur diagnostique des dessins des enfants difficiles. *Arch. Psychol. 27*, 285—Cited by Anastasi and Foley

Tyszkiewicz, M. (1975): Unexpected values in the art of mentally retarded children. In I. Jakab (ed.), *Psychiatry and Art*. Vol. 4, Transcultural Aspects of Psychiatric Art. Basel: S. Karger, pp. 242–247

Ueberschlag, H. (1936): Un délirant chronique, son historie, son langage, diagnostic. Thèse, Strasbourg—Cited by Ferdière, G., *Ann. Med. Psychol. 105, II*. 35 (1947)

Uhde, W. (1931): Painters of the inner light: Séraphine. Formes, 17, pp. 115-117. In J. MacGregor (ed.), *The Discovery of the Art of the Insane*. Princeton, N.J.: Princeton University Press, 1989.

Uhlin, D. M. (1964): *Recognition and Therapy of Neurologically Handicapped Children through Art*. Berkeley, Cal.: California Association of Neurologically Handicapped Children

Uhlin, D. M. (1969a): The basis of art for neurologically handicapped children. In I. Jakab (ed.), *Psychiatry and Art*. Vol. 2, Art Interpretation and Art Therapy. Basel–New York: S. Karger, pp. 210–241

Uhlin, D. M. (1969b): The descriptive character of symbol in the art of a schizophrenic girl. In I. Jakab (ed.), *Psychiatry and Art*. Vol. 2, Art Interpretation and Art Therapy. Basel–New York: S. Karger, pp. 242–248

Uhlin, D. M. (1971): Creative expression and the adolescent psycho-sexual paradox. In I. Jakab (ed.), *Psychiatry and Art*. Vol. 3. Basel: S. Karger, pp. 52–60

Ulman, E. (1971): The power of art in therapy. In I. Jakab (ed.), *Psychiatry and Art*. Vol. 3, Conscious and Unconscious Expressive Art. Basel: S. Karger, pp. 93–102

Van der Kolk, B. A. et al. (1985): Inescapable shock, neurotransmitters, and addition to trauma: Toward a psychology of posttraumatic stress. *Biol. Psychiatry, 20*, 314-325

Verworn, M. (1917): *Zur Psychologie der primitiven Kunst*. (2. Aufl.) Jena: G. Fischer

Vié, J., Suttel, R. (1944): Techniques morbides: exemples empruntés à des travaux féminins spontanés. *Ann. Med. Psychol. 102*, 357

Volmat, R. (1956): *L'Art psychopathologique*. Paris: Presses Universitaire de France

Volmat, R. (1961): Art et psychiatrie. In Gruhle et al. (eds), *Psychiatrie der Gegenwart*. Vol. 3. Berlin: Springer

Volmat, R. (1991): Van Gogh, la fortune et la gloire. In I. Jakab (ed.), *Art Media as a Vehicle of Communication*. Brookline, Mass.: American Society of Psychopathology of Expression, pp. 89–98

Volmat, R., Roumeguere, P. (1952): Analyse du film: "Images de la folie". *La semaine des hôpitaux de Paris*, Suppl. 32

Volmat, R., Wiart, C., Usal, J. (1967): Esquisse méthodique d'analyse des expressions plastiques: La couleur envisagée sous l'angle de la communication et de l'information. *Confinia Psychiatrica, 10*, 1

Wadeson, H., Bunney, W. E. Jr. (1969): Manic-depressive art: Tested graphic characteristics and psychodynamic implications. In I. Jakab (ed.), *Psychiatry and Art.* Vol. 2, Art Interpretation and Art Therapy. Basel–New York: S. Karger, pp. 249–252

Wadeson, H., Epstein, R. (1975): Intrapsychic effects of amphetamine in hyperkinesis as revealed through art productions. In I. Jakab (ed.), *Psychiatry and Art.* Vol. 4, Transcultural Aspects of Psychiatric Art. Basel: S. Karger, p. 290

Werner, W. (1952): *The Dream, Mirror of Conscience.* New York: Grune and Stratton

Weygandt, W. (1925): Zur Frage der pathologischen Kunst. *Z. Neurol. 94*, 421

Weygandt, W. (1926): Die pathologische Plastik des Fürsten Palagonia. *Z. Neurol. 101*, 857

Wiart, C. (1967): *Expression picturale et psychopathologie.* Paris: Doin

Winkler, W. T. (1966): Tiefenpsychologie und moderne Kunst. *Medizinische Welt, Stuttgart 17*, 987–995

Wyss, D. (1950): *Der Surrealismus. Eine Einführung und Deutung surrealistischer Literatur und Malerei.* Heidelberg: Schneider—Ref.: *Zbl. Neurol. 113*, 301 (1951)

Yahn, M. (1950): Sobre a criação de uma secção de Arte no Hospital de Juquieri. *Bol. Hig. Ment. São Paulo*—Cited by Bergeron and Volmat

Yamaguchi, T. (1995): Special presentation: Studies on atomic bomb survivors in Hiroshima by means of group art therapy. *J. Jpn. Assoc. Group Psychotherapy 11*, 1, 7–14

Yamaguchi, T. (1997): Hiroshima atomic bomb survivors: Group arts therapy approaches. In R. Pratt, Y. Tokuda (eds), *Arts Medicine.* Michigan: International Arts Medicine Association, pp. 53–59

Yamanaka, Y. (1966): The great Hanshin earthquake and the creativity of children. In I. Jakab (ed.), *The Influence of Recent Socio-Political Events on Fine Arts and on Patient's Art.* Brookline, Mass.: American Society of Psychopathology of Expression, pp. 259–266

Yessler, P. G. et al. (1961): On the communication of suicidal ideas. I. Some sociological and behavioral considerations. *Arch. Gen. Psychiatr. 3*, 12–29

Yoshida, A., Matsui, H., Sodenaga, M., Ueda, E., Shimogaki, H., Watanabe, N., Aizawa, S. (1994): Application trial of evaluation check list for group sessions in music therapy. First report. *Jpn. Bull. Arts Therapy 25*, 1. 5–11

Zeldenrust, E. L. K. (1951): L'art et la folie. Étude ontologique et anthropologique. *L'Evol. Psychiatr.* Paris 73–86

Zerbe, K. (1990): Berthe Morisot's bipolar illness: Art as therapeutic agent. In I. Jakab (ed.), *Stress Management through Art.* Brookline, Mass.: American Society of Psychopathology of Expression, pp. 71–86

Ziese, G. (1953): Die Bedeutung des affektiven Defektes in den sprachlichen und bildnerischen Darstellungen der Schizophrenen. *Psychiatr. Neurol. Med. Psychol. (Leipz.) 5*, 59

Zsakó, I. (1908): Graphologiai diagnosis. (Diagnostique graphologique.) *Orv. Hetil. 52*, 744

Zsakó, I., Jó, J. (1931): Budapesti angyalföldi elme- és ideggyógyintézet múzeuma (The museum of the mental institute of Budapest-Angyalföld). *Orv. Hetil. 75*, 629

# ABOUT THE AUTHOR

The author is a pioneer in the research of the pictorial expression of psychiatric patients. Her first book, *Dessins et peintures der aliénés* (Drawings and Paintings of the Mentally Ill), was published in French and German (1956, Akadémiai Kiadó), preceded only by the groundbreaking monograph *Bildnerei der Geisteskranken* by H. Prinzhorn (1922).

Irene Jakab received her medical degree from the University Franz Joseph in Kolozsvár, then Hungary, board certified in psychiatry and neurology in Hungary. Following her medical training, she earned her Ph.D. summa cum laude in psychology and education at the University Pázmány Péter in Budapest, Hungary.

Irene Jakab started her academic career in the United States in 1966 as Assistant Professor at Harvard Medical School in Boston. In 1969, following a postgraduate training at the Menninger School of Psychiatry in Topeka, Kansas, she was board certified in psychiatry by the American Board of Psychiatry and Neurology. From 1974 to 1992, she was Professor of Psychiatry, at the University of Pittsburgh, where she established and directed the John Merck Program for Mentally Retarded Emotionally Disturbed Children (the first such psychiatric inpatient program in the USA). Art therapy was introduced as an important and very successful treatment method for these children, serving as a bridge in addition to, or instead of, verbal communication.

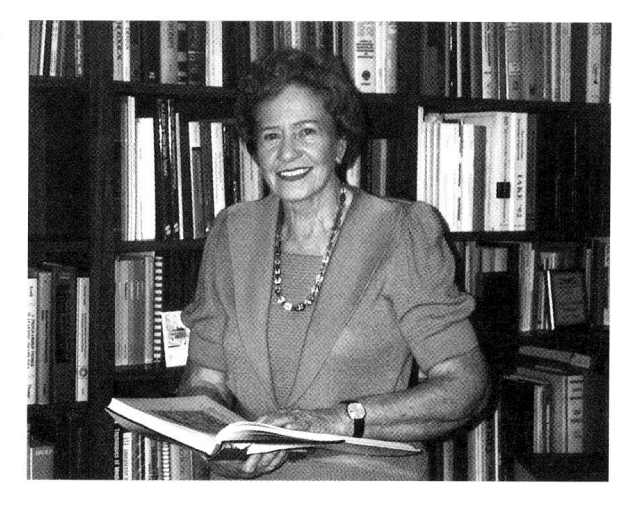

In 1992, Irene Jakab returned to Boston after retiring from the University of Pittsburgh as a Professor Emerita of Psychiatry. Presently, she teaches at Harvard Medical School as Lecturer on Psychiatry, and is Attending Psychiatrist at McLean Hospital.

Irene Jakab was the recipient of the Prinzhorn Prize from the *German Society of Psychopathology of Expression* (DGPH) in 1967 and of the Ernst Kris Gold Medal from the *American Society of Psychopathology of Expression* (ASPE) in 1973. She received the Benjamin Rush Gold Medal Award of the *American Psychiatric Association* (1980) for an exhibit: The Recognition, Diagnosis and Treatment of Brain-Damaged, Retarded, Emotionally Disturbed Children. In recognition of her contribution to psychiatry and to the research of art in psychiatric diagnosis and treatment, she was awarded a degree of Honorary Doctor of the University of Besançon, France, in 1982.

She is listed in Marqui's *Who is Who in America* (1997) and in Marqui's *Who is Who in the World* (1998).

She is founding member and vice president of the *International Society of Psychopathology of Expression* (ISPE, 1959) and founding member and president of the *American Society of Psychopathology of Expression* (ASPE, 1964). In this capacity she organized several national and international congresses in art and psychiatry. The proceedings of these meetings provide important contributions to the psychiatric literature in the field of art diagnosis, art therapy and research on creativity.

One of her hobbies is photography that she uses as tangible memories of her extensive travels. She visited many interesting places on all five continents where her sightseeings were always completed by visiting schools and psychiatric hospitals.

Irene Jakab plans to continue an active professional life, while not neglecting the leisure activities of retirement. She lives in Brookline, Massachusetts.